COMMENTS ABOUT THE 17 WALKS IN

This fun, well-informed book breaks the city down into 17 different curated walks, each of which offers fascinating perspectives on the many worlds of San Francisco.
Gary Kamiya, author of *Cool Gray City of Love: 49 Views of San Francisco*

Love it! There is no place like home, especially if home is the overwhelmingly gorgeous San Francisco! This book is a must read—the excited joy of it all is worth every second and makes a visit to San Francisco an unforgettable must do!
Angela M. Alioto, Esq., past member San Francisco Board of Supervisors

Poggioli and Eidson's *Walking San Francisco's 49 Mile Scenic Drive* pulls one out of his or her car or home and compels walking to the splendid sites that are illustrated in the book. The text is crisp and the production of the book superb—a must for Bay Area explorers as well as tourists.
**Charles A. Fracchia, author, lecturer, founder of the
San Francisco Museum and Historical Society**

Enticing photos, images and fun facts make me want to lace up my shoes and get walking!
Janet McBride, Executive Director, Bay Area Ridge Trail

I took my daughter on the Fisherman's Wharf Walk. During the walk, and then again at bedtime, she said, "Mom, I had a really good time." (I don't hear that a lot from my tween!)
Shannon Martinez – Pacifica, CA

A few months after walking Walk 1 I was back in the area with a friend telling him all the cool facts I'd learned – like Little Saigon, the Phoenix Motel, etc. He was so impressed and asked how I knew so much. I said, "Well there's a new book out…"
James Camarillo – San Francisco, CA

The whole area on the east side of 101 was new to us. Didn't know a pre-quake neighborhood even existed. Love 24th Street on the loop back with all the trees and small businesses. Can't wait to do all 17 walks.
Don Martin – Oakland, CA

We saw a lot more walking than driving or riding a bike would allow. And we took the time to wander in and out of places that were open (Asian Art Museum and St Mary's) and discovered all kinds of new things.
Jeff Becker – Oakland, CA

Thank you for exposing us to this incredible walk!!! What a wonderful experience, one I had never done end to end on foot! Loved it!!!

Paul Stoner & Abraham Hanif – San Jose, CA

I'm really working on walking in conjunction with Weight Watchers. That, combined with my general nerdiness and fascination with San Francisco history, makes this a favorite thing for me to do.

Amy Johnson – San Francisco, CA

My sweetie and I took the Golden Gate Park Walk today. It was a beautiful day and we really enjoyed the journey and the fun facts!

Deborah Schweizer – San Francisco, CA

I can't tell you how fun this was and what a good time I had. The book is TERRIFIC. I can hardly wait to do more of these walks. I loved all the tidbits of information you gathered and feel like I know this beautiful city so much better now.

Scott Walton – San Francisco, CA

What fun. We enjoyed our stroll and were surprised to discover so many things that we didn't know were there!

Dave Feldman & Vin Eiamvuthikorn – Daly City, CA

Just did Walk 13 – Twin Peaks. That was an awesome walk!

Michael Hamlin – San Francisco, CA

It's definitely a lovely walk, both for the simple pleasure of walking in nature, and for the many possible stops along the way.

Melissa Karam – San Francisco, CA

I would absolutely do Walk 11 again. It was a fantastic walk. The Stow Lake portion is a whole walk in itself and great for dogs. Loved the waterfall and view from the top of Strawberry Hill and all the historical facts.

Austin Mader-Clark – San Mateo, CA

I learned things about the city I didn't know, and saw parts I've never been to. I think it'd be a fun challenge to try to walk the whole thing.

Ben Keim – Berkeley, CA

Very interesting to walk the route vs. driving. For example, our companion had driven the route several times, but had never gotten out and hiked down to Sutro Baths – he was pleasantly surprised at the ruins. Looking forward to the next walk.

Larry Turner – Oakland, CA

Ocean Beach was an easy walk – the beautiful scenery made it all worthwhile.

Tom Sharp & Ellen Miller – San Francisco, CA

WALKING
San Francisco's 49 Mile Scenic Drive

EXPLORE THE FAMOUS SITES,
NEIGHBORHOODS, AND VISTAS IN
17 ENCHANTING WALKS

Kristine Poggioli
Carolyn Eidson

CRAVEN STREET
B O O K S

Fresno, California

WALKING San Francisco's 49 Mile Scenic Drive
Explore the Famous Sites, Neighborhoods, and
Vistas in 17 Enchanting Walks

Copyright © 2016 by Kristine Poggioli and Carolyn Eidson
All rights reserved

Published by Craven Street Books,
an imprint of Linden Publishing
2006 South Mary, Fresno, California 93721
559-233-6633 / 800-345-4447
QuillDriverBooks.com

Craven Street Books and Colophon are trademarks
of Linden Publishing, Inc.

ISBN 978-1-61035-279-6

Printed in the United States
Second Printing

Cover design: Maura Zimmerman
Interior design: Carla Green

Cover photos:
Top image ©Joe Christensen / www.iStockPhoto.com
Bottom image ©Ron Niebrugge / www.WildNatureImages.com

Library of Congress Cataloging-in-Publication Data on file

CONTENTS

FOREWORD

I think San Francisco is the most wonderful city in the world, and I've been pretty much everywhere. My love affair with the City began through my parents eyes. They met in San Francisco in 1947 on the corner of 9th and Market at the Bank of America. They loved the City.

My dad was from San Jose. Before he was drafted into the military for WWII he was a semi-pro baseball player. After the war, he figured he needed a new career so he moved to San Francisco and became a banker. My mom's family moved here from Wichita, Kansas, after her dad lost his job during the Depression. They owned the Chevron gas station in the Castro. My mom lived all over the City—from State Street in the Castro to Dolores Street in the Mission. She used to tell me stories about how she walked to work every day from Telegraph Hill to 9th and Market—in 4-inch spiked heels!

One day my friend Stephanie Lynne Smith was over. Knowing how much I love walking in the City, she told me about a book her friends were writing called Walking San Francisco's 49 Mile Scenic Drive.

"What's the 49 Mile Scenic Drive?" I asked. Yes, even though I consider myself to be "Mr. San Francisco," I didn't know what it was. I had seen the seagull signs all around town and wondered about them. I was intrigued. I came to find out I live on the 49 Mile Scenic Drive!

Many San Franciscans have had the same experience. Even the authors, Kristine (who grew up in the City) and Carolyn (who has lived here over 20 years), were not familiar with it. They discovered the Drive a few years ago when they were looking for a new exercise goal for the year. They decided to walk the historic 49 mile loop trail over the course of a year, a mile, or two, or three at a time. They had so much fun that they turned their experience into a book.

This is a book for both visitors and long time residents. For example: even though I walk all over Walk 3 (Fisherman's Wharf, the Marina, the Palace of Fine Arts) on a regular basis, Walking San Francisco's 49 Mile Scenic Drive taught me new things about my own neighborhood (people have been asking me about the Fontana Towers for years, and now I know the scoop—see page 50). As I read the book, I found myself searching for info about iconic landmarks that I've always been curious about, such as, what's the deal with those windmills along Ocean Beach? (The answer is in Walk 7.) Are there buildings still standing from the 1906 earthquake? (Hint: the Ferry Building, Walk 17.)

I especially like how this is a great handbook for how to get around in San Francisco. The book has instructions about how to ride Muni, how to ride a cable car, how not to get a parking ticket, how to curb your tires, and a lot more. I've often warned people when they are parking to curb their wheels, because the San Francisco meter maids actually take out a tape measure to see if a car is more than 18 inches from the curb!

But my absolute favorite thing about the book is that it gets people out walking. The book's challenge, to walk all 17 Walks (the entire route) in one year, sounds like fun, and I love the authors' suggestion to walk it as a family. For example: Every time your family or friends come to visit you, take one of the walks with them and create wonderful memories together.

I don't know if my parents ever drove the 49 Mile Scenic Drive, but I know its neighborhoods and sites have created memories that San Franciscans and visitors have shared for generations, and I'm glad Walking San Francisco's 49 Mile Scenic Drive is reintroducing the route to a new generation.

I can't encourage you enough to get out of your car, get out of your house or hotel room, and get walking in this beautiful, wonderful city. I hope you fall in love with it as much as I have.

—**Brian Boitano**, Olympic and world champion figure skater and proud San Franciscan

INTRODUCTION

Welcome to the joys of *Walking* San Francisco's 49 Mile Scenic Drive

Congratulations! Whether your goal is to see the best of San Francisco in a few days, or to be among the first people on the planet to walk the entire 49 Mile Scenic route, you have just taken the first step on a grand adventure.

San Francisco's historic, spectacular 49 Mile Scenic Drive has just been reinvented for the 21st century. This new-generation route is a green, healthy, gorgeous urban walk designed to give San Franciscans and people who love San Francisco a new intimate experience with one of the most beloved and most visited cities in the world.

Instead of zooming by San Francisco's most picturesque spots in a closed car, you are about to explore her breathtaking and quirky locales

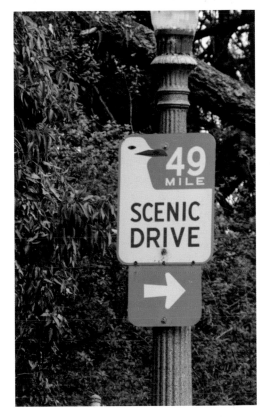

face to face, one step at a time—hiking through parks, along cliffs, through forgotten neighborhoods, and past treasured SF landmarks—with a little San Francisco history thrown in as a bonus.

By slowing down and walking the sidewalks of the City by the Bay, you may be surprised at how many new

Walks for First-Time Visitors
If this is your first visit to San Francisco, or you visit occasionally, you are welcome to dive in and see the city like a local. Check the table of contents for the several "must-see" walks that cover the most popular areas of the city. You will probably learn SF tidbits and quirky history factoids many locals don't know. Enjoy as many walks as you can, and trust that someday you will be back to see more.

things you discover on streets you may have traveled down dozens of times before. At this leisurely pace, your senses will have more time to engage with the sights, sounds, smells—and tastes—of many of San Francisco's distinct neighborhoods.

For those of you who accept the challenge to walk the entire route and eventually accomplish this feat— savor the fact that you will be one of the few people in the world, in history, who can say, "I walked San Francisco's 49 Mile Scenic Drive"—and the bragging rights will be all yours.

In whatever way you choose to enjoy the scenic route, these 17 well-crafted walks are designed so you can take this dazzling city tour at whatever pace, in whatever way, you find most enjoyable.

"So, what exactly is the 49 Mile Drive?" you may be wondering.

Chances are you've seen the drive's retro route markers on signposts all over town. A white seagull, wing outstretched against a field of blue sky with orange lettering pointing you toward . . . somewhere. You may have wondered what those signs are about. You may be among the thousands who've said, "I'm going to do that one day." You may even be one of the rare natives or visitors who has actually driven it. But what is it?

San Francisco's 49 Mile Scenic Drive is a nearly 80-year-old loop trail

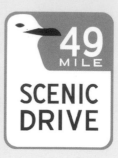

The Totally Cool Seagull Sign
The original 49 Mile route marker was a blue and gold triangle. In 1959 the Downtown Association held a contest to come up with a new design (another successful marketing gimmick—dang they are good). The winner—and still reigning champion— is a white seagull, wing outstretched against a field of blue sky, with orange lettering announcing the route. That graphic, designed by local artist Rex May, is so cool and popular that people keep stealing the signs. Stop it! You can buy plenty of cool seagull graphic 49 Mile Walk merchandise on the website, WalkSF49.com.

around the city designed to show off the city's most famous landmarks and varied neighborhoods. More than 50 top tourist sites and more than 100 local sites are on this route. It also takes you through the heart of real working neighborhoods all across town.

THE BIRTH OF THE 49 MILE SCENIC DRIVE

The 49 Mile Drive was born back in 1938 when the whole world had just been invited to visit San Francisco for the 1939–40 Golden Gate International Exposition. The Downtown Association wanted a way to get all those visitors out to see San Francisco's neighborhoods, marvel at her beauty, and think about doing business in San

Francisco. Originally they came up with a "50 Mile Scenic Drive" starting at City Hall and ending at Treasure Island, the site of the upcoming fair. Some fabulous, yet unknown, PR guy (or gal) even got President Franklin D. Roosevelt to take a tour of the drive. Then it occurred to someone (perhaps the original unsung PR whiz), "Hmmm . . . San Francisco is 49 square miles, the Gold Rush happened in 1849. Let's call it the 49 Mile Drive!" It was a hit.

Over the years the route and the distance have changed. When the exposition ended, the leg to Treasure Island was removed. New freeways and booming neighborhoods curved the route down new streets. During World War II security concerns closed the route through the Presidio for a while. The last major change was in 1999. But one thing has never changed: The glamour and beauty of this special city continue to draw visitors and locals alike to this 49 mile adventure over her steep hills, through her distinctive neighborhoods, and past her breathtaking vistas.

President Roosevelt at the beginning of the original 49 Mile Scenic Drive, the Golden Gate International Exposition on Treasure Island, 1938.
San Francisco History Center, San Francisco Public Library

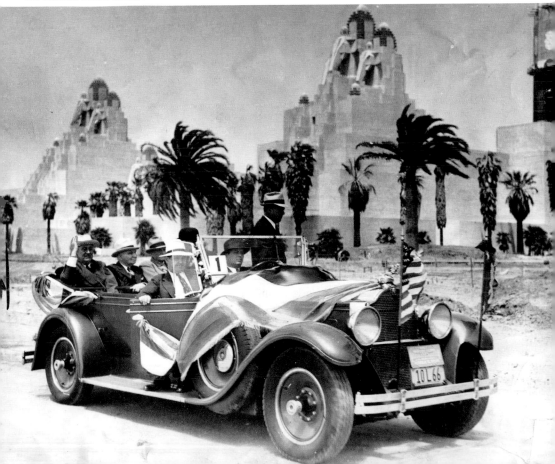

And Now the Drive Is Ready for a Green, Active, Healthy New Start

Yes, many, many people have enjoyed driving the iconic scenic route over the decades, which takes about four hours to drive by car . . . through SF traffic . . . searching for route markers while trying to read a guide book . . . craning your neck trying to get a quick glimpse out the right rear window of . . . "D'oh, missed it" . . . burning gas . . . sedentary . . . munching on snacks . . . did we mention four hours sitting in the car? Just kidding! The views on the route are magnificent, yet the route is so much more fun and better for your health and better for the environment when you're out walking it with friends, getting some exercise, and stopping at any spot that interests you.

> This urban hike breaks down the 49 Mile Scenic Drive into 17 walks, of two to four miles each—and challenges you to complete the entire 49 miles—on foot—*in a single year.*

Your Heart Will Love You for It

As you'll read in the bonus "Walking for Life" walking-for-exercise chapter, health experts consider walking to be one of the best forms of exercise in the world for your heart, your mood, your mind, and your overall health. Yet 80% of Americans don't do it very regularly. Why? A major factor is motivation—you know, something like having a big goal, like committing to

a one-year waking challenge through a gorgeous city, perhaps?

Walking the 49 Mile Scenic Drive is a great way to supplement your walking fitness with a motivational goal, an adventure, new experiences, and a lot of fun.

Whether You Take 1 Walk or All 17, These Walks Are So Wonderful, You May Just Fall in Love . . .

With a special someone

Feeling romantic? Want to get to know a friend better? Whether you are starting a new relationship, rekindling an old flame, or just hanging with your BFF, there are few more romantic or interesting cities to walk through than San Francisco. Can you imagine what might happen if you spent a year on a goal-oriented adventure walking and talking and hanging out together? But if you end up writing a book titled *Dating San Francisco's 49 Mile Scenic Drive*, we want some credit.

With your family

What would it be like to complete this challenge as a family? Each of these hikes gives you rare time to just walk—and possibly even talk—for a few hours, while accomplishing something together as a family. What if you started with your children in strollers, and through the years, bit by bit you had an adventure together, one hike at a time? Or what if every time your grandkids came to visit, you took them on a new walk? Maybe you could plan a special event as a reward to celebrate when you are done. (If you're spending a week in a hotel, walking is a great way to burn off some of the kids' energy.)

Post a map, choose a walk, and cross off street by street till one day you finish the entire route together. The streets of San Francisco will become a great memory of something you did together—a memory the children in your life will cherish for a lifetime, and one they may re-create with their kids and grandkids one day.

> TIP: The route runs in a counterclockwise direction, so the official 49 Mile route markers are visible only from the counterclockwise direction.

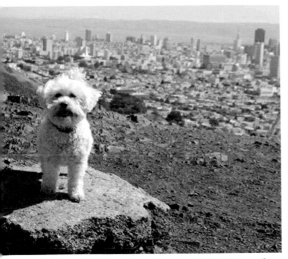

Charley the Bichon (seen here on Walk 13, top of Twin Peaks), hopes to be the first dog in history to walk the entire 49 Mile Scenic Drive.

With your inner athlete

Challenge seekers and athletes: Very few people on the planet, living or dead, have *walked* this entire route. You have the opportunity to be among the first and few to conquer this challenge. You can set the speed and time frame, decide whether it's a personal challenge or if you want to challenge your friends. It's not easy—that's why it's called a challenge. But when you've earned the right to wear the official badge, the bragging rights will be awesome.

Walkers and casual strollers: Make the walk part of your exercise program and go your own pace. Start with just one mile at a time and work your way up. If you took one full hike every three weeks, you would finish in a year. There is probably a Meetup group online right now that would love to have you join them. If not, create one that fits your schedule. (And it's a great way to work off the extra calories from San Francisco's exquisite cuisine.)

With yourself

Need space? All too often we dream of getting away. We need the solitude, relaxation, and stimulation of a vacation. Why not turn this challenge into a way to take time for yourself, a little staycation adventure once a month? It's amazing how rejuvenating it can be to get outside, walk, and explore. The rhythm of walking can actually alter our brain waves and put us into a creative or relaxed or meditative state. Pair that up with the beauty of San Francisco, the adventure of exploring a new place—and after a few hours hiking city streets, you might feel like you've just come back from a weekender.

With the city, all over again

San Francisco regularly wins the ranking of No. 1 popular tourist destination in the world. People from all over come for its beauty, culture, and history—and pay $200+ a night for the privilege. It's also ranked the fourth most expensive city in the country to live in. How much does it cost you per night to live in the city, or the greater Bay Area? Get out there and get your money's worth. And very soon—after a few gorgeous walks, and fun adventures, and surprising new sites, and rediscovered neighborhoods—you'll remember why you love it so much, and why you wouldn't live anywhere else.

Get Out and Enjoy This Beautiful City. You Paid for the Privilege of Being Here!

Whether you are a first-time visitor or native born, one of the wonderful things about this walking plan is it gives you lots of options to explore in the way that suits you best. Whether

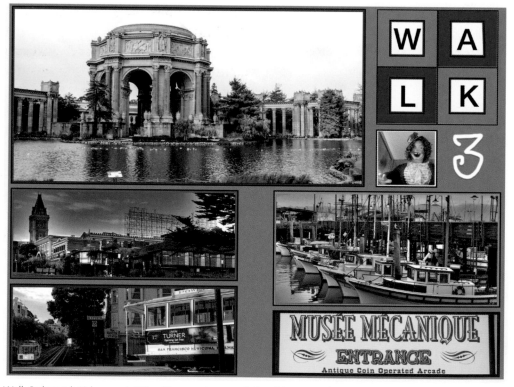

Walk 3 through Fisherman's Wharf is a must-see walk for visitors—and it's nice and flat.

you want easy walks while pushing your baby in a stroller, or you are an athlete who wants to be one of the first to walk it all—you have that option. If you live in the heart of the city, drive in on weekends, or visit only once a year—there are options for you, too!

This guidebook will give you all the information you need to walk San Francisco's 49 Mile Scenic route.

Each walk chapter covers a suggested walk of two to four miles and lists:

- The beginning and ending streets
- The bus lines you can take to get there and back
- Parking options
- A steepness rating for the hills
- Points of interest you will see along the route
- A history of the area
- Public bathroom locations along the route
- Warnings of "rough" neighborhoods
- An optional walk-back route

Plus:

- Suggestions for Because We Can shortcuts—little detours a car can't take, but *you* can
- Free museums along the way
- Must-see walks for out-of-town guests— if you can only fit in one or two walks, take one of the must-see walks, or send your visiting relatives on these walks. These focus on the city's most popular attractions.

The book also includes:

- Tabloid histories of San Francisco
- A full route map, so you can check off your progress
- Muni and SF parking basics
- Bonus chapters: including a lesson in identifying Victorian architecture

HOW TO USE THIS BOOK

This guide divides the 49 mile route into **17 walks of two to four miles each, some with optional side trips**. Each walk description gives you the starting and ending points, the length, the street-by-street directions, a map, a list of the sites you will be passing, some fun and obscure SF history factoids (which will make you the smartest person at the bar any night of the week). Each walk also includes the Muni connections, an optional walk-back loop, and much more. We've done all the hard work for you—well, except for the walking part.

You Don't Have to Sit Down and Read This Book All at Once Before You Start

The point is to get out and walk, so feel free to read the book one chapter at a time before each walk. Of course, if you find you enjoy the tabloid-style SF history tidbits so much you can't put the book down, that's okay, too. We hope that reading about the sites and history of the walk you are about to take will make the route more interesting. At the very least, the fun, obscure details of San Francisco's history will make you a better tour guide and will give you the opportunity to impress your friends with your knowledge.

You Don't Have to Walk the Route in Any Order

This is your walk, your adventure. The **Mile Markers and Walk segments** were chosen by what seem like logical neighborhood and topographical beginning and ending points, or because they are jam packed with gorgeous sites. The segments are just meant to make the route easier to plan and follow. Pick the walk that fits the weather or your mood that day. Walk one mile or six miles. Begin and stop where your preferred bus route has a stop. Speaking of which . . .

Strategies—How to Get Back to Your Car, Bus, or Hotel After Long Walks

If you are walking only one or two miles, it's easy to turn around and walk back to the beginning. However, if your goal is to follow the 49 mile route as far as you can in a day, three or six miles or more, you won't be beginning and ending in the same loca-

tion (known as a shuttle walk). But don't worry. We've built in some great strategies to get you back to your car, home, or hotel at the end of your day's adventure, such as the following:

- **Take Muni.** Each walk lists the bus you can catch at the end of the walk to return you to the beginning. Or check 511.org to see if there might be a better bus to catch at the end to take you where you want to go.

- **Use two cars.** If you and your friends are meeting for a long walk and traveling by car, consider parking one friend's car at the end of the walk to ferry you back to your car at the beginning of the route.

- **Take the walk-back loop.** For those who want longer five, six, or seven mile walks, we've designed alternate routes back to the beginning of each walk that show off other interesting sites in

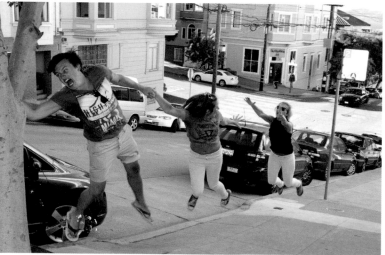

Muni travel helpers:
- 511.org
- MuniMobile app
- NextBus app

The Honess family, visiting from England, discovers San Francisco's hills.
PHOTO BY ANDY HONESS

the city. A few walk-backs are so good, they could be a great hike for another day.

- **Call a cab or Uber.**

Make it as big an adventure or as easy a stroll as you want.

A FEW 49 MILE ROUTE BASICS

The entire route is a giant loop running counterclockwise around the city. Thus the official route markers are displayed only in the counter-clock-wise direction. There is supposed to be a route sign at every turn, but while the city does a great job of maintaining the signs, they go missing now and then, so be sure to follow the guidebook directions.

The walks veer off the drive in a few places where it is illegal for pedestrians to walk, like the segment on Interstate 280, or where pedestrian safety is a concern. We have also noted a few places where you can choose to hike on trails parallel to the drive, or take the "Because We Can" shortcuts indicated in the guide that get you closer to San Francisco's treasures than a car can go.

Hills and Traffic

San Francisco has 48 (named) hills. The steepest 10 hills in the city climb at 25°–40° angles! Don't worry. We won't make you walk any of those, but you will climb many other hills.

Each walk has a 1–5 steepness rating so you know what you are getting into. 1=flat, 5=hire a Sherpa.

The goal is to walk the official 49 mile route, which runs on city streets, some of which are multilaned thoroughfares. Traffic is part of the city adventure—so are the more pastoral walks and return loops that trek through bushy paths or along the beach. (One of the bonus chapters, provided by pedestrian advocacy group **Walk San Francisco**, tells you about the innovative strategies San Francisco is putting into place to reduce traffic danger and make the city a safe walker's paradise.)

San Francisco Weather

You can comfortably walk in San Francisco year round. But our seasons can be confusing. June and July tend to be cold, foggy, and windy. Spring and fall actually have the clearest skies and warmest weather.

San Francisco			Weather
Averages	High °F	Low °F	Rain (in)
January	57	46	4.6
February	60	48	4.0
March	62	49	3.1
April	63	49	1.3
May	64	51	0.3
June	66	53	0.2
July	67	54	0.0
August	68	55	0.1
September	70	55	0.3
October	69	54	1.3
November	63	50	3.2
December	57	46	4.5

Packing List for Your Walk
- Long-sleeve shirt, jacket, hat
- Reusable water bottle
- Sunscreen
- Smartphone or cell phone
- BART / Muni pass, cash, quarters, or a credit card for parking or a taxi
- Directions
- List of bathrooms on the route (don't forget to "go" before you leave the house, just in case)

Except during droughts, it rains in January and February, but clear, warm days are possible, too. There is little chance of rain from late March through early December, when temperatures range from 55° to 75°.

However, you also have to consider the microclimates. San Francisco's many microclimates mean that on the same day and same hour, one San Francisco neighborhood can be sunny and warm (probably the Mission), while another can be foggy, windy, and chilly (like the Sunset). It's part of the charm—bring a jacket, wear layers, maybe throw in a waterproof layer and a hat, too. Really, always bring a light jacket. A surprise romantic walk in the rain or fog could be around any corner!

Bottomline: Check the weather before you go. WeatherUnderground. com networks amateur hobbyists with digital meteorology devices throughout the various SF neighborhoods and can help pinpoint the microclimates sometimes better than the local news.

Traveling by Bike, Car, Stroller, or Wheelchair? Or with Fido?

The route is on city terrain—beautiful, crowded, ragged, new, gritty, tree-lined, fascinating, varied terrain. That's part of the adventure. Some streets lack sidewalks so the walk reroutes pedestrians up stairs or along dirt paths. Some narrow sidewalks are also buckled by tree roots, making them too narrow for wheelchairs or strollers. Some gritty streets have broken glass you wouldn't want your puppy walking across. Not many, but a few. Downtown rush-hour sidewalks are too crowded for anyone to walk on! We can't fix city streets, so beware, some spots might be tough for people navigating the course on wheels or with pets. That said, city folk walk their dogs and traverse on wheels every day. Use your best judgment. Also be sure to check the steepness rating for each walk. Anything rated 3–5 may be challenging on wheels. (NOTE: Muni requires dogs to be muzzled.)

By car? Really? Okay, if you really just want to get in your car and drive the route, we won't judge you. Turn-by-turn instructions for driving are in the back of the book, plus we've created a shorter "highlights" route for those with limited time or patience.

Shhhh—don't tell anyone, but today's route is closer to 46 miles than 49. But you still get credit for walking all 49!

SF "TABLOID" HISTORY: WE'RE PRETTY SURE IT'S ALL TRUE

The walk celebrates SF history, heroes, and hilly sites—not all of them, just the ones found directly on the route. Along with basic neighborhood history, we've included a bonus section of SF tabloid history at the end of nearly every walk chapter. *The Daily Crab* serves up bite-size snippets of lesser known, quirky history told in a way to make you smile (or cringe) and may whet your appetite to Google for more details—or maybe even inspire you to read a history book. This city, founded by greedy gold-seekers, has never had a shortage of heroes, villains, adventurers, politicians, millionaires, and hundreds of thousands of average Joes and Janes working to keep it a creative, innovative, amazing place. We'll introduce you to a few, past and present.

WHAT IS NOT IN THE GUIDE

In some ways this is *not* a typical guidebook in that it doesn't list things like the hours of operation, phone numbers, and website addresses of every cool place you will pass along the way. (It's faster and more up to date to do a quick online search for that kind of info anyway.) The goal of this book is to get you out there walking the city streets, taking in the beauty, and having an adventure. But, please, feel

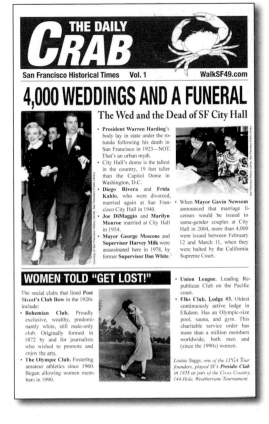

THE DAILY CRAB

San Francisco Historical Times   Vol. 1   WalkSF49.com

4,000 WEDDINGS AND A FUNERAL
The Wed and the Dead of SF City Hall

- **President Warren Harding's** body lay in state under the rotunda following his death in San Francisco in 1923—NOT. That's an urban myth.
- City Hall's dome is the tallest in the country, 19 feet taller than the Capitol Dome in Washington, D.C.
- **Diego Rivera** and **Frida Kahlo,** who were divorced, married again at San Francisco City Hall in 1940.
- **Joe DiMaggio** and **Marilyn Monroe** married at City Hall in 1954.
- **Mayor George Moscone** and **Supervisor Harvey Milk** were assassinated here in 1978, by former **Supervisor Dan White.**
- When **Mayor Gavin Newsom** announced that marriage licenses would be issued to same-gender couples at City Hall in 2004, more than 4,000 were issued between February 12 and March 11, when they were halted by the California Supreme Court.

WOMEN TOLD "GET LOST!"

The social clubs that lined Post Street's Club Row in the 1920s include:
- **Bohemian Club.** Proudly exclusive, wealthy, predominantly white, still male-only club. Originally formed in 1872 by and for journalists who wished to promote and enjoy the arts.
- **The Olympic Club.** Fostering amateur athletics since 1960. Began allowing women members in 1990.

- **Union League.** Leading Republican Club on the Pacific coast.
- **Elks Club, Lodge #3.** Oldest continuously active lodge in Elkdom. Has an Olympic-size pool, sauna, and gym. This charitable service order has more than a million members worldwide, both men and (since the 1990s) women.

Louise Suggs, one of the LPGA Tour founders, played SF's Presidio Club in 1935 as part of the Cross Country, 144-Hole, Weathervane Tournament.

free to stop, visit, shop, eat, or take pictures anywhere along the route because—yes, you've got it—it's *your* adventure, it's your city.

So get your gear together, call a friend, leash the dog, make a plan, look up the Muni route—and let's get started.

- *Tag and share your photos, new finds, and route hints at #WalkSF49.*
- *Connect with us and other walkers @WalkSF49.*
- *Plus get the WalkSF49 app and more at www.WalkSF49.com.*

MAP LEGEND

●	Start Here
———	49 Mile Walk Path
– – –	Optional Detour
••••••••	Optional Return Walk Path
———	Muni Return Route
‖‖‖‖‖‖	Muni Metro Route
P	Parking Lot
1	Point of Interest
18	Gone SF
a	Detour Point of Interest
MUNI	Muni Railway
8	Muni Route Number
👀	Take Caution
🚻	Public Restroom
▬	Public Park

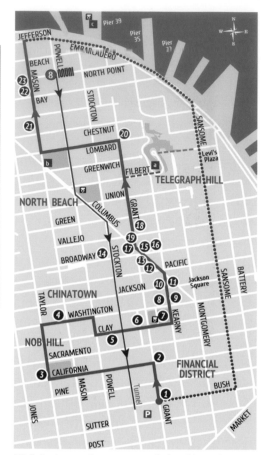

Walk 2, the no. 1 must-see walk for visitors, is packed with San Francisco icons—and lots of steep hills.

Of special note:

GONE SF

Denotes SF landmarks that are detailed on the route but have been torn down.

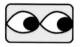

Denotes less safe parts of town where criminal activity has been known to occur, or homeless people might congregate, etc. Put your phone/wallet/valuables in your pocket, pay attention, walk quickly, and use your best judgment.

1 = flat terrain

5 = very steep hill

Miles—Steps—Hours

The miles per walk and length of walk are based on taking the direct route alone. If you stop and visit the stores, museums, and churches and take the detours—which we welcome you to do—you could double those estimates. Step counts are based on a 2,000-steps-per-mile average. Your step count will vary based on your height, stride length, and measuring device.

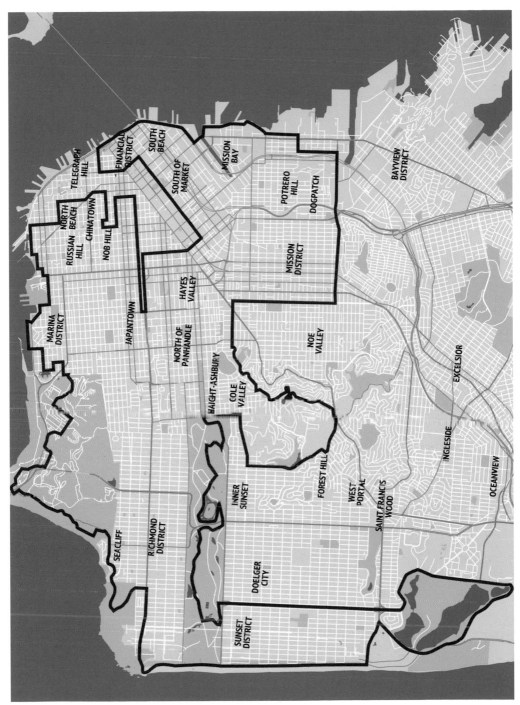

The entire 49 Mile route in a glance

49
MILE

SCENIC
DRIVE

Civic Center

Japantown

Union Square

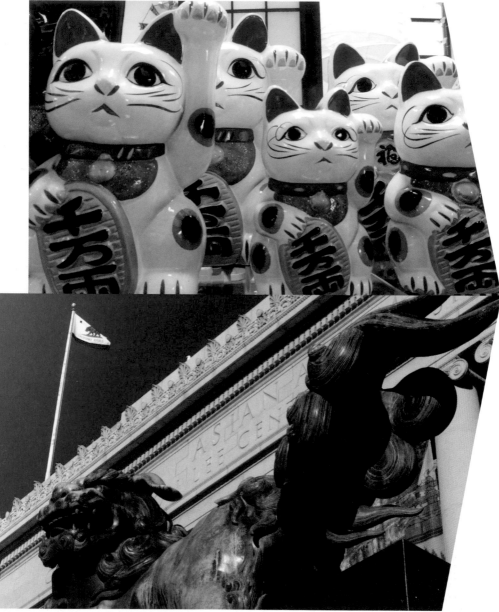

The maneki-neko lucky cats (top) are waiting to greet you in Japantown after your visit to the Asian Art Museum (bottom).

You are invited to start your 49 Mile Challenge anywhere along the route, but the official beginning is in front of San Francisco's Beaux-Arts City Hall, facing the grassy, one-square-block Civic Center Plaza. It's an easy walk up to City Hall from BART or Muni or you can park in the Civic Center underground parking lot.

You'll begin with a lap around the plaza's stately and historic buildings—the Bill Graham Civic Auditorium, the Main Library, U.N. Plaza, the Asian Art Museum, and the California Supreme Court building. Then you'll spend just a few blocks along the edge of the city's gritty and changing Tenderloin District, including a short walk through Little Saigon.

The uphill westward climb on busy Geary Boulevard takes you past a few of the sacred sanctuaries on Cathedral Hill as you head toward Japantown, where you'll flip back around eastward through the Union Square high-end shopping district and end at Chinatown's Dragon Gate. All in just three miles! Who needs Epcot Center when you have San Francisco?

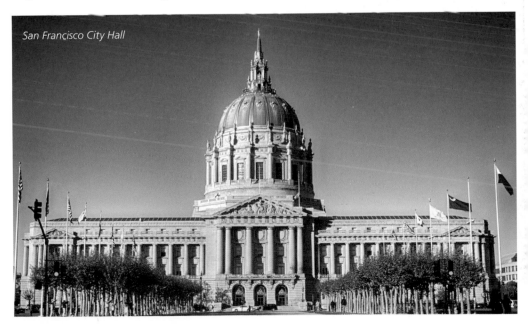

San Francisco City Hall

Begin:	City Hall Entrance, 1 Dr Carlton B Goodlett Place (Polk St) Hill Rating:
End:	Grant Avenue and Bush Street (Chinatown's Dragon Gate)
Distance:	ROUTE: 3.0 miles—6,000 steps—1 hour
	LOOP BACK: 1.8 miles—3,600 steps—35 minutes
Note:	Edgy neighborhood

Sites you will pass on today's walk include:

MILE 1

1. **City Hall**
   1 Goodlett Pl

2. **Bill Graham Civic Auditorium**
   99 Grove St

3. **Main Library**
   100 Larkin St

4. **United Nations Plaza**

5. **Asian Art Museum of San Francisco**
   200 Larkin St

6. **Giant Marquee**
   500 Turk St at Larkin St

7. **Phoenix Hotel**
   601 Eddy St at Larkin St

8. **Little Saigon**
   Eddy St at Larkin St

9. **Geary Boulevard**

10. **Tommy's Joynt**
    1101 Geary Blvd at Van Ness Ave

MILE 2

CATHEDRAL HILL

11. **Saint Mary's Cathedral**
    1111 Gough St at Geary Blvd

12. **Chinese Consulate**
    1450 Laguna St at Geary Blvd

13. **Kanrin Maru Trees**
    Geary Blvd at Laguna St

14. **Japan Center**
    1610 Geary Blvd

15. **Peace Pavilion** in Japantown

16. **Post Street**

a. **Relocated Victorians**

17. **Jack Tar Hotel**
    GONE SF Post St at Van Ness Ave

MILE 3

18. **Van Ness Avenue**

19. **Polk Street**

20. **Union Square**
    Post St between Powell St and Stockton St

21. **Victoria Monument**
    in Union Square

22. **Dragon Gate**
    Grant Ave and Bush St

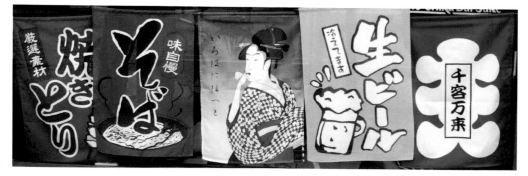

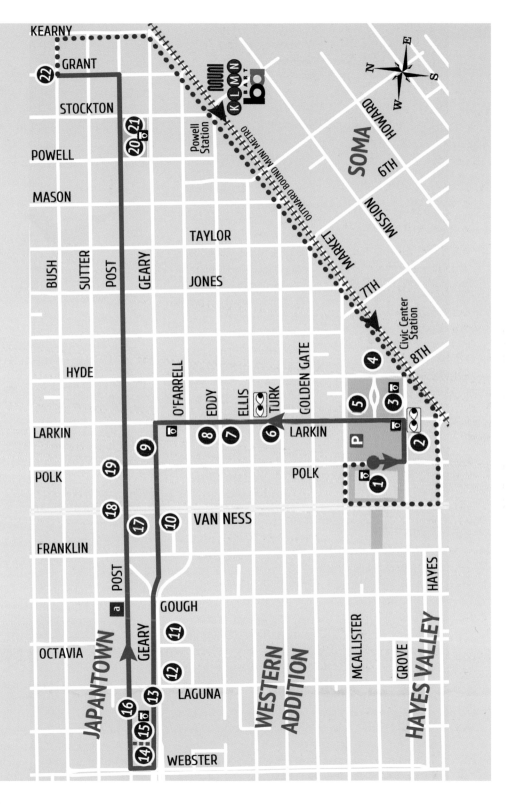

MILE 1

Begins on 1 DR CARLTON B GOODLETT PL

. . . .

Walk south on GOODLETT PL toward GROVE ST

. . . .

1. City Hall 1 Dr Carlton B Goodlett Pl

After the 1906 earthquake and fire destroyed the original City Hall, the job of the new Beaux-Arts-style City Hall was to show off San Francisco's glorious rebirth to fairgoers as they streamed into the 1915 Panama-Pacific International Exposition. With a little help from designer Arthur Brown Jr., SF outdid herself. Brown modeled the dome after St. Peter's Basilica in Rome and even sent an assistant to Washington, D.C., to measure the Capital Dome to make sure ours would be taller. After City Hall was damaged again in the 1989 Loma Prieta earthquake, it was closed for seismic retrofitting and emerged with a bonus $300,000 face-lift, including a shiny refurbished gold dome. Free tours: Mon.– Fri., 10 a.m., noon, 2 p.m.

. . . .

Cross GROVE ST
Left on GROVE ST

. . . .

California's First Black Governor—*Almost.* The street in front of City Hall is named for civil rights maverick Dr. Carlton B. Goodlett, a family doctor who built a small San Francisco weekly tabloid, the *Sun-Reporter*, into an influential newspaper chain, which he used to campaign for civil rights. His causes included the hiring of blacks by the San Francisco Municipal Railway, desegregation of the city's municipal labor unions, and improvements in public housing in the 1950s and '60s. In 1966, he became the first black American since Reconstruction to mount a serious candidacy for the governorship of California. He lost to Pat Brown in the Democratic primary.

2. Bill Graham Civic Auditorium
99 Grove St

This block-long, 6,000-seat arena to your right was built as part of the 1915 Panama-Pacific International Exhibition. Over the next century it went on to host events as diverse as the San Francisco Symphony Orchestra, the Democratic National Convention in 1920,

and the NBA Golden State Warriors from 1964 to 1966 before being renamed after rock-and-roll-promoting legend Bill Graham in 1991. (Not to be confused with evangelist Billy Graham.)

. . . .

Left on LARKIN ST

. . . .

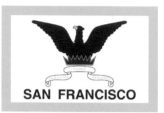

The city's official flag and motto, Oro en Paz. Fierro en Guerra. (Gold in Peace. Iron in War)

3. Main Library
100 Larkin St

On the 90th anniversary of the great quake, April 18, 1996, San Franciscans opened the doors of their brand-new main library, a block away from their old main library. Designed by I. M. Pei, who also designed the pyramid in front of the Louvre in France, this six-story building contains over 300 computer terminals, room for 1,100 laptops, and 1.1 million books written in 50 languages.

4. United Nations Plaza
(between the Main Library and Asian Art Museum)

The peace treaty that officially ended the Pacific War with the Empire of Japan and the United Nations Charter (1945)

Many people assume the city's rise from the ashes of the 1906 quake inspired the Phoenix symbol in San Francisco's city flag. *Not so.* SF burned down so often in the 1850s that the Greek mythological Phoenix bird rising from the fire seemed perfect for the city flag, which was designed in 1900.

were both signed here in San Francisco. Built in 1975 to honor the latter event, United Nations Plaza has become more known today for its entrance to Muni and BART, farmers' market, and hangout location for homeless people.

5. Asian Art Museum of San Francisco— Chong-Moon Lee Center for Asian Art and Culture 200 Larkin St

Moved from Golden Gate Park to the extensively remodeled old main library in 2003, San Francisco's Asian Art Museum graces us with one of the largest museums in the Western world devoted exclusively to Asian art— featuring over 17,000 works of art spanning 6,000 years of history. HINT: Free admission the first Sunday of each month.

6. Giant (Kahn & Keville) Marquee with Witty Sayings at Turk St and Larkin St

While serving as a soldier during World War I, Hugh Keville carried a little notebook of inspirational sayings to keep his spirits up. When he returned to his tire shop he decided to share the quotes that encouraged him with his customers. To the delight of San Franciscans the tradition has continued ever since. —as reported in *The Bold Italic*

7. Kitschy-chic Phoenix Hotel 601 Eddy St at Larkin St

The Phoenix Hotel is behind the fence on your left. Voted no. 1 Hippest Hotel by *Travel and Leisure* magazine in 2012, this former roadside "no-tell" hotel's funky vibe, retro 50s décor, and Southern California

palm tree-lined pool scene lures rock-and-rollers, hipsters, and artists—from David Bowie and Johnny Rotten to Vincent Gallo and Johnny Depp.

8. Little Saigon Dragon Gateway Eddy St at Larkin St

When the 2000 U.S. Census showed that more than 2,000 Vietnamese residents and 250 Vietnamese-owned businesses were packed into a two-block stretch of the Tenderloin neighborhood, the city responded by recognizing the corridor of Larkin Street between Eddy Street and O'Farrell Street as "Little Saigon" in 2004 and building a symbolic gateway in 2008.

> A Theory
> "Tenderloin" was the nickname given to the neighborhood in the days when policemen were paid more to work its mean streets, thereby affording the cops better cuts of meat, like tenderloin.

. . . .
Left on GEARY BLVD
. . . .

9. Geary Boulevard

Geary Boulevard began life as a dirt carriage track out to the Cliff House on the Pacific Ocean. Today, Muni's 38 Geary line, which services the modern commercial boulevard, is the most heavily used bus line in

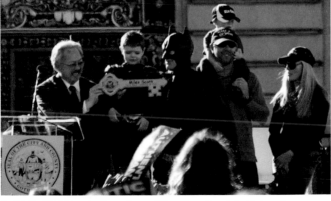

In 2013, 12,000 volunteers turned San Francisco into Batman's "Gotham City" to fulfill a "Make a Wish" request from child cancer survivor Miles Scott. After a day in the Batmobile stopping crime, "Batkid" Miles receives the Key to the City from Mayor Ed Lee in front of City Hall. PHOTO BY SHELLY PREVOST

the city, carrying over 50,000 passengers per day.

Geary Boulevard's sheer length and many lanes of traffic give it the unfortunate distinction of being one of the city's most dangerous streets for pedestrians—so pay attention at crosswalks!

10. Tommy's Joynt, Home of the Original Buffalo Burger, 1101 Geary St at Van Ness Ave

Arguably the most famous hofbrau in the city. Though they no longer serve deep-fried rattlesnake sandwiches, they've hardly changed since opening in 1947, and they like it that way: funky décor, good food, and cheap beer.

MILE 2

Begins on GEARY BLVD at GOUGH ST

CATHEDRAL HILL

Saint Mark's Lutheran Church (the oldest Lutheran church in the West) and **Saint Mary's Cathedral** are just a few of the churches on this holy hill. As you cross Franklin Street you'll pass the **Unitarian Universalist Church of San Francisco** on your left and the **Hamilton Square Baptist Church** on your right, which, some might say, reflect the spectrum of progressive and conservative religious belief, respectively.

11. Saint Mary's Cathedral
1111 Gough St

In the 1971 modern expressionist redesign of the **Cathedral of Saint Mary of the Assumption**, the four corners of the cathedral flow upward to form a cross. In the eye of some beholders, the top resembles a large washing machine agitator, which earned it the nickname "Our Lady of Maytag." On a more reverent note, Pope John Paul II celebrated papal mass in the cathedral in 1987.

12. Chinese Consulate, formerly the Salvation Army School for Officers Training
1450 Laguna St

The large campus of buildings on Geary Boulevard just

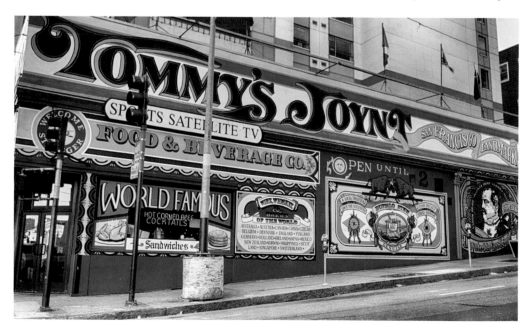

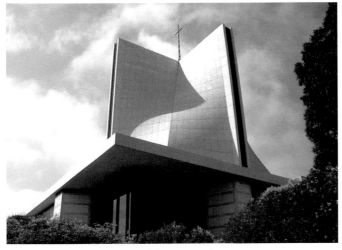

The Cathedral of Saint Mary of the Assumption

Japantown Origins

After the 1906 earthquake, tens of thousands of Issei (Japan-born immigrants), as well as Jewish people, settled in what is now called the Western Addition. By the outbreak of World War II it was the largest enclave of Japanese outside Japan. Horribly, the 40-block Japan-town neighborhood was emptied when President Roosevelt issued Executive Order 9066, sending the Issei and Nisei (American-born Japanese) to internment camps. African Americans arriving in San Francisco to work in the war industry moved into the vacated homes and into much of the adjacent Fillmore District. After the war, only a small portion of the Japanese residents moved back to the neighborhood.

past Saint Mary's houses the Consulate-General of the People's Republic of China in San Francisco (1450 Laguna Street). Visa and passport applications can be submitted here. Read more about the building's colorful past in the article at end of chapter: "Japanese Salvation Army Invades California."

. . . .

Cross to the even-numbered north side of GEARY BLVD

. . . .

13. Kanrin Maru Trees

Along the north side of Geary, at Laguna, as you approach Japantown you will see trees planted along the sidewalk in honor of the 150th anniversary of the 1860 arrival of the first Japanese ship ever to cross the Pacific, the *Kanrin Maru*.

14. Japan Center
1610 Geary Blvd

Comprising three square blocks, this complex celebrates Japanese culture with Japanese shops, restaurants, hotels, spa, and events, such as the Cherry Blossom, Soy and Tofu, Film, and J-POP festivals. It was completed in 1968 as part of the Western Addition Urban Renewal Plan.

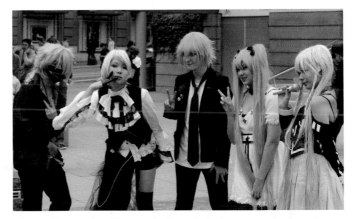

The J-POP summit celebrates the latest in Japanese pop music and culture. PHOTO: GARY STEVENS

15. Peace Pavilion
(or Peace Pagoda)
in Japantown

As a gesture of goodwill, San Francisco's sister city in Japan, Osaka, donated this five-tiered concrete shrine to us in 1968.

BECAUSE WE CAN
SHORTCUT

When you see the Peace Pagoda to your right, feel free to cut across the plaza here to Post Street (one-half block before the official turn at Webster Street).

Right on WEBSTER ST

Right on POST ST

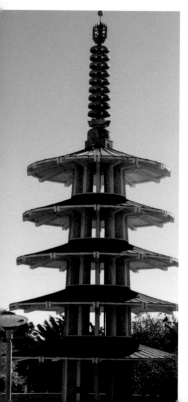

Peace Pagoda, Japantown

16. Post Street

We suggest you embrace your inner tourist all the way down Post Street. Look down alleys, stare up at the architectural features at the tops of buildings, and watch the neighborhoods change block by block. Wonder: How did these few Victorian houses on the 1400 block survive amidst the concrete rebuilding here? What was life like for turn-of-the-century workers in these cramped old apartment buildings? Find the circa 1916 date on the Poindexter Apartments (754 Post Street)—and one of the city's new parklets in front of it. Notice as the smorgasbord of Southeast Asian cuisine restaurants disappear and the art galleries, salons, and boutiques begin to appear in the theater district. See if you can spot any of the social clubs left from the 1920s Club Row: The Olympic Club, Bohemian Club, Union League, Elks Lodge.

a. Relocated Victorians
Post St at Gough St

When the Western Addition was declared "blighted" (a dangerous slum) and slated for urban renewal, approximately 2,500 Victorians were torn down, 883 businesses closed, and 30,000 residents displaced. Amazingly, 12 Victorian homes were jacked up onto trucks and relocated, including the four here on Post:

- 1400 Post, San Francisco stick
- 1402 Post, Edwardian
- 1406–1408 Post, San Francisco stick
- 1410 Post, slanted-bay Italianate Victorian

See fantastic photographs of these large homes being moved (including the ones you are passing on Post Street by Googling: David Glass House Movers. (The architecture chapter on page 184 explains the different styles of Victorians.)

GONE SF
17. Jack Tar Hotel, now the California Pacific Medical Center
Corner of Post St and Van Ness Ave

The cutting-edge Jack Tar Hotel, built on this site in 1960, boasted 403 modern rooms, a 450-car garage, attached 12-story office building—and the first air conditioning of any hotel in town. Most people hated the design; nonetheless, it became a city icon. In 1982, she became the Cathedral Hill Hotel and in 2009 closed after a devastating fire. The $2.1 billion, 274-bed CPMC Medical Center is slated to open in 2019.

MILE 3

Begins on POST ST at
VAN NESS AVE

18. Van Ness Avenue

The owners of the mansions that lined this wide residential street were not at all happy when the U.S. Army dynamited their exquisite homes as a firebreak to halt the inferno sweeping across the city in the aftermath of the 1906 quake. Happily, Van Ness returned as an upscale commercial district lined with grand apartment buildings. It is also officially part of U.S. Highway 101 as it runs through the city.

19. Polk Street

Polk Gulch, the neighborhood from Geary Boulevard to Union Square, was San Francisco's main gay neighborhood before 1970 and was the location of the first official San Francisco Gay Pride Parade, in 1972. Several LGBT bars and clubs remain in the area, but it is now a melting pot of cultures, restaurants, and nightlife. As you head north on Polk toward the Marina the street gets less "gritty."

20. Union Square

Post St between Powell St and Stockton St

Named for the pro-Union Civil War rallies held here during the early 1860s, the one-block Union Square plaza area now rallies shoppers to a 14-block radius of department stores, upscale boutiques, gift shops, art galleries, beauty salons, theaters, and upscale hotels. HINT: It's also home to the half-price ticket booth for shows throughout the city.

21. Victoria Monument —the power of sex appeal in Union Square

At the center of Union Square stands a tall Corinthian column commemorating the victory of Admiral George Dewey in 1898 at Manila Bay during the Spanish-American War. Sugar millionaire Adolph Spreckels personally chose six-foot-tall, buxom, loud Alma de Bretteville to pose for the statue of Victoria, goddess of victory, to top the column. Soon thereafter Alma became Mrs. Adolph Spreckels. Her pet name for her 23-years-her-senior hubby, "Sugar Daddy," joined the American lexicon.

When the society crowd shunned this former nude art model, she gave not a damn. Filthy rich "Big Alma" smoked cigars, swam nude at her pool

Union Square stores boast the world's most famous brands. The Spanish company Zara is a favorite of Kate Middleton, Duchess of Cambridge.

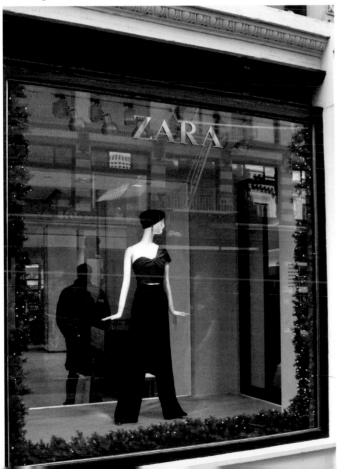

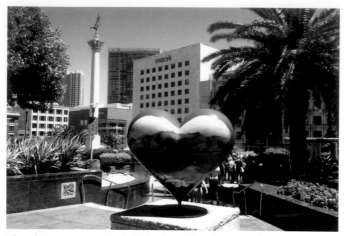

Victoria Monument stands high above Tony Bennett's heart sculpture at Union Square. PHOTO: LTLEELIM

WALK-BACK LOOP SCOOP

On this short, 35-minute walk-back route you can window-shop along Market Street, snap a pic of the cable car turnaround on Powell Street, and then, as you loop behind City Hall, gander up at some monumental Civic Center buildings on Van Ness Avenue: the Davies Symphony Hall, San Francisco War Memorial and Performing Arts Center (home of the San Francisco Opera), and California Public Utilities Commission. See the directions on page 25.

in front of her guests, guzzled martinis, had bisexual affairs, and used her wealth to buy art, donate to the city on a grand scale, and create her own bohemian salon. *You go, girl!*

· · · · · · · · · · · · · · · · · ·
Left on GRANT AVE
End on BUSH ST
· · · · · · · · · · · · · · · · · ·

22. Dragon Gate
Grant Ave and Bush St

Walk 1 ends here at the entrance to Chinatown. You can flip ahead a few pages to Walk 2 to continue on the next leg of your 49 Mile adventure; or head back to your car (via walking or bus); or walk over to Union Square for some shopping, food, theater tickets, and to watch hundreds of tourists lined up to catch the cable car at Powell and Market Streets. (We recommend catching the California Street cable car at Van Ness—see Fisherman's Wharf Walk 3 for details.)

TWEET YOUR SUCCESS

On the walk-back loop you can see the Twitter bird logo hanging off Twitter's headquarters on the corner of 10th and Market Streets. Tweet out your successful start of the 49 Mile challenge to the world—and tag us **@WalkSF49**—so we can celebrate with you!

Zero Traffic Deaths in San Francisco

Thanks to Vision Zero SF—a city and community effort to eliminate all traffic deaths in San Francisco by 2024—your stroll back along Market will be much safer than in previous years. How?

Until 2015, the stretch of Market between 3rd and 8th Streets was a teeming river of pedestrians, bikes, buses, trolleys, taxis, trucks, skateboarders—and as many as 500 cars an hour (during the busiest times of day). Right-hand turns made Market Street intersections the most dangerous in the city for cyclists and pedestrians.

Solution: Ban cars from turning onto Market between 3rd and 8th Streets. That 40% reduction in traffic not only will save lives, it also means smoother, quicker sailing for Muni and quicker delivery of goods by commercial trucks. Taxis (though not Uber or Lyft) and emergency vehicles are allowed. Private cars may cross Market but may not turn onto or drive down those five blocks.

This is one of 24 priority safety projects that the city has put in place as part of Vision Zero SF. *Thank you!*

WALK 1 NEED TO KNOW

TO GET THERE
BART/Muni

- Take any BART or underground Muni Train to CIVIC CENTER STATION
- Muni F-Line, 19, 21, 47, 49, 19 all stops near the start of this segment
- Check 511.org or NextBus.com for current bus schedules

PARKING
- Metered street (difficult)
- Civic Center Garage 355 McAllister at Larkin
- Check ParkMe.com for other area parking options

PUBLIC RESTROOMS
- City Hall
- Public Library (Grove)
- Grove (Larkin)
- Larkin (Myrtle)
- Japan Center (Geary)
- Union Square (252 Geary at Powell)

TURN–BY–TURN INSTRUCTIONS
Begin: Between MCALLISTER and GROVE STS where POLK ST turns into CARLTON B GOODLETT PL

- Walk south on GOODLETT PL toward GROVE ST
- Cross GROVE ST
- Left on GROVE ST
- Left on LARKIN ST

- Left on GEARY BLVD, 1.3 miles
- At LAGUNA ST cross to the even-numbered north side of GEARY BLVD
- Right on WEBSTER ST
- Right on POST ST, continue 1 mile, passed Union Square
- Left on GRANT AVE

End: BUSH ST at GRANT AVE

TO GET BACK
- Walk to MONTGOMERY ST and MARKET ST
- Enter underground MONTGOMERY STATION
- Take any outbound BART or Muni train to CIVIC CENTER STATION

or

- Walk to MARKET ST and GRANT AVE for other Muni 5, 21

OPTIONAL WALK-BACK LOOP DIRECTIONS
Distance: 1.8 miles, 3,600 steps, 35 minutes

Rating:

Begin: GRANT AVE and BUSH ST

- If you're facing Chinatown's Dragon Gate, turn Right down BUSH ST, 1 block to KEARNY ST
- Right on KEARNY ST, 3 blocks
- Right on MARKET ST
- Veer right onto HAYES ST
- Right on VAN NESS AVE
- Right on McALLISTER ST
- Right on POLK ST (GOODLETT PL)

End: CIVIC CENTER, City Hall

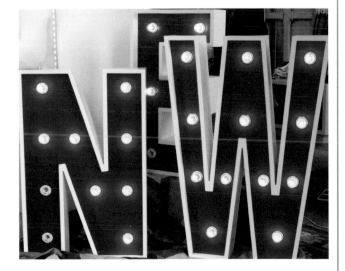

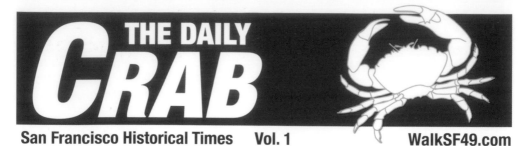

THE DAILY CRAB

San Francisco Historical Times   Vol. 1   WalkSF49.com

4,000 WEDDINGS AND A FUNERAL

The Wed and the Dead of SF City Hall

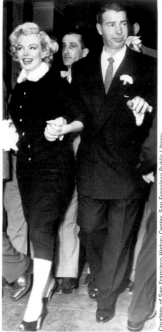

Courtesy of San Francisco History Center, San Francisco Public Library

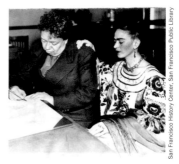

San Francisco History Center, San Francisco Public Library

- **President Warren Harding**'s body lay in state under the rotunda following his death in San Francisco in 1923—NOT. That's an urban myth.
- City Hall's dome is the tallest in the country, 19 feet taller than the Capitol Dome in Washington, D.C.
- **Diego Rivera** and **Frida Kahlo**, who were divorced, married again at San Francisco City Hall in 1940.
- **Joe DiMaggio** and **Marilyn Monroe** married at City Hall in 1954.
- **Mayor George Moscone** and **Supervisor Harvey Milk** were assassinated here in 1978, by former **Supervisor Dan White**.
- When **Mayor Gavin Newsom** announced that marriage licenses would be issued to same-gender couples at City Hall in 2004, more than 4,000 were issued between February 12 and March 11, when they were halted by the California Supreme Court.

WOMEN TOLD "GET LOST!"

The social clubs that lined **Post Street's Club Row** in the 1920s include:

- **Bohemian Club.** Proudly exclusive, wealthy, predominantly white, still male-only club. Originally formed in 1872 by and for journalists who wished to promote and enjoy the arts.
- **The Olympic Club.** Fostering amateur athletics since 1860. Began allowing women members in 1990.

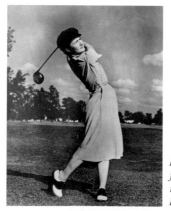

- **Union League.** Leading Republican Club on the Pacific coast.
- **Elks Club, Lodge #3.** Oldest continuously active lodge in Elkdom. Has an Olympic-size pool, sauna, and gym. This charitable service order has more than a million members worldwide, both men and (since the 1990s) women.

*Louise Suggs, one of the LPGA Tour founders, played SF's **Presidio Club** in 1953 as part of the Cross Country, 144-Hole, Weathervane Tournament.*

Japanese Salvation Army INVADES CALIFORNIA

After hearing a rousing **Salvation Army** minister speak at the 1915 Panama-Pacific Expo, charismatic Presbyterian minister **Masasuke Kobayashi** set out to bring the Army's ministries to **Nihonmachi** (Japantown).

Over 500 Japanese attended the official opening, and together the community created a Salvation Army rest home, medical clinic, orphanage, and day care center. The **Emperor of Japan** donated 5,000 yen ($1,700) for the new headquarters at **1450 Laguna** in 1937. Eventually, 12 Japanese Salvation Army ministers served the Japanese communities in Sacramento, Visalia, Seattle, Oakland, Stockton, Los Angeles, Fresno, and San Jose.

In 1942, after the attack on **Pearl Harbor**, the U.S. ordered the internment of people of Japanese descent. Salvation Army officials refused to cooperate. They filed appeals and even tried hiding the orphans on a farm in Marin County, but the government prevailed. Japanese Salvationists sent to internment camps held services there, but the larger

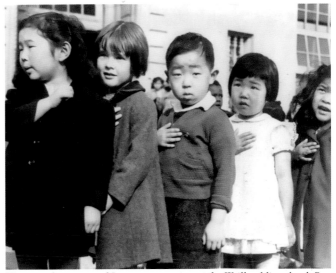

First-graders, some of Japanese ancestry, at the Weill public school, San Francisco, pledging allegiance to the United States flag (1942). Evacuees of Japanese ancestry were housed in war relocation authority centers for the duration of the war. Photo by Dorothea Lange

work in the Japanese community did not recover after the war.

The headquarters building became a training school for Salvation Army ministers. It was sold in 1975. Today the building houses the Chinese Embassy.
—from *The Bells of San Francisco,* by Judy Vaughn

WILL YOU SURVIVE?!
Tourist asks, "Is it safe to walk through the Tenderloin?"

A 2010 *New York Times* article described San Francisco's Tenderloin Neighborhood as "the ragged, druggy and determinedly dingy domain of the city's most down and out." A local online guide summed it up: "Sure, there are loads of drug dealers, addicts, prostitutes, and mentally unstable street people, but if you can get past that, you'll find it is also one of the city's most exciting and diverse locales."

Fortunately, you are walking by an outer edge during the day. Stay alert, keep walking, you'll be past it in a few short blocks.

MOVIE STAR SIGHTINGS AT UNION SQUARE

Francis Ford Coppola shot scenes of *The Conversation* (with actor **Gene Hackman**, 1974) in Union Square, where the bugged conversation, which forms the foundation of the movie, takes place.

Scenes of the square were also featured in **Alfred Hitchcock**'s thriller *Vertigo* (1958) and **Philip Kaufman**'s remake of *Invasion of the Body Snatchers* (1978).

In the opening scene of Hitchcock's *The Birds* (1963), the character Melanie Daniels (**Tippi Hedren**) looks up and sees hundreds of birds flying in a circular pattern around Victoria Monument.

49 MILE SCENIC DRIVE

MILE

This section of the historic 49 Mile route is jampacked with iconic San Francisco experiences. Your journey begins as you pass under the symbolic Dragon Gate and into the charming part of Chinatown that caters to out-of-town guests—chinoiserie pagoda architecture, colorful paper lanterns, and packed curio shops spilling jade, porcelain vases, silk, Buddha statues, and trinkets out into street stalls.

Then a sharp left takes you on a steep, steep climb to the remaining mansions, cathedral, and hotels of Nob Hill (where San Francisco's wealthy nobility, or "nobs," once lived). On the way back down, you'll pass the historic Cable Car Barn as you loop back to the other end of Chinatown—with its dizzying array of foods, sights, smells, shops, and restaurants on the crowded streets where the locals shop and work.

Take the time to gaze up at fire escapes and building architecture, peer down alleyways and mysterious stairwells leading belowground, and peek into shop windows—you will be rewarded! If you think you see bacon hanging on a clothesline, you do. It's a meat-curing method used in some Chinese homes.

As you pass the birthplace of San Francisco, Portsmouth Square, feel free to stop and practice your tai chi before traveling to your next historic neighborhood, North Beach, native land of the Beatniks, the sexual revolution, cappuccino, and Coit Tower. Since Walk 2 ends at Fisherman's Wharf, you are free to spend the next few hours exploring, shopping, and sampling the visual, historic, and gastronomic treats by the bay before you grab a cab home or take the walk-back loop down the Embarcadero and the Financial District.

The big question of the day: How many meals can you eat in one walk? And how will you choose among all the exquisite Chinese, Italian, and seafood delicacies on the way?

The copper-green triangular flat-iron building, the Columbus Tower, borders the Financial District, North Beach, and Chinatown (pictured at bottom).

		Hill Rating:
Begin:	Grant Avenue at Bush Street (Chinatown's Dragon Gate)	
End:	Lombard Street and Mason Street	
Distance:	ROUTE: 2.5 miles — 5,100 steps — 50 minutes	
	LOOP BACK: 2.0 miles — 4,000 steps — 40 minutes	

Sites you will pass on today's walk include:

MILE 4

1. **Chinatown Dragon Gate**
   Grant Ave and Bush St

2. **Old St. Mary's Cathedral**
   660 California St

NOB HILL

3. **Grace Cathedral**
   1051 Taylor St

4. **Cable Car Barn and Powerhouse**
   1201 Mason St

5. **Chinese Historical Society** 965 Clay St

6. **Waverly Place**
   off Clay St

"REAL" CHINATOWN

7. **Portsmouth Square**
   Clay St and Kearny St

8. **Buddha's Universal Church**
   720 Washington St

9. **CCSF Chinatown Branch**
   808 Kearny St

MILE 5

10. **Manilatown I-Hotel** 868 Kearny St at Jackson St

JACKSON SQUARE HISTORIC DISTRICT
Kearny St at Columbus St

11. **Columbus Tower/ Sentinel Building**
    916 Kearny St

12. **Vesuvio Café**
    255 Columbus Ave

13. **City Lights Bookstore**
    261 Columbus Ave

14. **Broadway**
    intersects at Columbus Ave

15. **Condor Club**
    560 Broadway

16. **Beat Museum**
    540 Broadway

17. *Language of the Birds* Broadway at Columbus Ave

18. **Grant Avenue**
    intersects at Columbus Av

19. **Caffe Trieste** 601 Vallejo St at Grant Ave

DETOUR

a. **Coit Tower**
   1 Telegraph Hill Blvd (use Filbert St stairs off Grant Ave)

20. **Lombard Street View** Grant Ave at Lombard St

b. **New North Beach Library**
   850 Columbus Ave

21. **Fior d'Italia**
    2237 Mason St

22. **Ginsberg's Dublin Pub**
    GONE SF 400 Bay St

23. **International Longshore and Warehouse Union**
    400 North Point St and Mason St

ON WALK-BACK LOOP

c. **Pier 39** Beach St and the Embarcadero

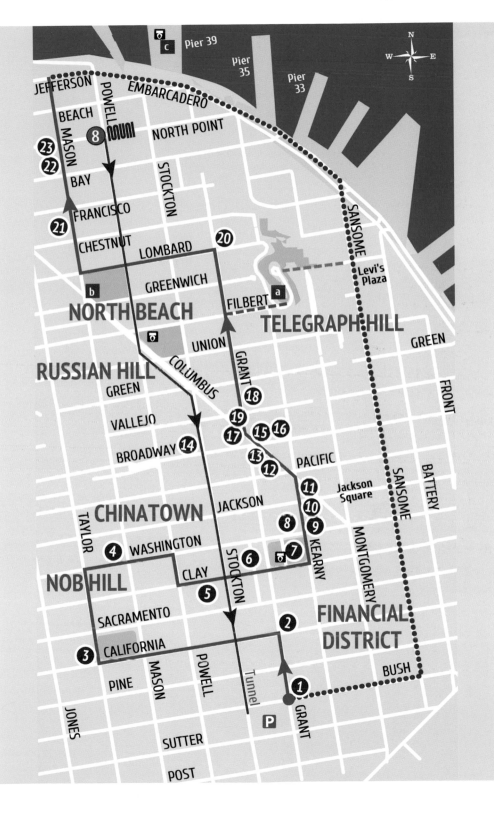

MILE 4

Begins at Chinatown's Dragon Gate, GRANT AVE at BUSH ST

Continue on GRANT AVE from Walk 1 (north)

1. Chinatown Dragon Gate
Bush and Grant Sts

"All under heaven is for the good of the people," says the inscription by Dr. Sun Yat-sen (founding father of the Republic of China) on Chinatown's two-tiered, green-tile-roofed arch. The captivating entryway, built in 1970, faces the correct feng shui-approved direction (south) and is flanked by two lion statues meant to thwart evil spirits.

2. Old St. Mary's Cathedral
660 California St

The oldest cathedral in California, Old St. Mary's, was built in 1854 by Chinese laborers using granite quarried in China and bricks shipped around Cape Horn from New England. In those wild, early days, bordellos surrounded the church. If men exiting those neighboring houses of ill-repute glanced up at the clock on the church bell tower they would be admonished by a Bible verse inscribed there, "Son, observe the time and fly from evil."

Chinese Lions

In China, the lion is regarded as the king of the forests and has thus long been used as a symbol of power and grandeur. It is even believed to offer protection from evil spirits. At the Dragon Gate a male lion sits with his right paw on a ball, the symbol of unity of the Chinese empire, while a female lion has a cub under her left paw, a symbol of offspring.

Left on CALIFORNIA ST (very steep uphill climb)

NOTE: If California Street looks too steep for you to climb, you can hop on a cable car. Ask to get off at Grace Cathedral.

How to Walk on Steep Hills
There's a natural tendency to lean forward when walking uphill and lean backward when walking downhill. However, leaning can put a lot of strain on your back and should be avoided when possible. So what's a walker to do? Remember your cues for posture and form. Maintain your posture as upright as possible, especially on mild and moderate hills. Steep declines may require slight leaning, but be careful not to put too much weight on your heels, which can cause your feet to slip out from under you on loose terrain. When walking up an incline, push upward and forward with your toes, pumping your arms to help you. When walking downhill, relax your knees a little bit to absorb some of the extra impact.

NOB HILL

San Francisco's nobility, aka nobs, are created by wealth, not birth. When the wealthiest

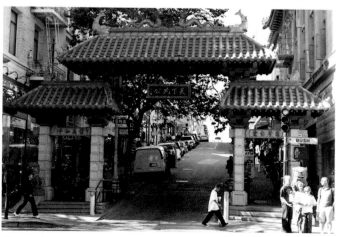

The southern entrance into Chinatown

of 19th-century nobs built their mansions high on a city hill, the hill was dubbed Nob Hill. The 1906 earthquake and fire swept nearly all of it away. Though Nob Hill remained affluent, every mansion owner relocated. Swank hotels were built over many of the ruins, named after the original mansion owner, such as the Mark Hopkins, Huntington, and Stanford Court.

! LOOK

. . . behind you and around you as you walk up California Street for surprise Bay Bridge and Coit Tower views.

BECAUSE WE CAN SHORTCUT

Feel free to cut right through Huntington Park (½ block before the official turn at Taylor St).

"I was one of the children told / Some of the blowing dust was gold."
from "*Peck of Gold*," by Robert Frost, who was born on Nob Hill in 1874 and lived here until age 11.

. . . .
Right on TAYLOR ST
. . . .

3. Grace Cathedral
1051 Taylor St

The original Grace Cathedral was destroyed in the fire following the 1906 earthquake. The railroad baron and banker Crocker family donated their fire-ravaged Nob Hill property to the church as a new location for the Episcopal cathedral. Visitors from around the world come to see her mosaics by De Rosen, replica of Ghiberti's *Gates of Paradise*, two labyrinths, Keith Haring's AIDS Chapel altarpiece, medieval furnishings, 44-bell carillon, three organs, and more.

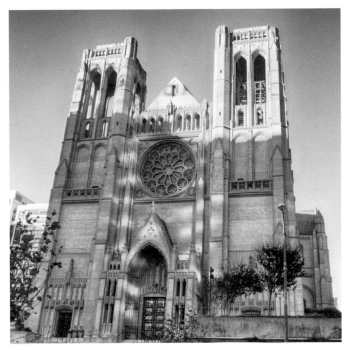

Early morning at Grace Cathedral

Grace Cathedral Shocking Revelations

• On June 25, 2010, the **Very Rev. Dr. Jane Alison Shaw** became both the first woman and the eighth dean of Grace Cathedral.

• The great-grandfather and great-great-grandfather of **U.S. former Presidents George H. W. and George W. Bush,** respectively, James Smith Bush, was a short-term rector of Grace Cathedral.

• The second-largest crowd ever at Grace Cathedral, about 5,000 people, mostly African American, came to hear **Rev. Dr. Martin Luther King Jr.** in 1965. Crowds filled the front stairs, plaza, Cathedral House, and parking lot.

• The largest crowd ever at Grace Cathedral, also about 5,000 people, attended the memorial service following the **September 11, 2001,** terrorist attacks.

•••••••••••••••••••••••••
Right on
WASHINGTON ST
•••••••••••••••••••••••••

4. Cable Car Barn and Powerhouse
1201 Mason St

Come look right down into the bowels of the beast! You are invited to view the cable-winding machinery and the actual underground cable as it pulls the cable cars. The Cable Car Barn Museum is not just a fun place to learn about cable cars, it's the actual working mechanical headquarters for the entire cable car network—and it's **free!**

•••••••••••••••••••••••••
Right on POWELL
Left on CLAY
•••••••••••••••••••••••••

5. Chinese Historical Society 965 Clay St

Free to the public on the first Thursday of every month (closed Sundays).

6. Waverly Place
off Clay St

The alleyway looks so adorable you might never guess this was the sight of a vicious Tong battle over a Chinese slave girl in 1879. Owing to the lack of women in early San Francisco, prostitutes were one of early Chinatown's most valuable assets. Tongs began as Chinese protective associations but became organized crime gangs, which still exist today.

"REAL" CHINATOWN

The locals live and work in the area you are walking through now. Every inch is visually, fantastically overstimulating so it may be hard to walk through without window-shopping. That is entirely up to you!

100,000 People in 20 City Blocks!
San Francisco's Chinatown is the largest Chinatown outside China and the oldest in the United States. Over 100,000 residents live within its 20 blocks of shops, restaurants, churches, grocers, historical landmarks, and more, making it San Francisco's most densely populated, as well as its *most visited*, neighborhood.

Hallidie's Horse Horror
Before cable cars were invented, rich people lived at the bottom of the hills and poor people climbed to homes higher up the hills.

In the 1870s engineer Andrew Hallidie witnessed horses being whipped while they struggled on the wet cobblestones to pull a horse-car up Jackson Street. The horses slipped and were dragged to their death. In response, Hallidie went to work, adapted a cable system he had developed to haul ore from mines, and built the Clay Street Hill Railroad. It was a hit.

The 53 miles of track laid over the next 30 years were damaged in the 1906 quake, and the city replaced most of them with cheaper electric cars. Since then many city bean counters have proposed eliminating the cable cars, but SF enthusiasts like Friedel Klussmann (in 1947) and then supervisor Dianne Feinstein (1984) led successful efforts to save them. Yay, us!
—*CableCarMuseum.org*

Getting a Grip
In 1998, a 52-year-old single mother from Oakland, Fannie Mae Barnes, became the first female cable car operator. The physical requirements of managing a 15-ton cable car include weighing 175 pounds and being able to lift a 50-pound sack of flour over your shoulder. Fannie Mae, a longtime Muni driver, worked out in the gym for nine months and passed the test with flying colors—*80% of men fail the test.*

BECAUSE WE CAN SHORTCUT

Cut left through Portsmouth Square to see the plaque for the first public school in California, a replica of the *Goddess of Democracy* used in Tiananmen Square, and dozens of impromptu card and domino games played and enjoyed by Chinatown residents.

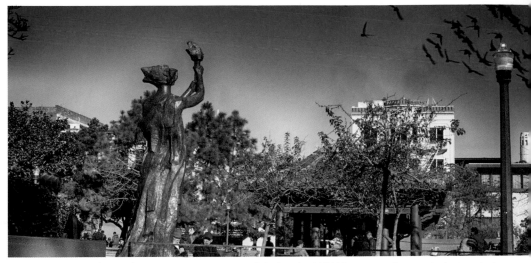

A replica of the Goddess of Democracy statue created during the 1989 Tiananmen Square student protest stands guard over Portsmouth Square and enjoys a nice view of Coit Tower (upper right).

7. On This Spot! History-Packed Portsmouth Square
Clay St and Kearny St

In 1846, Captain John B. Montgomery of the sloop of war *Portsmouth* marched into the then-Mexican town's central square, raised the American flag, and declared

Yerba Buena and its few hundred inhabitants part of the United States. A year later, the city was renamed San Francisco. The square was still a mere cow pen surrounded by tents in 1848 when the discovery of gold was announced here. By 1850 an entire city of 25,000 residents had built up around the square.

. . . .

Left on KEARNY ST
. . . .

Ten months after gold was discovered in California, Rev. T. Dwight Hunt held his first service in the schoolhouse at Portsmouth Square. Though tens of thousands of immigrants were flooding into the city, only eight people attended that first service. Membership grew very, very slowly in the early years, but by the time of the 1906 quake, the First Congregational Church of San Francisco was the largest Protestant church in SF.

8. Buddha's Universal Church 720 Washington St

Built with a decade of volunteer labor from congregants, this is one of the largest Buddhist churches in the United States (dedicated in 1963). Before that, the dilapidated brick building at *720 Washington Street* was most famous as the factory that sparked the 1938 garment workers strike.

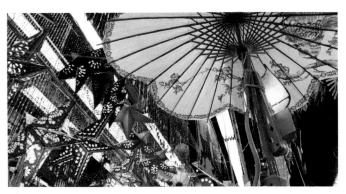

Chinatown Souvenir Shop. PHOTO: CHRISTINA SPICUZZA

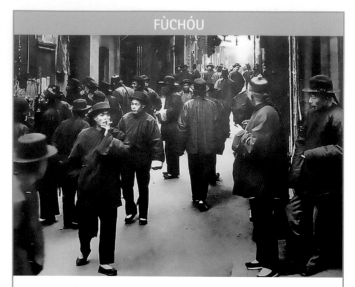

FÙCHÓU

The Street of Gamblers (Ross Alley), *by Arnold Genthe, 1898. The population was predominantly male because U.S. policies at the time made it difficult for Chinese women to enter the country.*

Chinatown Historical Hoodwink History

Even though the Chinese immigrants arriving in San Francisco in the mid-1880s were needed to work on the railroads, they were met with hostility and anti-Chinese legislation—including restrictions on immigration, interracial marriage, and where they could live.

When Chinatown was leveled in the 1906 earthquake and fire, city leaders thought they were finally rid of the "Chinese problem" and could reclaim the valuable Chinatown area next to the Financial District. However, the earthquake turned out to be a double boon for the Chinese. Ironically, because the immigration records at City Hall had been destroyed, many Chinese were able to claim citizenship, then send for their children and families in China.

In addition, while the city leaders were pondering where to relocate the Chinese (many favored Hunters Point), a wealthy businessman named Look Tin Eli quickly obtained a loan from Hong Kong and hired white architects to rebuild Chinatown with an "Oriental" look—adding theatrical chinoiserie to the buildings—to draw tourists. Chinatown was reborn out of the ashes, quickly filled with children, and has flourished through good and bad times into a vibrant, courageous, and proud community for Chinese Americans and greater San Francisco. (Fùchóu = Chinese for Revenge) —PBS, *The Story of Chinatown*

Barbary Coast

When tens of thousands of sailors and young male gold seekers flood into a town, can predatory saloons, bawdy dancing halls, and all manner of violent and illicit behavior be far behind? San Francisco entrepreneurs gladly responded to the need by creating a nine-block red-light district named for the notorious pirate-strewn North African Barbary Coast.

Walks 1, 2, and 3 of the 49 Mile route tramp through much of the historic Barbary Coast area. In fact, on your walk today, if you look down occasionally you will likely notice bronze Barbary Coast medallions embedded in the sidewalk. Historian Daniel Bacon in collaboration with the San Francisco Historical Society has created a 3.8-mile Barbary Coast Trail® walking guide to show off the history of that raucous era and area—and did the amazing, worthwhile, and hard work of designing, funding, permitting, and placing 170 medallions along the route. *Good job!*

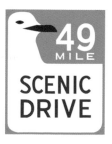

9. CCSF Chinatown Branch 808 Kearny St

Founded in 1935, today City College of San Francisco is one of the largest community colleges in the country. Multicultural and multi-campus, offering 50 academic programs and 100 occupational disciplines and serving 70,000 students, CCSF provides an invaluable service to the citizens and industries of SF.

MILE 5

Begins on KEARNY ST at JACKSON ST

10. Manilatown I-Hotel 868 Kearny St at Jackson St

The International Hotel was built in 1907 as low-cost housing in the heart of Manilatown, but it became ground zero for social revolution in the late 1960s. As often happens, urban developers—who feel they are doing good by tearing down "slums"—clash with the communities that have family, home, and affordable living (e.g., 50¢ a month at the I-Hotel) in the "blighted" neighborhoods. The mass evictions at the I-Hotel turned it into a symbol for every group fighting for rights in the turbulent '60s and '70s and inspired massive protests. Three decades later the Manila Heritage Foundation and 100 or so affordable housing units

were constructed, and the I-Hotel was born anew. Step inside and learn more: Wed.–Sun., 1–6 pm.

JACKSON SQUARE HISTORIC DISTRICT
KEARNY ST AT COLUMBUS AVE

These brick buildings stand as part of SF's oldest commercial neighborhood. When preachers proclaimed that God sent the 1906 earthquake to punish a sinful city, a ditty was written about the whiskey warehouse that survived the quake:

If, as they say, God spanked the town
for being over-frisky,
Why did he burn the churches down
and spare Hotaling's Whiskey?

11. Columbus Tower/ Sentinel Building 916 Kearny St

The seven-story, copper-green, Flat-Iron building on Columbus and Kearny survived the 1906 earthquake and fire, then allegedly went on to be the place where: Caesar salad was invented, the Kingston Trio recorded, Barbra Streisand sang (at the hungry i nightclub), and Francis Ford Coppola's Zoetrope Studios was headquartered. The Coppola story is probably true.

. . . .
Left on COLUMBUS AVE
. . . .

12. Vesuvio Café 255 Columbus Av

Popular Beat-era hangout known for poetry and jazz.

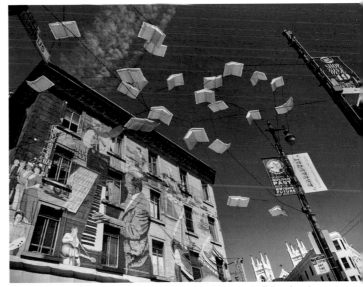

The Jazz Mural seen behind the Language of the Birds flying book art was created by Bill Weber, whose ancestors arrived with Juan Bautista de Anza in 1775 and helped found San Francisco.

13. City Lights Bookstore 261 Columbus Ave

The first paperback-only bookstore in the U.S. Owner Lawrence Ferlinghetti was charged with obscenity for publishing Allen Ginsberg's *Howl and Other Poems*. He won the court battle, and his support of Beat poets launched the Beat movement.

· · · · · · · · · · · · · · · · · · ·

Cross Columbus Ave at Broadway to get to the right-hand (south) side of Columbus

· · · · · · · · · · · · · · · · · · ·

14. Broadway intersects at Columbus Av

North Beach—San Francisco's Little Italy, former center of Beatnik culture, and red-light district strip club mecca—was established during the Barbary Coast days (1848–1858). Back then North Beach actually was a beach. The cove was filled in with soil and landfill after the 1906 earthquake and fire.

15. Condor Club 560 Broadway

The Condor Club fired a major salvo in the sexual revolution when it became the first topless (1964) and bottomless (1969) entertainment venue in the country. The 40-foot neon-lit cartoon image of stripper Carol Doda with two red lights on her bikini top came down in 1992 (but if you are brave enough to peek inside, you will get a glimpse of it right inside the front door!).

16. Beat Museum 540 Broadway

Offers a bookstore and a memorabilia section ($8 fee).

❗ LOOK UP

17. *Language of the Birds* Broadway at Columbus

The illuminated books flying past the traffic island at Columbus and Broadway are the first of two public art installations by Brian Goggin and Dorka Keehn found on the 49 mile scenic walk (see Walk 17, Caruso's Dream, for their other work).

· · · · · · · · · · · · · · · · · · ·

Right on GRANT AVE

· · · · · · · · · · · · · · · · · · ·

18. Grant Ave intersects at Columbus Ave

Columbus Avenue is the typical guidebook route through North Beach, but Grant Avenue is North Beach for the locals. Boutiques, bakeries, music, antiques, and art. Check to see if you can spot the 49 Mile Drive graffiti wall on the right-hand (east) side of the street.

19. Caffe Trieste 601 Vallejo St

Founder Giovanni Giotta claims that Caffe Trieste was the first espresso house on the West Coast and that he taught Americans to love cappuccino. In the 1950s and '60s this was Beatnik Central.

DETOUR

Yes, it's so steep you'll have to climb stairs to get there, but you've walked halfway up Telegraph Hill already, so why not go all the way up and see Coit Tower in person?

- From GRANT AVE, turn Right on FILBERT ST; this is STEEP.

- You'll see a green sign pointing to "Stairs to Coit Tower" at the end of FILBERT ST.

- For a break, stop halfway up, turn around, and admire the views.

- Sightsee Coit Tower.

- Return back down to GRANT AVE to rejoin the route.

I'll Make You a Cappuccino You Can't Refuse
TRUE: Francis Ford Coppola wrote much of the screenplay for *The Godfather* while sitting in Caffe Trieste on *Grant Avenue.*

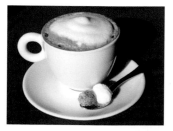

a. Coit Tower
1 Telegraph Hill Blvd

Fire-truck chasing, fireman loving Lillie Coit bequeathed one-third of her estate to beautify San Francisco. Whether the tower named in her honor represents a fire hose, a Greek column, or some other type of erection honoring the strapping young pioneer firefighters of Engine Company No. 5 is in the eye of the beholder. $8 admission to murals inside the tower, but views and selfies from Pioneer Park are free.

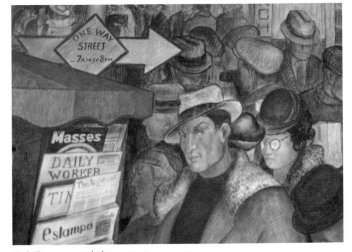

Coit Tower mural close-up. Photo: SAILKO

. . . .
Left on LOMBARD ST
. . . .

! LOOK

. . . at the Lombard St intersection west (downhill) through the trees, across the valley to catch a sliver view of the city's "crookedest street" at the top of the hill in the distance.

20. Lombard Street— Not Crooked Enough?
View from Grant Ave at Lombard St

Though Lombard Street has eight turns, Potrero Hill residents argue that the seven turns on Vermont Street on Potrero Hill are steeper, giving it a higher sinuosity index (1.56 vs. Lombard's 1.2 index). Therefore, Vermont Street is truly the city's "Crookedest Street."

Coit Tower Commies
In 1933 the New Deal federal employment program for artists put 26 Bay Area artists to work adorning the interior of Coit Tower with murals of California life. After viewing the suffering around them during the Great Depression, many artists had become radicalized and felt a responsibility to use their art to depict the harsh realities of the day. They drew scenes showing the exploitation of the poor, the indifference of the wealthy, angry workers reading socialist papers, and an ethnically diverse labor march. The murals caused a great deal of controversy and threats of censorship, but in the end, only a hammer and sickle (communist symbol) was removed. $8 admission.

Sinuosity
Sinuosity or sinuosity index measures the deviation of a path between two points from the shortest possible path. It is given by the ratio of:

$$\frac{\text{actual path length}}{\text{shortest path length}}$$

! LISTEN

As you pass Joe DiMaggio Playground to your left on Lombard Street, named for the San Francisco Seals (and NY Yankees) baseball legend. You may hear the bells from Saints Peter and Paul Church.

b. New North Beach Library
850 Columbus Ave

. . . .
Right on MASON ST
. . . .

21. Fior d'Italia
Opened 1886
2237 Mason St

Fior D'Italia bills itself as the oldest Italian restaurant in the United States.

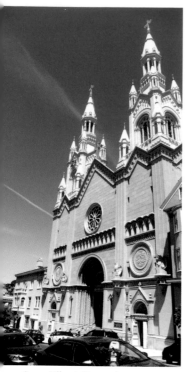

Soon Filbert Street, between Saints Peter and Paul Church and Washington Square Park, will be closed to traffic and turned into a grand-style Italian piazza—the Piazza St. Francis, the Poet's Plaza—dedicated to art, poets, and peace, where you can relax, meet friends over a caffè freddo, and listen to open-air opera.

GONE SF
22. Ginsberg's Dublin Pub 400 Bay St

Corner of Bay and Mason. A haunt for many generations of sailors. Built in 1906, closed in 2011. Still boarded up at time of printing.

23. International Longshore and Warehouse Union (ILWU) 400 North Point St and Mason St

Beginning in 1902 on the docks of the Pacific coast, ILWU workers "built a union that is democratic, militant and dedicated to the idea that solidarity with other workers and other unions is the key to achieving economic security and a peaceful world" and the best way "to achieve a better life for themselves and their families." —www.ILWU.org

· · · · · · · · · · · · · · · · · · · ·
End on JEFFERSON STREET
· · · · · · · · · · · · · · · · · · · ·

ON WALK-BACK LOOP

c.   Pier 39 Beach Street and the Embarcadero

Sea lions, waterfront dining, street performers, Aquarium of the Bay, live music, shopping, views of Alcatraz, and more have been welcoming and entertaining visitors at Pier 39 since the 1970s.

But people mocked Warren Simmons when he first presented his ideas to create it. In fact he was so far behind budget and schedule that then Board of Supervisors president, Dianne Feinstein made a bet with Simmons saying if he finished on time she would show up in a bikini to dedicate it. He finished on time. A good sport, Feinstein showed up in an old-time, one-piece Sutro Baths swimsuit.

WALK-BACK LOOP SCOOP

After that uphill hike, you deserve a little break! We suggest you turn right on Jefferson and, in just two long blocks, you will be at Pier 39—with lots of visual and gustatory delights with which to end your day's hike. Afterward you can continue on Walk 3, Fisherman's Wharf, or hop a cab/Uber/bus to your next adventure of the day. If you want to walk back, see the directions on page 41.

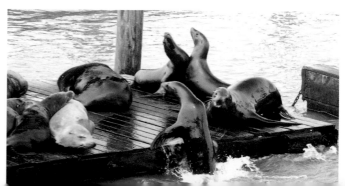

If you take the walk-back loop past Pier 39, stop and wave at the sea lions.

WALK 2 NEED TO KNOW

TO GET THERE
BART/ MUNI TRAIN

- Take any BART or underground Muni Train to MONTOMERY STATION
- Walk 2 blocks to Post AND Grant

or

- Muni 1, 2, 3, 8, 30, 45, 81X
- Check 511.org or NextBus.com for current bus schedules

PARKING
- Sutter-Stockton Garage recommended
- Metered street parking (difficult)
- Check ParkMe.com for other area parking options

PUBLIC RESTROOMS
- Portsmouth Square (Kearny and Clay)
- Washington Square Park (Columbus and Filbert)
- Pier 39 (Embarcadero and Beach)

TURN–BY–TURN INSTRUCTIONS
Begin: GRANT AVE at BUSH ST

- Continue on GRANT AVE from Walk 1 (north)
- Left on CALIFORNIA ST (very steep uphill climb)
- Right on TAYLOR ST
- Right on WASHINGTON ST

- Right on POWELL ST
- Left on CLAY ST
- Left on KEARNY ST
- Left on COLUMBUS AVE
  - Cross BROADWAY on right-hand side of street
- Right on GRANT
  - Detour option:
    > Right on FILBERT ST
    > Go up FILBERT ST stairs
    > Visit Coit Tower
    > Return the way you came
    > Right on GRANT AVE to rejoin route
- Left on LOMBARD ST
- Right on MASON ST

End: JEFFERSON ST

TO GET BACK
Muni:

- Board BUS 8X at SW corner POWELL ST and NORTH POINT ST
- Get off at SUTTER ST and STOCKTON ST
- Other Muni routes: Hyde St. cable car, F-Line, 39, 47

OPTIONAL WALK-BACK LOOP DIRECTIONS:

WALK-BACK LOOP

After your optional (but recommended) stop at Pier 39, continue southeast along the Embarcadero (toward the Bay Bridge) past Pier 33 (the Alcatraz Island ferry terminal) to Sansome St. Sansome will take you through a former warehouse district, past the hidden, cliff-side backstairs to Coit Tower (look right at Greenwich St) and the back of Levi's Plaza. You'll continue through Media Gulch (TV stations and ad agencies), the Jackson Square Historical District (oldest commercial section of SF, between Pacific and Washington Sts) into the Financial District with both modern skyscrapers and grand columned edifices, including the former Stock Exchange Tower, now a gym, at 155 Sansome.

Distance: 2.0 miles, 4,000 steps, 40 minutes

Rating:

Begin: JEFFERSON ST and MASON ST

- Turn right, head east, on JEFFERSON ST
  - Merge with EMBARCADERO
- Continue on EMBARCADERO
  - In two blocks, optional stop at Pier 39, on your left
- Continue on EMBARCADERO
- Right on SANSOME ST
- Right on BUSH ST

End: BUSH ST and GRANT AVE

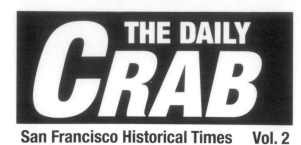

THE DAILY CRAB

San Francisco Historical Times   Vol. 2

"TEAR DOWN COIT TOWER"

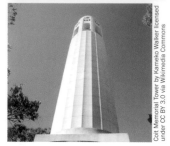

DODA'S DOUBLE DD DYNASTY

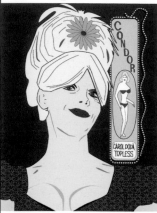

The fearless dancer **Carol Doda** admits to enhancing her 34Bs to create the 44DD/24/35 figure she illegally exposed to the patrons of the **Condor Club** in the 1960s. Yes, she was arrested, but she was "back on stage in two shakes of a stripper's tail," she says. Overnight, the other San Francisco clubs followed suit (or, similarly removed suits?). California declared bottomless dancing illegal in venues that served alcohol in 1972, but Doda continued dancing topless at the Condor Club until 1986. You go, girl!

Until her death in 2015, Doda owned a plus-size lingerie boutique, Champagne & Lace, in San Francisco.

GRAND OLD PARTY

TRUE: Many delegates from the 1964 Republican National Convention in San Francisco visited the Condor Club to watch the topless action.

"San Francisco has three great attractions. The other is a bridge." —SF Chronicle, 1964

Over 500 people signed a protest letter against the original creation and design of Coit Tower in the 1930s—some calling it a "glorified smoke stack," "an ugly shaft that would ruin Telegraph Hill," and a "grave aesthetic error." But **Herbert Fleishhacker** of the newly formed **San Francisco Art Commission** pushed on. The design uses three nesting concrete cylinders, requiring 5,000 barrels of cement and 3,200 cubic yards of concrete, which—hmmmm—were all purchased from Fleishhacker's Portland Cement Company. Well, it's a fabulous city icon today, and the cement had to come from somewhere. Fleishhacker, a philanthropist and civic leader, also built the 10,000-person-capacity Fleishhacker Pool at the beach and founded what became San Francisco Zoo.

CHINESE LADIES KICK FROCK

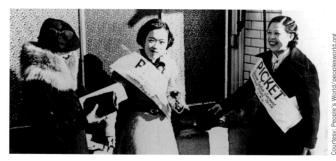

In the 1930s women working in Chinatown's filthy, dangerous sweatshops began demanding safe working conditions and fair pay. The largest garment manufacturer, Dollar National Store, refused. Historically, Chinese people had been excluded from unions, but now the **International Ladies' Garment Workers' Union** (ILGWU), desperate to cut down on the competition posed by low-paid workers, saw the benefit in uniting with Chinese workers. Together they formed Local 341 **Chinese Ladies' Garment Workers' Union**. They declared a strike, picketed for a grueling 14 weeks, and finally won enforcement of health, fire, and sanitary conditions and a 40-hour workweek!

CROCKER'S SPITE FENCE CRIME

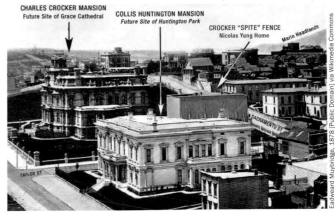

CHARLES CROCKER MANSION
Future Site of Grace Cathedral   COLLIS HUNTINGTON MANSION
Future Site of Huntington Park
CROCKER "SPITE" FENCE
Nicolas Yung Home   Marin Headlands
SACRAMENTO ST
TAYLOR ST

Eadweard Muybridge, 1878 [Public Domain] via Wikimedia Commons

Six-foot-tall, 300-pound Charles Crocker, one of the "Big Four" multi-millionaire partners in the Central Pacific Railroad, was used to getting what he wanted. What he wanted was the best mega mansion, on the best spot, with the best views, on the best hill in SF, Nob Hill. The problem was, other people owned homes on that block of land. Crocker managed to buy up all the lots except the one owned by undertaker **Nicolas Yung**. Yung couldn't think of any reason to give up his wonderful, quiet family cottage with great views of the entire bay.

According to Crocker, he eventually offered double market rate and claimed Yung was trying to extort more money from him. With Yung's final refusal to sell, Crocker was quoted as saying, "I'll seal him in as if he was in one of his own coffins!" Crocker hired his railroad engineers to surround Yung's home with a 40-foot wall on three sides. With all sunlight, air, and views blocked from the Yung home, it became unlivable. The family had to move out, but in retaliation, Yung mounted a coffin on his roof facing Crocker's new mega mansion—with skull and crossbones and the phrase **RIP C.C.** on it.

Crocker's Spite Fence, as it was known, became one of the city's most popular sightseeing attractions—a symbol of capitalist power over the "little man." The newspapers, echoing the ire of most San Franciscans, began calling the fence "Crocker's Crime."

Eventually, Yung's heirs sold out to Crocker's heirs just before the 1906 quake and fire leveled both homes. The Crocker heirs then donated the land to build Grace Cathedral.

—FoundSF.org

ROBBER BARON BASTARDS

The business practices of San Francisco's Big Four—**Mark Hopkins, Collis P. Huntington, Charles Crocker,** and **Leland Stanford**—made them some of the most hated people of their time and earned them the title "Robber Barons." They made their fortunes by building the first Central Pacific Railroad, using exploited Chinese laborers, shoddy material, monopolistic practices to drive out competitors, $200,000 in bribes to politicians, laying unnecessary extra tracks, and double billing through dummy companies—which garnered them $36 million in overpayments from the U.S. government—and 9 million acres of free land for their private use. All four built themselves large mansions on top of Nob Hill. All four mansions burned down in the earthquake and fire of 1906. *Karma's a bitch, boys!*

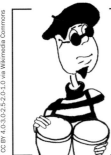

BEATS CAN'T BEAT BEATNIK NICKNAME

Many writers and young people in the 1950s became worn out disillusioned, "beat" by the social and political systems left behind after World War II. This self-named **Beat Generation** embraced alternative music, sexualities, religions, and more. In 1958, the heyday of the *–nik* suffix made popular by the Russian spaceship *Sputnik*, San Francisco columnist **Herb Caen** coined the word Beat*nik* to make fun of the Beats. Rumor has it the Beats were not amused.

49 MILE

MILE

SCENIC DRIVE

Fisherman's Wharf

Marina

Palace of Fine Arts

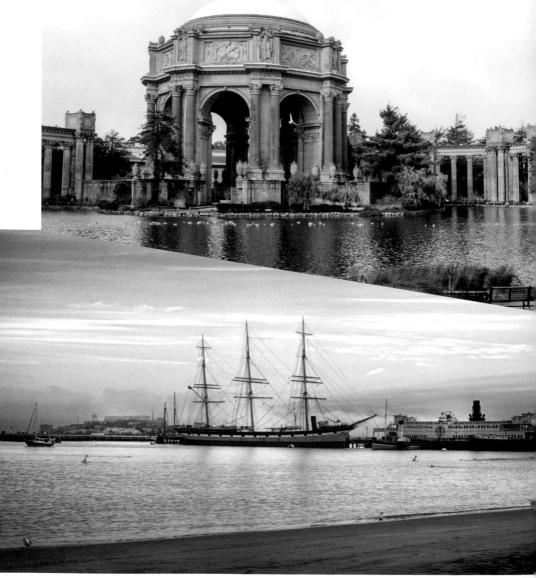

Top: Palace of Fine Arts
Bottom: Aquatic Park at dawn with the ships of Hyde Street Pier in the foreground and Alcatraz in the distance

It takes only 20 minutes to walk through Fisherman's Wharf, but with so much to see, eat, buy, and explore here, you may want to give yourself some extra time to complete this walk. Stop to enjoy some fresh Dungeness crab or clam chowder served in a sourdough bread bowl. Spend a few minutes exploring the antique mechanical games at the Musée Mécanique. If you like old ships, you can tour the World War II submarine USS *Pampanito* or Liberty Ship SS *Jeremiah O'Brien*, or detour down Hyde Street Pier to board an old car ferry or sailing vessel. The free museum at the Maritime National Park's Visitor Center gives a wonderful overview of the area. And if you like shopping and SF souvenirs or want to visit Alcatraz or wait in a very long line for a cable car ride . . . well, you may want to come back another time and spend a whole day!

If your goal is to complete another leg of the 49 Mile Scenic Drive, try to walk by, take it all in, and note what you want to do next time.

Then, as you pass the cable cars, catch your breath, grab a quick bite of Ghirardelli chocolate to boost your strength, and push on to the second half of this walk through the Marina District. Feel free to gawk at the fabulous million-dollar homes built on top of a former washerwoman's lagoon and tons of 1906 rubble (the Marina District). Wave at the Wave Organ as you wind your way over to take must-have photos at the Palace of Fine Arts. And wait, the duel! Who died in the duel? And which house did Marilyn Monroe live in? And, wow! There's a lot of history to take in along with the views on this walk. Enjoy!

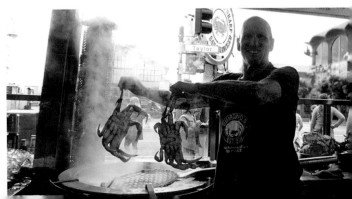

Mike Guardino's family has been serving up crab along Taylor Street since 1908.

Begin: Mason Street and Jefferson Street
End: Lombard Street and Lyon Street (Presidio Gate)
Distance: ROUTE: 3.0 miles — 6,000 steps — 1 hour
LOOP BACK: 2.4 miles — 4,800 steps — 47 minutes

Hill Rating:

Sites you will pass on today's walk include:

MILE 6
FISHERMAN'S WHARF
1. **Wax Museum**
145 Jefferson St
2. **Boudin Sourdough Bakery**
160 Jefferson St
3. **8 Alioto's** No. 8 Fisherman's Wharf

DETOUR
a. **Musée Mécanique**
Pier 45 (Taylor St)
4. **The Cannery**
2801 Leavenworth St

MUST-SEE
5. **Maritime National Park Visitors Center**
499 Jefferson St

DETOUR
b. **Hyde Street Pier**
Hyde St at Jefferson St

MILE 7
6. **Cable Car Turnaround**
Hyde St at Beach St
7. **Buena Vista Café**
2765 Hyde St
8. **Ghirardelli Chocolate Company** Beach St between Larkin St and Polk St
9. **Aquatic Park Bathhouse Building (Maritime Museum)** 890 Beach St
10. **Fontana Towers**
1050 North Point St
11. **Fort Mason** Bay St between Van Ness Av and Laguna St

MILE 8
THE MARINA
12. **Laguna Street— Washerwoman's Lagoon** *GONE SF*
13. **Fort Mason Center**
Laguna St and Marina Blvd
14. **Marina Green**
15. **Marina Green Parking Lot**

DETOUR
c. **Wave Organ View Point**

MILE 9
16. **Palace of Fine Arts**
3301 Lyon St (Beach St at Baker St)
17. **Lombard Gate**
Lombard St at Lyon St

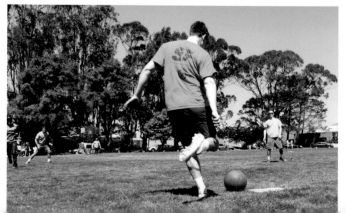

Twenty-something men and women play KickballSF at the Marina Green. They take their motto seriously, "Where booziness happens."

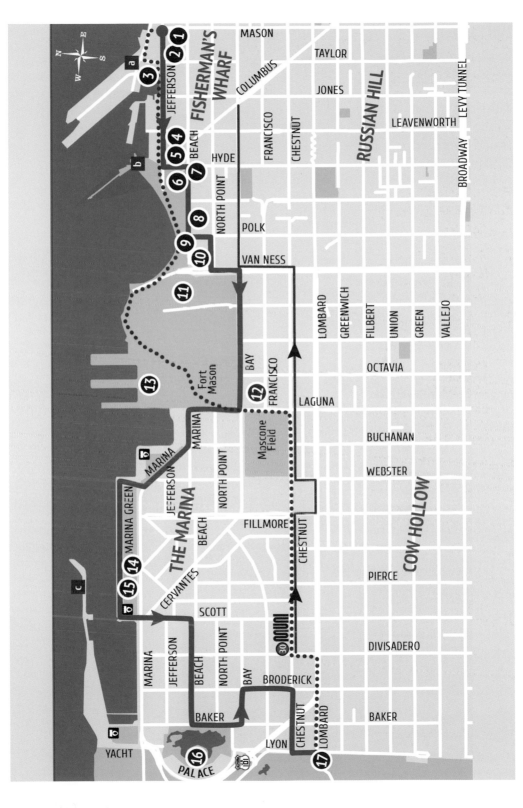

MILE 6

Begins on MASON ST at JEFFERSON ST

· · · · · · · · · · · · · · · · · · ·

Continuing from Walk 2, turn left (head west) on JEFFERSON ST

· · · · · · · · · · · · · · · · · · ·

FISHERMAN'S WHARF

Once home to over 500 (mostly Italian-owned) fishing boats, today the wharf attracts nearly 16 million tourists a year to both historic and new restaurants, shops, views, and attractions. A few third-generation fishermen still go out fishing from here—in both old-time Monterey Hull boats and diesel-powered, state-of-the-art commercial fishing boats.

> The city first began promoting the wharf as a tourist attraction to the visitors of San Francisco's 1939 Golden Gate International Exposition.

1. (Original) Wax Museum (closed, now replaced)
145 Jefferson St

Thomas Fong fell in love with the wax figures he saw at the 1962 Seattle World's Fair. Knowing his hometown's goal of turning Fisherman's Wharf into a tourist attraction, Fong purchased an old grain mill at the wharf and begin hand-making wax figures. His son and grandson kept up the tradition, to the delight of 12 million visitors, until 2013. The site reopened as Madame Tussauds Wax Museum in 2014.

2. Boudin Sourdough Bakery
160 Jefferson St

Isidore Boudin, the son of a family of master bakers from Burgundy, France, was one of 30,000 French people who ventured to California for the Gold Rush. In 1849, the Boudin family discovered that wild yeasts in the San Francisco air gave a unique tang to their traditional French bread, giving rise to "San Francisco sourdough French bread." Every sourdough loaf they've made since has had a piece of the original 1849 "mother dough" added to it.

3. 8 Alioto's
No. 8 Fisherman's Wharf (just to your right, down Taylor St)

Family owned and run for four generations, Alioto's was just "fish stall no. 8" in 1925, but in the 1930s it became one of the first restaurants on the wharf. Owner Rose Alioto invented cioppino here—a spicy tomato shellfish stew.

DETOUR

a. Musée Mécanique (Mechanical Museum) Pier 45, end of Taylor St

Turn right on Taylor Street, walk past the crab vendors, and head into the big building on Pier 45— then pull out a pocketful of quarters and enjoy this whacky, remarkable collection of old-time mechanical entertainments from your grandpa's era. Have your fortune told, test your strength, watch an antique peep show—and see if your kids are brave enough to stand under large, looming, down-at-the-heels Laffing Sal as she cackles at them.

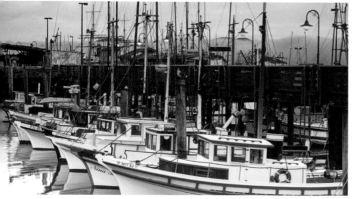

Monterey Clipper fishing boats in the Fisherman's Wharf Marina

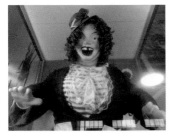

Laffing Sal at Musée Mécanique

Opera Fog Horns
The Italian fisherman's love of singing — including Verdi operas — was a form of communication on the water. You could not see a nearby boat in the fog, but from the song of its captain, you knew it was there.

4. The Cannery
2801 Leavenworth St

When the 1906 earthquake and fire destroyed the California Fruit Canners Association plants, they built this new facility on the wharf next to the shipping and rail lines. By 1909, The Cannery was the largest fruit and vegetable canning plant in the world, producing over 200,000 hand-soldered cans per day and employing 2,500 people. In 1937 Del Monte (the association's new name) ceased production here. In 1963 Leonard Martin saved the brick structure from the wrecking ball and turned it into a marketplace reminiscent of romantic Europe. Three cheers for Leonard! Today it is the campus for the **Academy of Arts University** School of Sculpture.

! MUST SEE

5. Maritime National Park Visitors Center
499 Jefferson St at Hyde St

View a Fresnel lighthouse lens, walk down a see-hear-touch SF waterfront replica, touch an excavated Gold Rush anchor, listen for Yelamu native peoples readying their tule reed canoe, watch a show, such as one about Tugboat Annie working in maritime industries and lots o' cool stuff. Stop and get the scoop. 9:30 a.m.–5:00 p.m. Free, but donations accepted.

MILE 7
Begins on HYDE ST at JEFFERSON ST

. . . .
Left on HYDE ST
. . . .

6. Cable Car Turnaround
Hyde St at Beach St

Hella long lines. Don't get on here. (When your relatives come to town have them catch the California Line at Van Ness, which will take them through Chinatown before it ends at the Embarcadero Center just a block away from the Ferry Building. $7 a ticket)

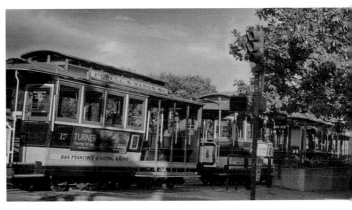

Cable car turnaround

DETOUR

b. Hyde Street Pier Hyde St at Jefferson St

If you lived across the bay before the Golden Gate and Bay Bridges opened, you had no choice but to take a ferry to get you or your automobile to San Francisco. Formerly the main ferry terminal, today Hyde Street Pier is part of the San Francisco Maritime National Historic Park, where you are welcome to explore some old steam-powered ferries and tugs and an 1886 square-rigged sailing ship, the *Balclutha*. Entrance fee: $10 (good for 10 days).

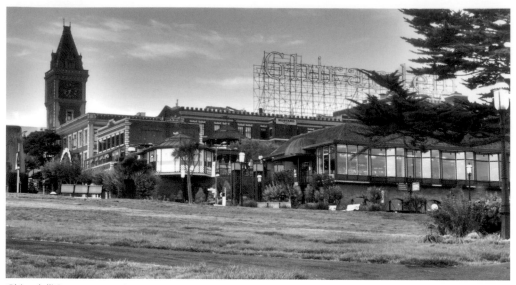
Ghirardelli Square at sunrise

7. Buena Vista Café
2765 Hyde St

A saloon since 1916, the Buena Vista Café introduced Irish coffee to America in 1952 and today claims to be the largest single consumer of Irish whiskey in the country—18,720 liter-size bottles a year.

Right on BEACH ST

8. Ghirardelli Chocolate Company
Beach St between Larkin St and Polk St

Built on this block in 1893, Domingo Ghirardelli's Chocolate Company stands as one of the oldest chocolate manufacturers in the nation. (HINT: pronounced with a hard 'g': gear-ar-delly) In 1962, San Franciscan William Roth and his mother bought the land to prevent the square from being replaced with condos. *Bless you, Roths!*

9. Aquatic Park Bathhouse Building (Maritime Museum)
890 Beach St

No, that's not a beached ocean liner, it's an Art Deco–style, New Deal, Works Progress Administration (WPA) bathhouse built in 1939. After occupation by WWII-era troops from 1941 through 1948, the building eventually became home to the San Francisco Maritime Museum and the country's first Senior Center. The SF Maritime Association operated the museum until transferring it to the National Park Service in 1978.

Left on POLK ST
Right on NORTH POINT ST

10. Fontana Towers
1050 North Point St

Built in 1960. When San Franciscans saw how these twin 17-story towers blocked the view of the waterfront, the angry outcry caused the Board of Supervisors to enact a 40-foot-height limit along the rest of the waterfront. Every few years developers try to sneak in a city ballot measure to get the building height limit removed. Unless you want the entire wharf and waterfront area views blocked by luxury condos, don't fall for it!

Left on VAN NESS AVE, Right on BAY ST

11. Fort Mason Bay St between Van Ness Ave and Laguna St

Fort Mason served as an army post for more than 100 years, including during World War II, when it was the principal Port of Embarkation for the Pacific campaign. Today, as part of the Golden Gate National Recreation Area, it includes museums, restaurants, a youth hostel, a music school, open green space for concerts, event space, and much, much more.

MILE 8

Begins on LAGUNA ST at BAY ST

Right on LAGUNA ST to the MARINA

GONE SF
12. Laguna Street's name-sake: Washer-woman's Lagoon

The area from Laguna Street down to Greenwich Street and over to Gough Street once held Washerwoman's Lagoon—the city's main laundry spot. Laundry businesses were run on her banks, but thrifty housewives held Sunday picnics there for their families while they scrubbed for free on her shores. —*FoundSF.org*

13. Fort Mason Center Laguna St and Marina Blvd

The lower warehouse portion of Fort Mason houses about 30 nonprofit organizations. Nearly 1.5 million people visit the site each year for more than 15,000 gatherings, performances, and special events. The entrance archway sits catty-corner from the Marina Safeway (which is fabled to be the best grocery store in SF for singles to meet and find a date).

Left on MARINA BLVD

Bear right to stay on MARINA BLVD

14. Marina Green on Marina Blvd

Today, dogs, kite flyers, joggers, picnickers, and sightseers all enjoy this outdoor sea of grass on the edge of the bay, but from 1920–1944 it was actually Montgomery Airfield, the first terminus of the United States Post Office's Transcontinental Air Mail Service route.

> Joe DiMaggio and Marilyn Monroe lived for a time at the DiMaggio home in San Francisco at 2150 Beach Street.

Right into MARINA GREEN PARKING

AREA. Follow road around edge of parking area to exit at the other side. NOTE: The 49 Mile sign is missing.

15. Marina Green Parking Lot Marina Blvd

The most scenic parking lot in the world? Perhaps. Scan the bay from left to right to see the St. Francis Yacht Club, the Golden Gate Yacht Club, Golden Gate Bridge, the Wave Organ, Fort Baker and Sausalito across the bay, and Angel Island and Alcatraz Island on the bay.

DETOUR

c. Wave Organ: Hear the ocean make music!

On the very end of the jetty you see from the Marina Green, the **Exploratorium**'s Pete Richards placed 25 pipes into the water at various heights. Whenever the Pacific waves flow into and out of them the Wave Organ pipes make noise—a different tone for each pipe length. You'll hear more "music" during high tides, less as the water level drops. (To get out there you would have to take Marina Boulevard all the way down to Yacht Road and walk past the yacht clubs out to the end of the jetty.)

Restrooms

By the small craft harbor at the northwest corner of the Green

. . . .

As you exit the parking lot, continue straight across the street (MARINA BLVD) onto SCOTT ST

. . . .

MILE 9

Begins on SCOTT ST at BEACH ST

. . . .

Right on BEACH ST

Left on BAKER ST

. . . .

! CLASSIC PHOTO OP

16. Palace of Fine Arts
Beach St at Baker St

Built as one of 11 great exhibit palaces for the 1915 Panama-Pacific International Exposition, this fictional Greek-Roman-inspired "ruin" was a crowd favorite. When it came time to demolish the fair, Phoebe Hearst stepped in and rescued the colonnade and rotunda. The Palace stands as one of the fair's few surviving structures, and one of only two buildings still on its original spot. She has served as an art gallery, tennis court, military motor pool, warehouse, and fire department headquarters. The Palace received a desperately needed complete renovation

Shake, Quake, and Make

After the 1906 earthquake, the city dumped tons and tons of rock and brick rubble onto the tidal marshlands west of Fisherman's Wharf. Later, to provide land for the 1915 Panama-Pacific International Exposition, the city built the (present-day) Marina District on top of that rubble landfill. After the expo buildings were demolished, apartment buildings, homes, and businesses sprouted up rapidly and in great numbers over the next few decades until the Marina, with her front-row view of the Golden Gate Bridge, had become one of San Francisco's most desirable places to live, work, and visit.

Until 1989, that is, when another earthquake rocked the city and sparked 27 fires citywide, including the devastating Marina blaze. Many of the area's poorly supported buildings collapsed atop the unstable 1906 earthquake rubble landfill. The reconstruction effort after the Loma Prieta quake brought with it new standards of earthquake-sturdy construction, and within a decade the Marina had been rebuilt and revamped with a shiny new face and stronger bone structure—reclaiming her status as an active, affluent, desirable SF neighborhood.

in 1965 and a seismic retrofit in 2009. The **Exploratorium** moved out in 2013. The next lease awarded for the Palace will last up to 55 years, and the tenant will ultimately be responsible for nearly $20 million in improvements to the 143,996-square-foot space.

Disney's California Adventure honored the Palace of Fine Arts' status as a beloved city icon by building a miniature replica of her in Anaheim.

. . . .

Left on BAY ST

Right on BRODERICK ST

Right on CHESTNUT ST

Cross RICHARDSON AVE

Left on LYON ST

END on LOMBARD ST

. . . .

17. Lombard Gate
Lombard St at Lyon St

To continue walking through the Presidio to the Golden Gate Bridge, flip over to Walk 4 for directions. Or, since this is the second-longest walk on the route, take a bus, cab, or Uber back to the wharf for something great to eat. However, if you still have a little extra energy, the walk back is just as gorgeous as the walk here, and includes a bonus detour along the green paths at the back of Fort Mason onto the beach at Aquatic Park.

WALK-BACK LOOP SCOOP

The gorgeous walk back should take about an hour. See the directions on page 53.

WALK 3 NEED TO KNOW

TO GET THERE
- Muni 39, 47, Hyde St cable car, F-Line
- Golden Gate Transit 58

PARKING
- Street parking (difficult)
- Pier 39 Garage recommended (Beach and Stockton—not shown on map)
- Metered street parking very difficult, 1–2 hour limits, strictly **enforced 7 days a week**
- Check ParkMe.com for other area parking options

PUBLIC RESTROOMS
- Jefferson and Powell
- Marina Green Triangle
- Marina Green Yacht Harbor (NW corner of parking lot)
- 3650 Yacht Road (near Palace of Fine Arts)

TURN–BY–TURN INSTRUCTIONS
Begin: MASON ST at JEFFERSON ST
- Continuing from Walk #2, turn Left (head west) on JEFFERSON ST
- Left on HYDE ST
- Right on BEACH ST
- Left on POLK ST
- Right on NORTH POINT ST
- Left on VAN NESS AVE
- Right on BAY ST

- Right on LAGUNA ST
- Left on MARINA BLVD
  - Bear right to stay on MARINA BLVD
- Right into MARINA GREEN PARKING AREA
  - Follow road around edge of parking area to exit at the other side
  - NOTE: The 49 Mile sign is missing
- As you exit the parking lot, continue straight across the street (MARINA BLVD) onto SCOTT ST
- Right on BEACH ST
- Left on BAKER ST
- Left on BAY ST
- Right on BRODERICK ST
- Right on CHESTNUT ST
  - cross RICHARDSON AVE
- Left on LYON ST

End: LOMBARD STREET (Presidio Gate)

TO GET BACK
Muni:
- Walk to NW corner of DIVISADERO ST and CHESTNUT ST
- Board bus 30 (toward 4th St)
- Get off at COLUMBUS AVE and BAY ST

Other transit routes:
- Muni 28, 30, 43, 45
- Golden Gate Transit 10, 70, 101

OPTIONAL WALK-BACK LOOP DIRECTIONS
Distance: 2.4 miles, 4,800 steps, 47 minutes

Rating:

Begin: LOMBARD ST and LYON ST
- Left on LOMBARD ST to DIVISADERO ST
- Left on DIVISADERO ST
- Right on CHESTNUT ST
- Left on LAGUNA ST
- At BAY ST enter park at Fort Mason
- Follow trail on the left
  - Stay left as trail continues across park
  - Head downhill at the end of the park to the waterfront (VAN NESS AVE)
- Right on VAN NESS AVE
- Take first Left onto trail toward Aquatic Park Beach
  - Continue veering left to Aquatic Park Beach
  - Trail ends at JEFFERSON ST
- Take JEFFERSON ST
- Left on TAYLOR ST
- Right on EMBARCADERO
- Right at POWELL ST
- Right at JEFFERSON ST back to MASON ST

End: JEFFERSON and MASON ST

THE DAILY CRAB

San Francisco Historical Times   Vol. 3

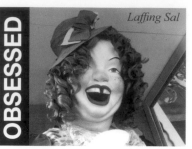

Laffing Sal

OBSESSED

JOE DIMAGGIO'S FATHER *BANNED* FROM FISHERMAN'S WHARF

At the outbreak of World War II, the U.S. government required over a million people of Italian, German, and Japanese ancestry to register as "enemy aliens"—making them subject to arrest, FBI investigation, and seizure of property. Over 110,000 Japanese, 11,000 Germans, and 10,000 Italians were interned in camps. Because of fear of submarine attacks on the coasts, fishermen and sailors were especially targeted, including baseball legend **New York Yankee Joe DiMaggio's father, Giuseppe**.

While Joe, like the children of many Italian, Japanese, and German immigrants, was serving in the U.S. Army, his father was banned from fishing in San Francisco Bay and the family was barred from running their restaurant on Fisherman's Wharf.

By 1942, the growingly absurd attacks on prominent Italian Americans, such as accusing **SF mayor Angelo Rossi** of giving a fascist salute, illustrated the absurdity and illegality of the restrictions. **New York mayor Fiorello La Guardia** demanded an end to the process, and on Columbus Day, 1942, the government removed Italians from enemy alien status.

Ed Zelinsky's fascination with game machines started when he was a child in the 1930s. As his private collection grew to nearly 300 items, it became one of the world's largest. His mechanical wonderland has entertained San Franciscans for decades, first at **Playland-at-the-Beach,** then in a basement of the **Cliff House**, and since 2002 at **Pier 45 on Fisherman's Wharf.**

"OO-KOO-LAY-LAY"

The **ukulele**, hula, and Hawaiian steel guitar debuted on the mainland at the **1915 Panama-Pacific International Exposition,** setting off a stateside ukulele craze.

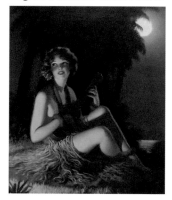

Girl in Moonlight with Banjo Ukulele! *by Edward Mason Eggleston, oil on canvas, 1925–30*

I Got Crabs—*but it wasn't easy*

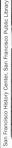
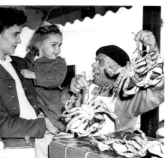

San Francisco History Center, San Francisco Public Library

A century ago, crabs flourished throughout SF Bay. Over the years, as clams, the natural food of the crab, disappeared from the bay, so did the crab. Today, crabbers must drop their crab pots far out, near the **Farallon Islands** in 18 to 35 fathoms of ocean water to catch SF's native seafood favorite.

TAR AND FEATHERS ESCAPE

In 1853 hustler Henry Meiggs speculated on a new wharf in a new part of San Francisco. The first "Fisherman's Wharf" ran from the end of Powell Street 1,600 feet out into the bay with the intention of serving the lumber trade, fishermen, and weekend sunbathers. Sadly, the new wharf did not catch on as he had expected—and he had to flee town just ahead of a posse acting on behalf of his creditors.

Eventually, the industrial needs of the **Ghirardelli Chocolate Factory, the Cannery,** and **Woolen Mill** (which clothed the Union Army) pushed shipping west of Pier 35, creating the need for today's **Fisherman's Wharf**.

PANAMA-PACIFIC PARTY PARADISE

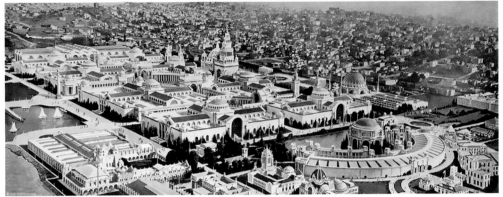

The Marina District is built on the former SF Pan-Pacific Expo site. Aeroplane view lithograph, 1915.

San Francisco worked hard to beat out New Orleans as the host for the **1915 Panama-Pacific International Exposition**. We invited the world to come celebrate the completion of the Panama Canal and reflect on the ascendancy of the United States to the world stage—but at heart we saw it as a chance to show the world how the largest and wealthiest city on the West Coast had risen triumphantly from the ashes of the 1906 quake and fire.

Our ambitious endeavor included pouring landfill into **630 acres** of bay-front tidal marsh—from Fort Mason through the Presidio waterfront—to create the fairgrounds.

On this new land, **21 nations** and **48 U.S. states** built exhibit halls connected by 47 miles of walkways. "It would take an individual years to visit all the attractions," proclaimed the press. The expo hosted **18,876,438 visitors** during the nine months of the expo.

For the first time ever, a plane flew through a building—the Palace of Machinery, the largest structure in the world at the time. The glass dome of the Horticulture Palace was larger than St. Peter's Basilica in Rome and the 40-story Tower of Jewels shone with **102,000 pieces of multicolored cut glass.** A full-scale replica of the Old Faithful Inn at Yellowstone National Park invited overnight guests.

The "famous" flooded in. Visitors included presidents **William Howard Taft** and **Theodore Roosevelt**, future president **Franklin Delano Roosevelt**, World War I flying ace **Eddie Rickenbacker**, **Buffalo Bill Cody**, **Henry Ford**, **Thomas Edison**, **Luther Burbank**, author **Laura Ingalls Wilder**, and silent-film star **Charlie Chaplin**.

Like any movie set, all those magnificent physical structures were built to be temporary and, at the fair's close, were torn down.

HOUSING HUSTLERS

New residents crowding into the city after the Gold Rush caused a housing and land shortage. The U.S. military owned Black Point (Fort Mason's original name) but hadn't built on it, so some entrepreneurial developers built luxury homes on the empty bluff and sold them to SF notables. When the military returned in 1861, the "gentleman squatters" were evicted.

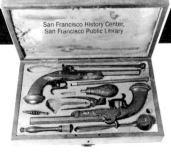

On Walk 8, the 49 Mile Drive passes the site of the infamous **Broderick–Terry** duel of 1859. Mortally wounded, Broderick died at a home in

PRICEY PISTOLS

Fort Mason with like-minded abolitionists three days later.

The two Belgian .58 calibre pistols used by Broderick and Terry (pictured here) sold at a **Butterfield & Butterfield** auction in San Francisco in 1998. An unidentified private collector purchased the cased single-shot pistol set, including a copper powder flask, loading rod, and mallet, for $34,500.

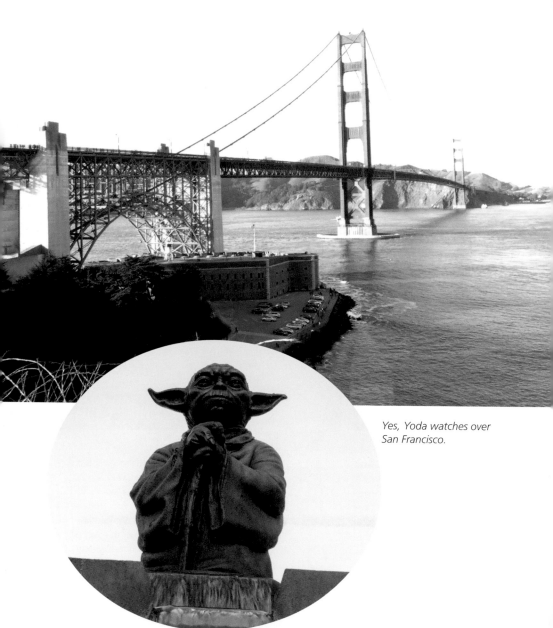

49 MILE

SCENIC DRIVE

The Presidio to Golden Gate Bridge

Yes, Yoda watches over San Francisco.

The views you'll see today explain why 16 million people visit San Francisco every year. The historic buildings, the bay, the city skyline, the natural landscapes, the Golden Gate Bridge—this walk is almost too spectacular to describe. And lucky locals like many of you can visit anytime you want!

The walk begins at the Presidio's Lombard Gate, entryway to the patch of ground where San Francisco was born. Native people lived here for thousands of years. In 1776 Spain claimed the land, and over the next two centuries three countries used it as a fort to protect the Golden Gate.

When the Presidio became part of the Golden Gate National Recreation Area in 1994 it began an ongoing transformation into a new kind of national park in the heart of a bustling urban area.

The Presidio's streets you will walk today have been groomed to show it all off—new trails, peekaboo views, history plaques, The Walt Disney Family Museum, earthquake shacks, the second-oldest adobe in the city— even the street signs detail the origin of the street names.

At the Crissy Field Overlook, be prepared to catch your jaw dropping as the panoramic view of the city, the water, and the East Bay hills open up before you and then, after all that beauty, you'll step onto the Golden Gate Bridge. Wow!

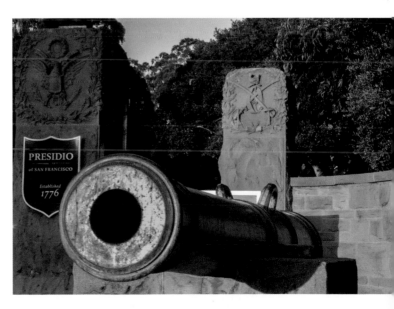

The Presidio Gate

Begin: Lombard St and Lyon St (Presidio's Lombard Gate)   Hill Rating:
End: Golden Gate Bridge Welcome Center
Distance: ROUTE: 2.5 miles — 5,000 steps — 50 minutes
           LOOP BACK: 2.5 miles — 5,000 steps — 50 minutes

/3\

Sites you will pass on today's walk include:

MILE 10

1. **The Presidio of San Francisco**

   DETOUR
a. **Lucasfilms, the Letterman Digital Arts Center**
   1 Letterman Dr

2. **Old Post Hospital and Officers' Row**
   Funston Ave

   DETOUR
b. **Earthquake Shacks**

3. **Inn at the Presidio**
   42 Moraga Ave

4. **Presidio Officers' Club** 50 Moraga Ave

5. **Parade Grounds**
   between Anza Ave and Montgomery St

6. **Presidio Performing Arts Center**
   386 Moraga Ave

MILE 11

7. **San Francisco National Cemetery**
   1 Lincoln Blvd

8. **Presidio Cavalry Horse Stables**
   663 McDowell Ave

   DETOUR
c. **Presidio Pet Cemetery**
   McDowell at Crissy Field Ave

9. **Crissy Field Overlook**
   Lincoln Blvd

   DETOUR
d. **Crissy Field**
   1199 E Beach

10. **Golden Gate Bridge**

ON WALK-BACK LOOP

e. **Fort Point**
   Marine Dr

f. **Palace of Fine Arts**

NOTE: For safety reasons, this hike veers off the street away from a vehicle-only underpass and directs you instead onto a path that parallels the 49 Mile Scenic Drive and leads to the pedestrian walkway under the Golden Gate Bridge. (As a bonus, you will see military ruins, trails, and bridge views you would miss from a car window at the beginning of Walk 5.)

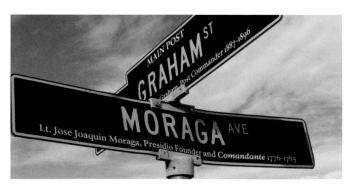

Note how the Presidio street signs detail the origin of the street names.

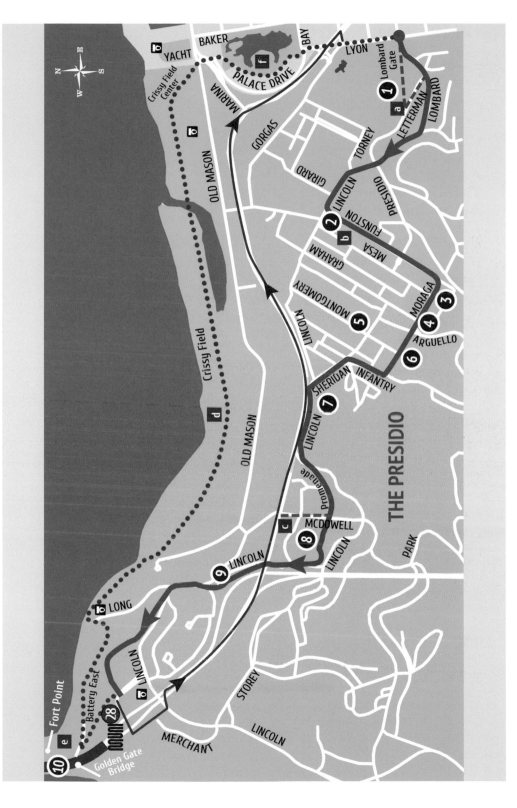

MILE 10

Begins on LOMBARD ST at LYON ST

1. The Presidio of San Francisco

First for Spain, then Mexico, and finally the U.S., the Presidio served as an active military fort from 1776 to 1994. The Presidio Trust now manages most of the park's 800 buildings and 1,491 acres in partnership with the National Park Service. The Presidio Trust Act calls for "preservation of the cultural and historic integrity of the Presidio for public use." Another main objective, achieving financial self-sufficiency by fiscal year 2013, was reached in 2006!

· · · · · · · · · · · · · · · ·

Go through Presidio entrance, LOMBARD GATE

· · · · · · · · · · · · · · · ·

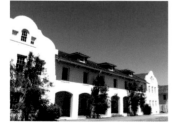

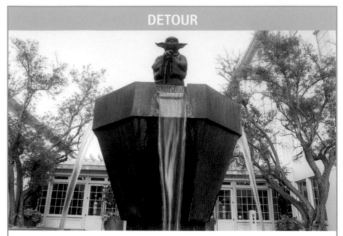

DETOUR

a. Lucasfilms, the Letterman Digital Arts Center
1 Letterman Dr

Yoda Fountain: Yoda sits outside the front door of the **Letterman Digital Arts Center** guarding the combined home of **Industrial Light & Magic**, **LucasArts**, and **Lucasfilm**'s marketing, online, and licensing units.

· ·

- As soon as you walk through the Presidio entrance gate you'll see a red-brick building to your right.

- At the brown PRESIDIO sign turn right onto the trail.

- Follow the trail past the red-brick buildings.

- As you begin approaching a third red-brick building, head into the courtyard straight ahead where you will find Yoda guarding a fountain.

  ◦ Waiting for you he is.

  ◦ Seek Yoda's advice.

- Turn around and head out of the courtyard.

- Take your first right up a little road to LETTERMAN DR.

- Left on LETTERMAN DR.

- Right on LOMBARD ST to rejoin the route.

Military Architecture at the Presidio
The vast array of military architecture in the Presidio reflects 200 years of development under three different nations, Spain, Mexico, and the United State. More than 470 of its buildings are historic. The iconic **Mission revival** style (1910–1940) we most associate with the Presidio today reflects our Spanish colonial history—and grew out of a desire to have a distinctive West Coast identity rather than to import designs from the East Coast.

• • • • • • • • • • • • • • • •

Follow LOMBARD ST

Right onto PRESIDIO BLVD (crossing the street for continual sidewalk)

PRESIDIO BLVD turns into LINCOLN BLVD

Left (south) on FUNSTON AVE

• • • • • • • • • • • • • • • • • •

Coming 2018: New Presidio Parklands Project
The New Presidio Parklands Project's ambitious goal seeks to create a new, magnificent 14-acre landscape that will link the heart of the Presidio to the shoreline and offer panoramic Golden Gate views.

Original 1906 earthquake cottages

2. Old Post Hospital and Officers' Row
Funston Ave

You are standing on the oldest intact streetscape in San Francisco! Read the history plaques about these 19th century married officers quarters and relics of the old Presidio as you walk by, and look closely at the new signs on each building. Modern-day businesses now rent these old quarters. But first—

DETOUR

> Take the stairs, which are between the Old Post Hospital and the large piece of artillery to its left.

> Walk behind the hospital.

> Return.

b. Earthquake Shacks

After the 1906 earthquake, the U.S. Army housed 16,000 refugees in military-style tent camps around the city. As winter approached, 5,610 wooden earthquake refugee "shacks" were built. Rent was $2 a month. Two remaining shacks are on display behind the Old Post Hospital.

Painted green to better blend into the parks and public squares in which they were erected, all had cedar-shingle roofs, Douglas fir floors and redwood walls. As you can see, they were pretty basic: one room, no kitchen, no bathroom. When the camps began closing in August 1907, refugees hauled cottages to private lots, where they often cobbled together two or more to form larger residences.

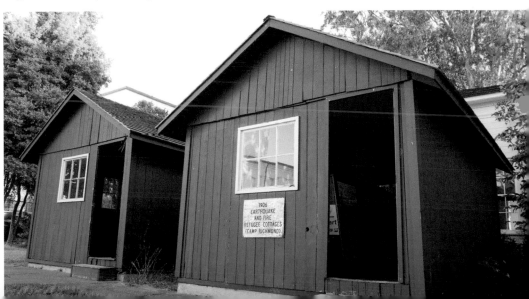

Right on MORAGA AVE

3. Inn at the Presidio (historic Pershing Hall) 42 Moraga Ave

Built in 1903, the elegant Georgian revival–style building originally served as the barracks for unmarried officers. In 2011, the Presidio Trust completed a historic rehabilitation of Pershing Hall, transforming it into the park's first lodge, Inn at the Presidio.

4. Presidio Officers' Club 50 Moraga Ave

Built in 1776, this building is one of only two remaining adobe structures in San Francisco (Mission Dolores is the other—and they argue over which came first). The building once housed Mexican and Spanish post commanders. The meeting that established the government of the town of Yerba Buena was held here. (Yerba Buena was later renamed San Francisco.) To protect it, sections of the surviving adobe were covered over in wood in 1812 and further restoration was attempted in 1934. After extensive rehabilitation, the **Presidio Officers' Club** reopened in 2014, featuring two spectacular event spaces and a history section where you can view a section of the original adobe walls.

5. Parade Grounds between Anza Ave and Montgomery St

The lush six-acre expanse of lawn framed by prominent buildings still summons up the pomp of military reviews. Today civilian celebrations and gatherings have taken the place of the military exercises, ceremonies, and drills, and the buildings surrounding the central parade ground are filled with wonderful museums to explore, such as **The Walt Disney Family Museum**.

> **Presidio Visitor Center**
> If it hasn't yet been moved to its new home on the Main Post, the Visitor Center will likely be located at **36 Lincoln Boulevard**, across from the Presidio Transit Center (where visitors can pick up the free **PresidoGo** Shuttle to explore the park). Google it. Open Thurs.–Sun., 10 a.m.–4 p.m.

6. Presidio Performing Arts Center 386 Moraga Ave

PPAC celebrates dance, music, and theater from across the globe—and welcomes artists to rent its multipurpose studio with 3,000 square feet of newly laid Harlequin Allegro Marley.

The Presidio's Main Parade Ground is now a grassy green gathering space.

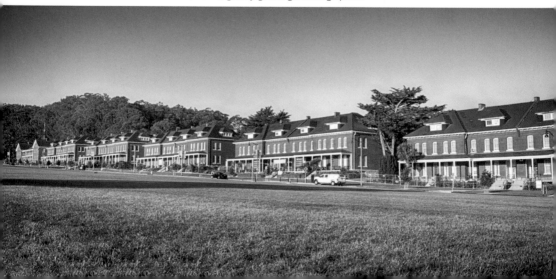

Herb Alpert, Grammy Award–winning bandleader of the Tijuana Brass, played in the 6th Army Band at the Presidio during the 1950s. Alpert says the structure and discipline of the army helped him with his music.

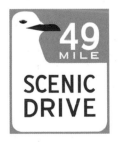

San Francisco National Cemetery

Bear right onto INFANTRY TERRACE

Bear left onto SHERIDAN AVE (crossing the street for continual sidewalk)

MERGE onto LINCOLN BLVD

MILE 11

Begins at SHERIDAN AVE at LINCOLN BLVD

7. San Francisco National Cemetery
1 Lincoln Blvd

The cemetery "offers a breathtaking final resting place for the nation's military veterans and their families." Among the 30,000 Americans laid to rest here since 1854 are Civil War generals, Medal of Honor recipients, Buffalo Soldiers, and a Union spy. In 1973, the cemetery officially closed to new interments except in reserved gravesites. The Department of Veterans Affairs attends to the gardening of the cemetery's 28.34 acres as well as the cleaning of tombstones.

—National Parks Service

The National Cemeteries Act of 1863 established 13 cemeteries to inter veterans of the armed forces and their families.

To get help locating a gravesite:

- Visit the office within the cemetery grounds
- Visit the Veterans Affairs website www.cem.va.gov
- Search a grave-finding website
- Write to U.S. Dept of Veterans Affairs, 1300 Sneath Lane, San Bruno, CA 94066

On your right, at YELLOW BIKE PATH SIGN on LINCOLN BLVD, leave the sidewalk to follow PRESIDIO PROME-NADE PATH (also called PATTEN RD)

ON THE BIKE PATH

8. Former Presidio Cavalry Horse Stables 663 McDowell Ave

The stables at the Presidio were built in 1914 for the 9th Cavalry. In the later years, cavalry regiments of the Buffalo Soldiers (soldiers in the all-black U.S. Army regiments) used these stables on their rotations to and from the Philippines. (NOTE: Many Buffalo Soldiers chose to stay in SF; 400 are buried at the Presidio in the SF National Cemetery.)

49 MILE

SCENIC DRIVE

DETOUR

> Turn right on MCDOWELL AVE, head downhill.

> Under the freeway to your left is the Pet Cemetery

> Return to route

c. Presidio Pet Cemetery
McDowell Ave at Crissy Field Ave

It probably began as a burial ground for cavalry horses in the 19th century. Sometime after World War II, when about 2,000 military families were stationed here, it became the final resting place for over 420 dogs, cats, birds, hamsters, lizards, and goldfish that once "served" at the Presidio.

Continue on PRESIDIO PROMENADE PATH

The path runs along LINCOLN BLVD and crosses the Crissy Field Lookout

9. Crissy Field Overlook— STUNNING
Lincoln Blvd

Mount Diablo, UC Berkeley Campanile, San Francisco skyline, Palace of Fine Arts, Alcatraz, Angel Island, the new Bay Bridge—wow! From the Crissy Field Overlook you can truly appreciate the Presidio's breathtaking location at the entrance to the Golden Gate.

You can view Crissy Field from the outlook and walk through it on the walk-back loop.

DETOUR

d. Crissy Field
1199 E Beach (Old Mason Rd, SF Bay Trail)

Once an asphalt-covered military airstrip, today Crissy Field is an extraordinary public recreational space for joggers, walkers, bikers, windsurfers, dogs, and picnickers—right alongside 20 acres of restored original tidal marshland nurturing 100 species of birds, 14 species of fish, and thousands of native plants. Another crowning success of the Golden Gate National Recreation Area!

$15 Million View
The Crissy Field Overlook was made possible by a $15 million gift from the Evelyn and Walter Haas, Jr. Fund. The overlook is part of a program to nearly double the size of the Presidio's trail system and create new ways for the community to experience the Presidio's great outdoors. (NOTE: The fund's philanthropy in the Golden Gate National Parks—more than $30 million total (as of 2014)—is the largest cash contribution ever received for America's national parks. *Thank you!*)

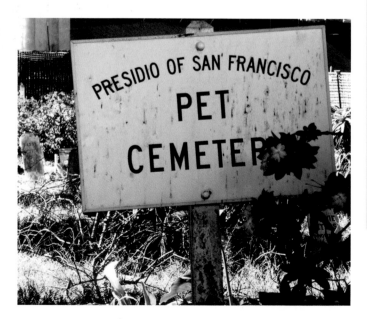

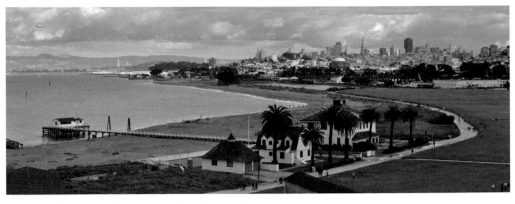

View from the Crissy Field Overlook. Photo: Paxson Woelber

Stay on paved bike path heading toward bridge
END at Golden Gate Bridge

. . . .

10. Golden Gate Bridge

Over 75 years old and she still looks gorgeous in red. You go, girl! When completed in 1937 the Golden Gate Bridge claimed title as the world's longest and tallest suspension bridge—with exquisite 820-foot-tall twin Art Deco towers as a bonus. About 41 million vehicles cross her 1.7-mile span annually.

ON WALK-BACK LOOP
e. Fort Point (view from above or hike down)

Strategically placed to defend San Francisco Bay against hostile warships, this fort was completed just before the American Civil War. No hostile warships, Confederate or foreign, ever arrived. No shots were ever fired from the fort. (HINT: Look up at the bridge structure above it. The Golden Gate Bridge designers had to build a special arch on the southern shore to accommodate the fort.)

f. Palace of Fine Arts

See Walk 3 for details

WALK-BACK LOOP SCOOP

Gorgeous. Do it. This walk-back loop is on unpaved trails and has some steep downhill walks and stairs—but worth it for the views! See the directions on page 66.

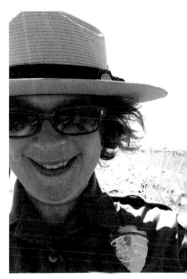

Ranger Robinson says, "Get out and enjoy your parks!"

WALK 4 NEED TO KNOW

TO GET THERE
- Muni 28, 30, 43, 45
- Golden Gate Transit 10, 70, 101

STREET PARKING
Free, 3 hour limit

PUBLIC RESTROOMS
- Golden Gate Bridge

On walk back:
- Warming Hut
- Crissy Field
- 3650 Yacht Road (near Palace of Fine Arts)

TURN-BY-TURN INSTRUCTIONS
Begin: LOMBARD ST at LYON ST

- Go through Presidio Entrance, LOMBARD GATE

DETOUR TO YODA

- ◦ As soon as you walk through the Presidio entrance gate you'll see a red-brick building to your right
- ◦ At the brown PRESIDIO sign turn right onto the trail
- ◦ Follow the trail past the red-brick buildings
- ◦ As you begin approaching a third red building, head into the courtyard straight ahead where you will find Yoda guarding a fountain.
- ◦ Turn around and head out of the courtyard

- ◦ Take your first right up a little road to LETTERMAN DR
- ◦ Left on LETTERMAN DR
- ◦ Right on LOMBARD ST to rejoin the route
- Follow LOMBARD ST
- Right onto PRESIDIO BLVD (crossing the street for continual sidewalk)
- PRESIDIO BLVD turns into LINCOLN
- Left (south) on FUNSTON AVE
  - ◦ Detour up the stairs behind the Old Post Hospital to see two earthquake shacks
- Right on MORAGA AVE
- Bear Right onto INFANTRY TERRACE
- Bear left onto SHERIDAN AVE (crossing the street for continual sidewalk)
- Merge onto LINCOLN BLVD
- Pass the National Cemetery
- On your right, at YELLOW BIKE PATH SIGN on LINCOLN BLVD, leave the sidewalk to follow PRESIDIO PROMENADE PATH (also called PATTEN RD)
  - ◦ Pass the horse stables (detour to Pet Cemetery if you wish), cross MCDOWELL AVE, keep following the path

- ◦ Stay on paved bike path heading toward bridge
- Veer right to head into Golden Gate Bridge Lookout area

End: GOLDEN GATE BRIDGE WELCOME CENTER (main bridge parking lot and plaza)

TO GET BACK
Muni
- At the Golden Gate Bridge parking lot, board Muni bus 28 (toward VAN NESS)
- Get off at RICHARDSON and FRANCISCO

Other Transit routes:
- Golden Gate Transit 10, 70, 101

OPTIONAL WALK-BACK LOOP DIRECTIONS:
Distance: 2.5 miles, 5,000 steps, 50 minutes

Rating:

Gorgeous—it's worth taking this route as its own hike some other time if you don't have time today. It's all trails, so if you feel lost, in general head downhill away from the bridge, toward the bay and Crissy Field, in the direction of the Palace of Fine Arts.

You can also hike all the way down to Fort Point if you want. Enjoy the amazing up-close under-the-bridge views, stop and read interpretive signs along the trail, walk out to the beach and stare at

Alcatraz, explore the stores and warehouse businesses along Crissy Field, look at the scrub grass and lagoon to get an idea of what early SF looked like. What's not to like? Gorgeous. Enjoy.

Begin: GOLDEN GATE BRIDGE WELCOME CENTER

- Walk to large statue of Joseph Strauss (chief engineer of the Golden Gate Bridge)
- Veer left around Strauss and walk up two sets of stairs
- Come down a set of stairs to the bike path (PACIFIC PROMENADE)
- Turn right to walk along the paved bike path
  - Though there are switchbacks, in general you will be heading away from the bridge, back toward the beginning of the walk
- Watch for the CRISSY FIELD sign on your left— follow it on the steep downhill walk
  - Just past the overlook you will go through a low brick tunnel
  - Watch for unpaved trail to CRISSY FIELD
- Veer left onto CRISSY FIELD trail, down the stairs
  - At the bottom of the stairs, you'll find restrooms, the Warming Hut (café and store), fishing pier
- Follow the SF BAY TRAIL along Crissy Field
- At the Crissy Field Center (big spinning metal things in front), cut right onto the paved side trail back out to the city streets
- At the crazy intersection (YACHT-LYON, MASON-MARINA), figure out how to use the lights to cross MARINA BLVD to the Palace of Fine Arts
- OPTION:
  - Shorter route: Turn right onto PALACE DR to walk behind the Palace of Fine Arts
  - Scenic route: Veer left to walk in front the Palace of Fine Arts on BAKER ST or on the Palace walkway
- Head down LYON ST
- Cross RICHARDSON AVE, turn left
- Right on FRANCISCO ST, which becomes LYON ST

End: LYON ST at LOMBARD ST (LOMBARD GATE)

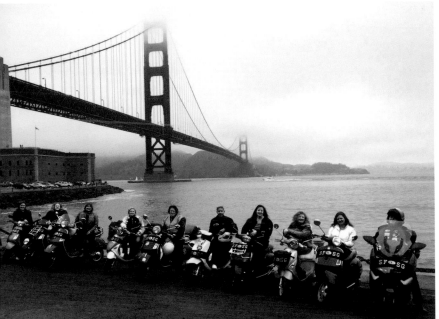

Carolyn (fourth from left) with the San Francisco Scooter Girls on their celebratory 10-year anniversary ride.

Note Fort Point in the background. The Golden Gate Bridge engineers had to construct an arch over the fort to preserve it.

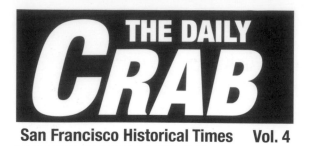

THE DAILY CRAB

San Francisco Historical Times Vol. 4

HALFWAY-TO-HELL CLUB

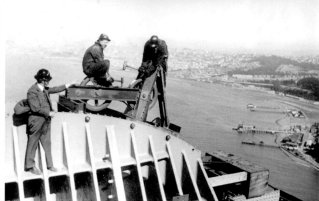

Courtesy of San Francisco History Center, San Francisco Public Library

One man killed for every million dollars spent had been the norm for bridge building in the early 20th century. So the **Golden Gate Bridge** builders added extra safety precautions, such as adapting miners' hard hats for use by bridge workers and, more noticeably, suspending a giant safety net from end to end under the floor of the bridge. The net saved the lives of 19 men who became known as the Halfway-to-Hell Club. In four years of construction only one fatality occurred, setting a new all-time safety record. Sadly, on February 17, three months before the bridge opened, a section of scaffold carrying 12 men fell, crashing through the safety net, and 10 more men lost their lives.

Paint stores can create the bridge color with the formula:

    C=Cyan: 0%
    M=Magenta: 69%
    Y=Yellow: 100%
    K= Black: 6%

The closest premixed color codes are PMS 173 and 174, and Pantone 180. Currently, the paint is specially mixed and supplied for the bridge by **Sherwin-Williams**. Their closest off-the-shelf paint match: **Fireweed** (SW 6328).

1,000,000 PLASTIC BAGS

In 2010, nonprofit group **Save The Bay** estimated that about 1 million plastic bags entered San Francisco Bay every year, choking our wetlands and smothering the bay's wildlife. Today all nine counties that touch the bay have voted to establish restrictions on plastic bags. *Yay, us!*

To help, contact SaveSFbay.org

NAVY PAINTS GOLDEN GATE BRIDGE IN YELLOW & BLACK STRIPES

Horrifying! When the bridge was being built, the U.S. Navy wanted her painted in yellow-and-black stripes—while the Army Air Corps argued for red-and-white candy stripes!

Thankfully, consulting architect **Irving Morrow** knew full well that the need for increased visibility on foggy days does not require ugliness. He selected the distinctive, warm International Orange color because it blends well with the surrounding warm colors of the landmass while contrasting with the cool colors of the sky and sea. Harmonious with its natural setting—while still enhancing visibility for passing ships. *Fabulous, Irving!*

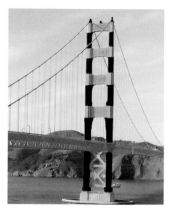

Who Lives? Who Dies? Who Decides?

Throughout most of history, wounded soldiers were left lying on the battlefield for days, even weeks. Those lucky enough to be carried to (filthy, crowded) field hospitals were more likely to die from infection than their wounds. Thank god for **Dr. Jonathan Letterman**.

Letterman's innovations, organization, and insistence on modern medical practices in the military saved thousands of soldiers from dying horrible deaths and earned him the title **"Father of Battlefield Medicine."**

For example, as surgeon and medical director of the Army of the Potomac during the **American Civil War**, he created an ambulance corps and invented the system of battlefield triage

still used today: prioritizing patients' treatment based on severity of condition and resources available. The bloodiest day in U.S. history, the Civil War battle of **Antietam**, left 10,000 wounded. Within 24 hours all the soldiers were in a hospital.

The Presidio hospital, established in 1898 to care for sick and wounded soldiers returning from the Philippine Islands during the **Spanish–American War**, was renamed for Letterman in 1911. In **World War I**, staff physicians there developed orthopedic devices, including the "Letterman Leg," and pioneered the field of physical therapy.

During **World War II**, Letterman became the largest army

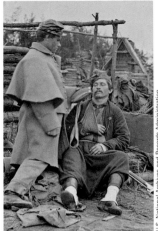

Deserted camp and wounded soldier. Photo by Mathew Brady.

U.S. National Archives and Records Administration

hospital in the country, treating 76,000 patients in 1945 alone. By the end of WWII, Italian and German prisoners of war provided the hospital's labor. Letterman Hospital closed in 1992.

WE WIN!!

What should the citizens do with thousands of acres of unused military bases on pristine scenic lands all around the bay? Sell them to condo developers, of course. *NOT!* Congressman Phillip Burton along with many extraordinary people of vision, fought to turn our endangered public lands into the world's largest urban park, **the Golden Gate National Recreation Area** (GGNRA).

Since 1972, **75,000 acres** of former military bases, watersheds, historic sites, and open spaces spanning **70 miles** have been preserved, restored, and combined to create the GGNRA. Over **16 million people** a year visit hundreds of sites around the Bay, from **Tomales Bay** and **Muir Woods** in Marin to **Alcatraz** and the **Presidio** in SF to the beach cliffs of San Mateo County.

Golden Gate Bridge Destroyed

Movies in which the GG Bridge meets a horrifying fate. How many have you seen?

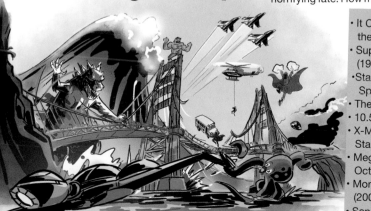

- It Came from Beneath the Sea (1955)
- Superman: The Movie (1978)
- Star Trek: Deep Space Nine (1999)
- The Core (2003)
- 10.5 (2004)
- X-Men: The Last Stand (2006)
- Mega Shark vs. Giant Octopus (2009)
- Monsters vs. Aliens (2009)
- San Andreas (2015)

by Jett Atwood

WALKING FOR LIFE—HOW TO BE A HEALTHIER, HAPPIER, SMARTER YOU By Amy Gladin, PT, DPT, OCS

When it comes to exercise you probably already know this: To be healthier and live longer you have to get up and get moving *every day*. It doesn't take a lot of work, or equipment, or money, or time. In fact, just 30 minutes of moderate activity five times a week (or 150 minutes total per week) can change your life. And you are worth it.

The good news is you are already an expert at the no. 1 doctor-recommended form of exercise: walking. You've been doing it since childhood, yes? Though it's the easiest exercise to do, it gives you an extraordinary number of benefits.

Walking is not only good for your heart, lungs, bones, muscles, balance, and overall health; it improves your brain, fights disease, and helps you live longer.

The U.S. Surgeon General, the American Heart Association, the American College of Sports Medicine, and countless other researchers report that moderate-intensity walking for 150 minutes a week will reduce the risk of many chronic diseases that result in early death.

Walking reduces the risk of:
- heart disease and stroke
- diabetes mellitus type 2
- osteoporosis—if your walks include going up and down hills
- breast and colon cancer
- falling
- cognitive decline

Walking improves:
- blood pressure
- blood sugar levels
- mental well-being

Gear: Get a Good Pair of Walking Shoes
Keep your feet happy—this is supposed to be enjoyable. The body's whole alignment starts with the support of your foot over your ankle and knee and hip and so on. It's worth spending a little money on the right shoes. It's generally recommended that you replace your shoes every six months. So even if you have great walking shoes, make sure they are still in good condition. Finally, **the most important consideration when chosing a shoe is comfort**. There is no such thing as needing to break in your shoes. They should be comfortable from the moment you put them on.

Walking Makes You Smarter, Keeps You Younger

Researchers from the University of Illinois at Urbana-Champaign have shown that walking not only contributes to new growth of adult brain cells, it also builds up the connectivity between brain circuits. Which means walking improves memory, attention, and cognitive function skills—things like planning, scheduling, dealing with ambiguity, working memory, and multitasking. These are the very skills that tend to decline with aging. Walking may be the wonder drug to prevent aging!

On top of that, the endorphins released from brisk walking can help fight depression, boost your energy, reduce stress, and improve your sleep.

And if all of that doesn't make you run out and buy a pair of new walking shoes . . . .

Take a walk in San Francisco—you never know what you might see.

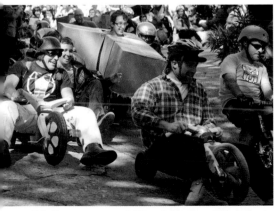

This "leave-no-trace," $5, neighborhood Big Wheel race happens every year on San Francisco's actual crookedest street. PHOTO: NICKI DUGAN POGUE

Walking Makes You Sexier

As you walk you tone your muscles, you reduce your body fat, you start looking fit and healthy, and you will likely feel more confident and be more positive. Yes, beauty is in the eye of the beholder, but "fit, confident, and positive" sure sounds like the definition of sexy! (And admit it, sitting on the couch griping about your aches and pains and what you just saw on TV is the opposite of sexy.)

So How Much Walking Does It Take?

To meet contemporary exercise guidelines for recommended *minimum* exercise levels, you need to take 5,000 to 7,000 steps a day. Taking 1,200 steps per day is considered inactive. A good goal is 10,000 steps a day (approximately five miles of walking per day). Unless you have an active job such as waitressing or nursing, it would be difficult to log 10,000 steps just with daily activity. Most Americans would have to add a brisk 30-minute walk or two to reach that. But every bit helps. For example, just adding 2,000 steps a day helps lower high blood pressure.

When was the last time you set aside a little hunk of time each day just to take care of yourself?

With All Those Benefits Why Aren't Americans Out There Walking?

While it seems so simple to do, and hosts all these benefits, the Surgeon General reports that only about 20% of Americans get the minimum recommended amount of moderate exercise per week. The toughest thing about starting a fitness program is developing a habit. **Step one: Get started.** If you don't walk at all, start with walking out the door five times a week for a 10-minute walk. Then to keep going, you need to throw in some success and some fun.

Walk to a parade

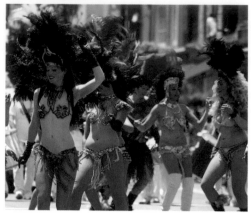

or better yet, join a dance group and prance in a parade, such as Carnaval, San Francisco's free two–day annual family festival held in San Francisco's Mission District over Memorial Day weekend.
Photo: JialiangGao, www.peaceonearth.org

How to Boost Your Motivation

In our busy lives it's easy for exercise to creep down our list of priorities, especially when the fun factor is low. Here are some factors shown to improve motivation and success:

» **Set a realistic goal**
The key is to set a challenging but reasonable goal that you can achieve and build on. For example:
- Short term: Walk around the block at lunchtime five times a week for one month

Be Prepared for Changing Weather—Wear Lightweight Layers
In San Francisco, you may start out on a damp morning and then the fog burns off and suddenly you're peeling down to your shirtsleeves and wishing you had your sunscreen. Or visa versa. It's also a good idea to wear a hat for warmth, or shading your face when the sun comes out.

- Performance based: Increase daily steps by 500 steps a day
- Choose an event: Do the Bridge to Bridge walk, or complete the entire 49 mile walk.

» **Measure Your Goals**
State your goal in a way that can be measured. Walk 10,000 steps per day. Walk the entire 49 mile walk in one year. **And track your progress.**

» **Write it down**
When something is written in the calendar you are more likely to do it. Set a date.

» **Count your steps**
A pedometer, old school or high tech like a Fitbit, is a simple way to count your steps—and studies show people who wear step counters average an additional 2,000 steps per day.

» **Share your goal**

When you share your goal with others, it's more likely that you'll achieve your goal. Announce your goal to your social networks, such as your intention to hike the 49 mile walk this year. You will not only elicit their support, but you may also recruit others to join you. Then announce your success or progress once a month and enjoy the praise.

» **Find a workout buddy**

We are more likely to stay consistent when we are accountable to another person.

Celebrate your successes
and reward yourself!

» **Join a group**

There are walking groups galore that will be happy to have you along—try searching on Meetup. com. Joining a group (or creating one of your own) will keep you accountable and provides an outside source of encouragement to keep going. As a side benefit, you'll likely create some new relationships along the way. Creating a group with your family and friends is a fun way to get moving together and build a lifetime habit of walking and exploring the city.

» **Keep it fun**

Any walk you can take with new sites, sounds, and adventure—or with a good friend—can take your mind off exercise and put a smile on your face. Plus, getting out and enjoying the sheer beauty of the San Francisco Bay Area fills the spirit and makes you feel good about life.

> Thirty minutes of moderate activity five times a week *can change your life*. And you are worth it!

The Best Motivation of All: You Deserve a Happy, Healthy Life!

Bottom line: This is your life. When was the last time you set aside a little hunk of time each day just to take care of yourself? You deserve to be healthy and happy. Just 30 minutes of moderate activity five times a week, or 20–60 minutes of vigorous activity three times a week, can change your life. However you choose to exercise, please get started and keep it up. Do it for you.

Amy Gladin, PT, DPT, OCS, is a senior physical therapist, an orthopedic clinical specialist (OCS), and a clinical researcher.

Walk to a pillow fight...

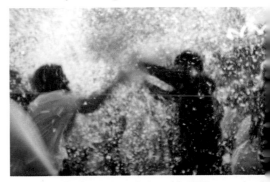

and burn off a few extra calories with 1000+ people at the annual (unpermitted, flash mob) Valentine's Day Pillow Fight at Justin Herman Plaza.
PHOTO: CHRISTOPHER MICHEL

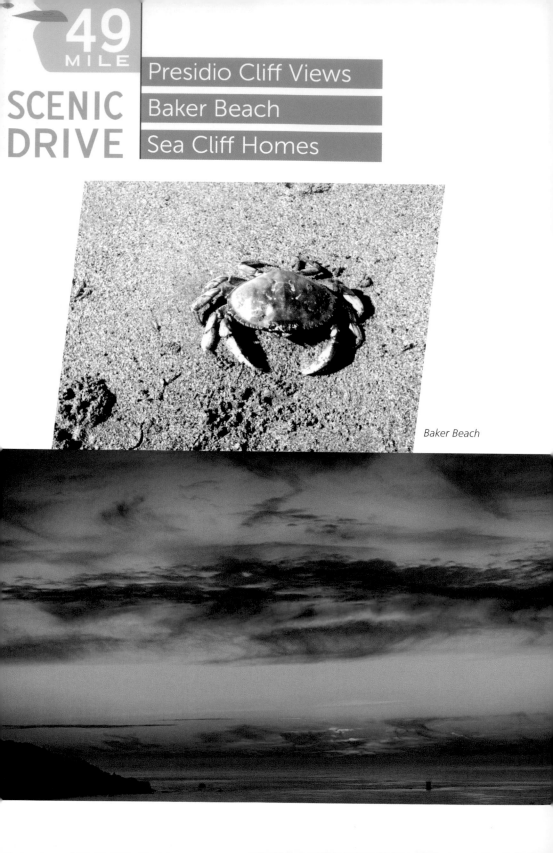

49 MILE
SCENIC DRIVE

Presidio Cliff Views

Baker Beach

Sea Cliff Homes

Baker Beach

Walk and Gawk.

This hike begins above the coast on the rugged cliffs and bluffs of San Francisco's Presidio. Even if you've *driven* the west-of-the-bridge stretch of Lincoln Boulevard a thousand times, you will see so much more when you *walk* it: trails, cliff-side stairways, native plant life, artillery, magnificent bay views, rugged beauty—and possibly a naked person or two on the hidden beach coves below the bluffs. The Presidio Trust is determined to build world-class trails and natural experiences for visitors here. They are succeeding.

After you wander downhill between the Presidio traffic bluffs for a while, the trail takes you across the sands of Baker Beach passed an old artillery battery before it emerges into one of the city's most manicured, affluent neighborhoods, Sea Cliff. Stately El Camino Del Mar will lead you past the estates, chateaus, Spanish colonial–revival mansions, and swaying palms that belie the area's humble origins as a fishing camp for Chinese fishermen at China Beach. The road winds along the historic route of the Lincoln Highway directly into Lincoln Park through the edge of Lincoln Golf Course's ocean-side cliffs and ends at the Palace of the Legion of Honor.

The 3.5-mile beach-and-cliffs walk-back loop is worth taking as its own walk another day if you can't make it today—highly recommended!

Whether you are walking one-way or round-trip, have your camera ready for postcard views of the ocean meeting the bay, the Marin Headlands, and the Golden Gate Bridge throughout the walk. Amazing.

NOTE: There are *no stores* along this route or return walk at which to grab a snack or bottle of water. Bring your own or purchase what you need at a store in the Golden Gate Bridge main parking lot.

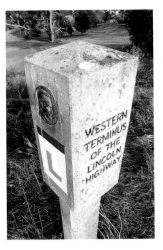

The Lincoln Highway terminus marker is well hidden. Walk past the fountain and look behind the bus stop at the Legion of Honor.

Begin: Golden Gate Bridge Welcome Center
End: El Camino Del Mar and 34th Avenue (Legion of Honor)
Distance: ROUTE: 2.9 miles — 5,800 steps — 1:00 hour
LOOP BACK: 3.1 miles — 7,000 steps — 1¼ hours

Hill Rating: 3

Sites you will pass on today's walk include:

MILEs 12–13
1. **Presidio Coastal Bluffs**
2. **Baker Beach**
3. **Battery Chamberlin**
4. **Lobos Creek**

MILE 14
SEACLIFF
5. **El Camino Del Mar**

RICHMOND DISTRICT'S FIVE NEIGHBORHOODS
a. **China Beach**
6. **Lincoln Park**
7. **Lincoln Highway Western Terminus Marker**

NOTE: For safety reasons, walk on the trail that parallels Lincoln Blvd until *after* Baker Beach. Do not walk on Lincoln Blvd. The street is very dangerous for pedestrians here. The path next to Lincoln detours off toward Baker Beach, then brings you out to the final stretch of Lincoln, which has a sidewalk for you to walk on.

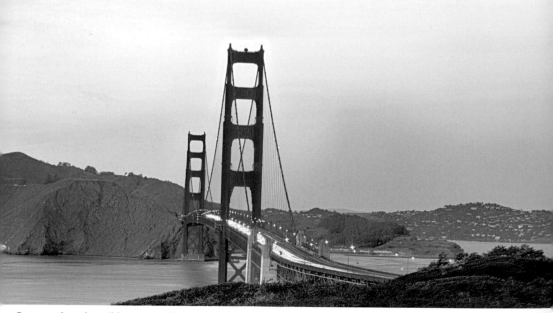

Come explore the wild western side of the Golden Gate Bridge. Photo taken at sunset.

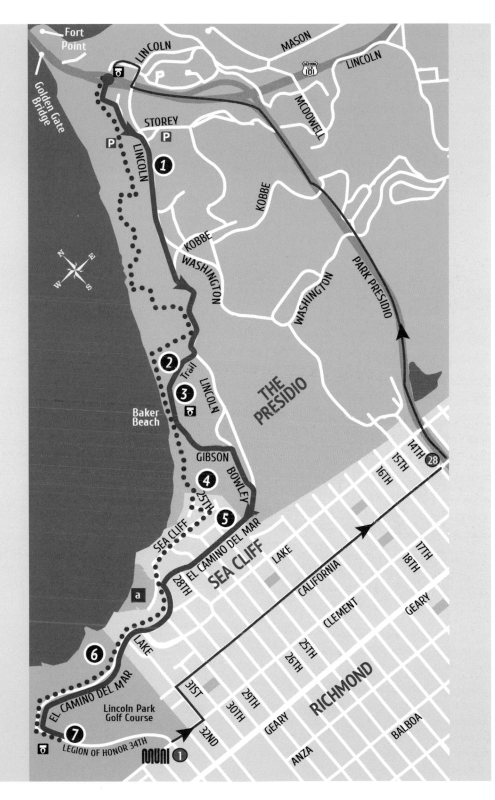

MILE 12-13

Begins at Golden Gate Bridge main parking Lot

· · · · · · · · · · · · · · · · · ·

Next to the café and gift shop is a tunnel under the bridge that includes a pedestrian walkway

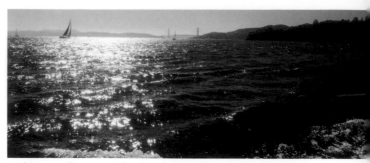

Nighttime sailing past Baker Beach toward the Golden Gate Bridge

Take PEDESTRIAN UNDERPASS west under the bridge

Turn left

Right at MERCHANT RD

Follow MERCHANT RD around to LINCOLN BLVD

At LINCOLN BLVD turn right (west) up stairway to PACIFIC COASTAL TRAIL

Follow the trail as it parallels LINCOLN BLVD

· · · · · · · · · · · · · · · · · ·

1. Presidio Coastal Bluffs

As wonderful as the Lincoln Boulevard stretch of this hike is, it's totally worth a return trip to explore the neighboring Batteries to Bluffs Trail (or better yet take the Batteries to Bluffs Trail as your optional walk-back loop today). It guides you along the ocean's untamed side, past rugged cliffs, blue-green streaked serpentine rock, historic gun batteries, hidden springs, dramatic outlooks, an isolated beach, and unparalleled views of the bridge. Some of the most intact natural habitat in the Presidio grows on these bluffs—rare plants adapted to serpentine soil and cool foggy conditions.

Hiking and Biking

A great way to explore the Presidio is on the park's extensive 24-mile hiking and biking trail network, which has a dozen distinctive routes and eight scenic overlooks. More trails are added yearly.

· · · · · · · · · · · · · · · · · ·

Stay on PACIFIC COASTAL TRAIL as it veers right, downhill toward BAKER BEACH

Before you reach the beach, turn left through chain-link fence

· · · · · · · · · · · · · · · · · ·

2. Baker Beach

Frisbees, frolicking, fishing, and spectacular views of the Pacific Ocean, Marin Headlands, and container ships navigating under the Golden Gate Bridge! Woohoo! Plus, this mile-long stretch of sandy beach includes picnic areas, parking, bathrooms, trails, bird watching, and natural coastal bluffs. NOTE: Dogs and naked people are restricted to the northern end of the beach.

Shorts, Shovels, Sunscreen, and Smiles

Love the park? Come share your time and talent! For just one day, or once a week, or with a group. Volunteers needed for archeology, forest and tree care, gardening and landscaping, habitat restoration, nursery work, trail maintenance, docents, compost and salvage. NOTE: You aren't required to be good-looking to volunteer, but we've noticed that most of the volunteers are hot! Presidio.gov/volunteer

Where Burning Man Began
The annual desert art event now known as Burning Man began as a summer solstice celebration in 1986 when Larry Harvey, Jerry James, and a few friends met on Baker Beach and burned an eight-foot tall wooden man as well as a smaller wooden dog.

3. Battery Chamberlin—Free Demonstration

If you take a peek through the chain-link fence at Baker Beach—you'll see a 50-ton coastal defense gun hiding there. Stranger still, you can come help load it and aim it—during the free monthly demonstrations. Built in 1904, this is the last artillery installation of its type on the West Coast. Demonstrations are typically held between 11 a.m. and 3 p.m. on the first Saturday and Sunday of each month. There's a bunker museum, too.

Military Batteries
Back in the 1890s, the military began fortifying California's coast with military batteries: concrete structures on which they could mount and hide artillery (guns). They became obsolete and were abandoned after World War II, but the remnants still dot the coast.

Continue past concrete bunkers into parking lot

Walk through the parking lot onto GIBSON RD

Take GIBSON RD back up the hill toward LINCOLN BLVD

Right at BOWLEY ST (Baker Beach upper parking lot), which merges back onto LINCOLN BLVD

4. Lobos Creek

Once the source of water for the Presidio and early San Francisco, Lobos Creek is the last free flowing stream in San Francisco. Lobos Creek Valley gives native plants and wildlife a survivable habitat in an otherwise urban area. Restoration work is helping to bring rare plant species back to the area.

LINCOLN BLVD turns into EL CAMINO DEL MAR at 25th AVE

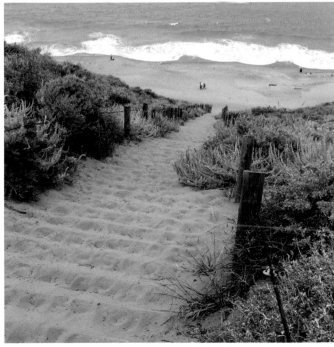

Those little dots you see at the bottom of the Baker Beach sand ladder are people.

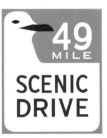

49 MILE

SCENIC DRIVE

MILE 14

Begins on EL CAMINO DEL MAR at 25th AVE

· · · · · · · · · · · · · · · · ·

Follow EL CAMINO DEL MAR

· · · · · · · · · · · · · · · · ·

SEA CLIFF

After the earthquake and fire of 1906, wealthy San Franciscans wanted to build their homes far away from the rubble and charred remains of places like Nob Hill. To keep our prosperous citizen from fleeing the city, we hired Mark Daniels, the famed landscape architect who created the 17-mile drive around Pebble Beach, to help create a new upscale neighborhood in SF: Sea Cliff. This quiet affluent neighborhood abounds with multimillion-dollar homes, manicured landscaping, celebrity hideaways, and some of the most coveted views of the city and the Golden Gate Bridge. Tour buses and vans are largely banned.

$18 MILLION VIEW
In the post–market crash year of 2009, a splendid Sea Cliff mansion perched on the cliffs overlooking the Golden Gate sold for $18 million. Median home price in 2014: $4.725 million.

5. El Camino Del Mar

"The road of the sea" began in the 1910s as part of a grand boulevard connecting the Panama–Pacific International Exposition through the Presidio to Ocean Beach. The main portion—running from the Presidio to Lincoln Park—was completed in 1915 and has been enjoyed ever since. The magnificent second stretch of El Camino Del Mar—running around the Legion of Honor below Fort Miley to Sutro Baths—slid into the sea so many times, it was finally closed in 1958.

· · · · · · · · · · · · · · · · ·

Veer left with EL CAMINO DEL MAR at the T in the road

· · · · · · · · · · · · · · · · ·

Ansel Adams Survives 1906 Quake
When the childhood home of American photographer and environmentalist Ansel Adams was built in 1903 (at what is today 129 24th Avenue in Sea Cliff to your left, just before you reach 25th Avenue) it stood among just a handful of houses on a sandy dune overlooking the Presidio. Both young Ansel and his home survived the earthquake of 1906, though Ansel suffered a broken nose when an aftershock threw him against a brick wall.

In 1929, two years after he took his famous photograph of Half Dome in Yosemite, he built a photographic studio next to his childhood home. He sold both in 1962.

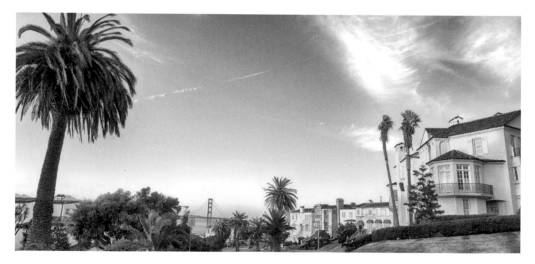

RICHMOND DISTRICT'S FIVE NEIGHBORHOODS

Sea Cliff, Lake Street, and Inner, Central, and Outer Richmond make up the five residential neighborhoods of the Richmond District. The Richmond, as locals call it, is bounded on three sides by natural features or green space: the Presidio and Lincoln Park to the north, the Pacific Ocean to the west, and Golden Gate Park to the south. Arguello Boulevard defines the eastern border.

a. China Beach

Tucked between Lands End and Baker Beach, this tiny sheltered cove at the bottom of a steep slope features a secluded beach for sunbathing and picnicking with good play spots for children, and spectacular views of the Marin Headlands and Golden Gate. Legend has it that local residents named China Beach for the Chinese fishermen who, long ago, anchored their junks (fishing boats) in the cove and camped on the beach.

· · · · · · · · · · · · · · · · · ·

As you hit LINCOLN PARK, continue on steep hill up to LEGION OF HONOR

· · · · · · · · · · · · · · · · · ·

6. Lincoln Park

This 100-acre park in the city's northwest corner began as a Gold Rush–era paupers' cemetery, fittingly named Potter's Field. The graves were removed in 1908, and the Parks Department took over the site, built a golf course, and dedicated the new park to Abraham Lincoln in 1909. The California Palace of the Legion of Honor, built to honor soldiers killed in WWI, broke ground in 1923, and the San Francisco Holocaust Memorial, designed by George Segal, was dedicated in 1984. (All of which you'll pass on Walk 6.)

7. Lincoln Highway Western Terminus Marker

In 1913, the first transcontinental highway for cars across the United States, the Lincoln Highway, pulled into San Francisco and chose Lincoln Park as a fitting end point. The route starts in New York City at Times Square, traverses 14 states, and then in SF, snakes from the Hyde Street Pier to North Point Street, Van Ness Avenue, California Street, 32nd Avenue, and El Camino del Mar to reach its terminus in front of the Palace of the Legion of Honor.

· · · · · · · · · · · · · · · · · ·

END: EL CAMINO DEL MAR at LEGION OF HONOR (Palace of the Legion of Honor)

· · · · · · · · · · · · · · · · · ·

WALK-BACK LOOP SCOOP

This off-road, beach-and-cliffs hike along the Presidio Battery to Bluffs Trail is worthy of coming back for to do as its own hike some day. But if you have a bit of energy left, we recommend it as a great hike back to the Golden Gate Bridge. Challenging 3.1-mile trail with gorgeous views!

"Some of the earliest 'inhabitants' of the Richmond were the dead." —RichmondSFBlog.com

Nineteenth-century San Franciscans called the wild, empty, western part of the city the Outside Lands. At the time, this remote area seemed the perfect place for the four cemeteries built there: Laurel Hill, Calvary, Masonic, and Odd Fellows, plus the paupers' cemetery in Lincoln Park.

Eventually, the cemeteries got in the way of housing expansion in the area so the San Francisco City and County passed the Cemetery Removal Ordinance of 1937. Most bodies were moved by 1941, most reinterred in Colma. The Columbarium, originally part of Odd Fellows Cemetery, still remains today, run by the Neptune Society. NOTE: The headstones of unclaimed bodies were recycled into construction projects such as lining Buena Vista Park pathways and creating the Ocean Beach Seawall—they can still be found today by savvy seekers.

WALK 5 NEED TO KNOW

TO GET THERE
- Muni 28
- Golden Gate Transit 10, 70, 101

PARKING
Parking is extremely limited; we highly recommend taking public transportation to get there.

- East side of the Golden Gate Bridge (these lots fill up quickly)
  - Golden Gate Bridge parking lot, metered parking next to the bridge
  - Larger lot farther down Lincoln Blvd
- West side of the bridge (less known, less crowded)
  - National Park Service lots: Merchant Rd, Story Rd, and along Lincoln Blvd.
  - Check signs for rates and time. Some lots are free; some are pay-to-park and may have time limits.

PUBLIC RESTROOMS
- Golden Gate Bridge
- China Beach
- Baker Beach parking lot
- Behind the Legion of Honor

TURN–BY–TURN INSTRUCTIONS
Begin: GOLDEN GATE BRIDGE main parking lot. Next to the café and gift shop is a tunnel under the bridge that includes a pedestrian walkway

- Take PEDESTRIAN UNDERPASS west under the bridge
- Turn left
- Right at MERCHANT RD
  - Follow MERCHANT RD around to LINCOLN BLVD
- At LINCOLN BLVD turn right (west) up stairway to PACIFIC COASTAL TRAIL
- Follow the trail as it parallels LINCOLN BLVD
- Stay on COASTAL TRAIL as it veers right, downhill toward BAKER BEACH DETOUR
  - Before you reach the beach, turn left through chain-link fence
  - Continue past concrete bunkers into parking lot

- Walk through the parking lot onto GIBSON RD
- Take GIBSON RD back up the hill toward LINCOLN BLVD
- RIGHT at BOWLEY ST (Baker Beach upper parking lot), which merges back onto LINCOLN BLVD
- LINCOLN BLVD turns into EL CAMINO DEL MAR at 25th AVE
- Follow EL CAMINO DEL MAR
- Veer left with EL CAMINO DEL MAR at the T in the road
- As you hit LINCOLN PARK, continue on steep hill up to LEGION OF HONOR RD

End: EL CAMINO DEL MAR at LEGION OF HONOR RD (Palace of the Legion of Honor)

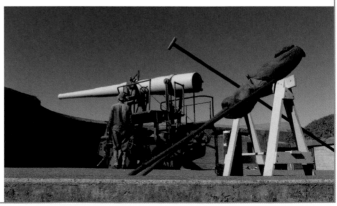

Artillery demonstration at Battery Chamberlin, Baker Beach

TO GET BACK
Muni

- Board bus 1 at SE corner of 33RD AVE and CLEMENT ST (toward downtown)
- Get off at CALIFORNIA ST and PRESIDIO BLVD
- Go to NE corner to transfer to b 28 (toward Fort Mason)
- Get off at Golden Gate Bridge

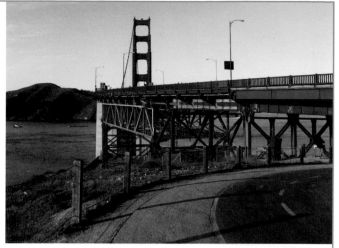

Pedestrian/bike trail under the bridge

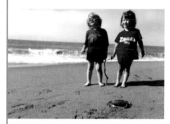

OPTIONAL WALK-BACK LOOP DIRECTIONS
Off-road, beach, and Presidio trails

Steep, 60-floor-step-climbing challenge up and down and up and down cliff-side stairs and trails! Great, gorgeous workout.

Distance: 3.1 miles, 7,000 steps, 1¼ hours

Rating: 5

Trail hint: When in doubt keep heading east toward the Golden Gate Bridge.

Begin: Return back down EL CAMINO DEL MAR

- As EL CAMINO DEL MAR veers right, stay left (toward the ocean)
- Right onto SEACLIFF AVE
- Left at 25TH AVE
- At T in the road turn right
- Take cul-de-sac entrance onto BAKER BEACH
- Head left toward the ocean and turn right to walk along BAKER BEACH, nearly to the end, about ½ mile
  - You will pass the restrooms, the artillery battery, a trail down to the beach, a yellow solar-powered emergency phone
- On your right you will see a steep SAND LADDER
- Take SAND LADDER up to LINCOLN BLVD

- Turn left on LINCOLN BLVD, watch on your left for BATTERY TO BLUFFS trail entrance sign
- Take TRAIL, watch for and follow the signs
  - You will go up and down and up and down the cliffs on wood-and-sand stairs (you shouldn't reach the beach again)
  - Occasionally the trail splits; just keep heading toward GG Bridge. The trails to the left tend to have great cliff views, but most trails lead back to the bridge
  - You will pass a number of batteries and, toward the end, begin seeing parking lots
- Head to your car or bus stop

End: GOLDEN GATE BRIDGE WELCOME CENTER

THE DAILY CRAB

San Francisco Historical Times   Vol. 5

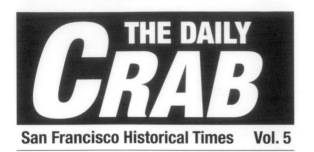

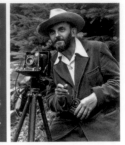

Native San Franciscan Ansel Adams 1902–1984

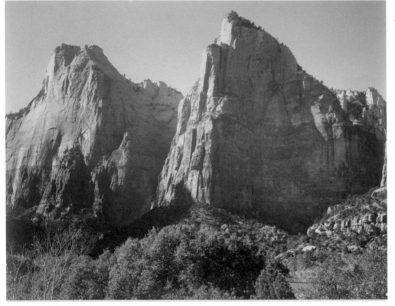

Court of the Patriarchs, Zion National Park, Utah; April 1933. From the series "Ansel Adams Photographs of National Parks and Monuments."

Ansel Adams took to the beauty of nature at an early age, exploring his neighborhood— **Lobos Creek** to **Baker Beach** and the sea cliffs leading to **Lands End**. In 1915, Ansel's father gave him a yearlong pass to the **Panama-Pacific Expo**. Enthralled, 13-year-old Ansel returned daily. Was it this exposure to modern painting, sculpture, and photography in his adolescence that led him to become a world-famous photographer and environmentalist? *It couldn't have hurt.*

The Best Thing That Ever Happened in the History of Baker Beach

Three days before our November wedding on San Francisco's Baker Beach, the biggest rain in three years hit—with more storms predicted on the wedding day. The guests worried, the minister called to suggest we move to an indoor venue—but we had faith, and held firm.

Early morning of the wedding day, the rain was blowing sideways. Then half an hour before the wedding, the rain stopped, the clouds parted, and the newly washed bridge glistened. We proceeded along the empty beach to the sound of a ukulele and a tenor voice singing the "Iz"

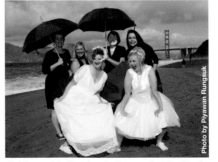

Bridesmaids Stephanie Lynne Smith, Cindy Reich, Katharine Holland, and Amy Gladin stand behind authors, Kristine and Carolyn

Photo by Piyawan Rungsuk

version of "Somewhere Over the Rainbow."

We beamed and cried, standing under a canopy embroidered with the names of our mothers and passed-on loved ones we knew were smiling down on us. With 50 of our closest friends and family standing near, the minister sent our wedding rings around for each of them to hold and add their blessings. By the powers vested in her by God, the United Church of Christ, the State of California, and the United States of America, we were pronounced legally married. ***Woohoo!***

—*Kristine and Carolyn*

GRAVEYARD GOLF

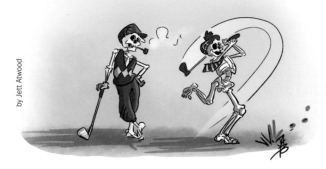

by Jett Atwood

Like many cemeteries of that era, **Potter's Field** (located in what would become Lincoln Park) was ethnically divided. In addition to the paupers' section, the societies that used the cemetery included Italian, French, Jewish, German, Knights of Pythias, Slavonic Illyric, St. Andrews, Orthodox Easter Greek Church, Grand Army of the Republic, Ladies' Seaman Society, Old Friend's Society, Colored IOOF, Chinese Six Companies, Chinese Christian, and Japanese.

In one year, 1893, the interments included 11,000 indigent and 7,000 from societies.

In 1902, golfing enthusiasts, seeking to create a course for those who couldn't afford private club fees, obtained permission to map out a three-hole municipal golf course at Potter's Field. The course proved so popular the Parks Department took over the site in 1908 and city supervisors asked the different organizations that had burial plots there to remove them to make way for a new city park and expanded golf course: **Lincoln Park**.

The clever, well-written Lincoln Park Golf Club website has no qualms about letting us know that Italians once rested under the eighteenth fairway, Chinese ancestors graced the depths of the first and thirteenth fairways, and Serbians took final refuge under the high terrain at the fifteen fairway and thirteenth tee.

Hopefully, all our Italian, Chinese, and Serb relatives made the final trip to the cemeteries in Colma, but sadly many of the paupers' graves were overlooked. Occasionally, during heavy rains, a deceased resident pops up in the park—well, no, that's just an urban legend. But it is true that during a major renovation of the **Legion of Honor** in the 1990s, workers uncovered 700 unmarked graves—whose occupants were turned over to the Medical Examiner and properly reinterred. From looking at excavation maps, some experts estimate there could be 11,000 more bodies under the museum. It was unclear whose responsibility it would be to search for more graves so no more digging was done. Any remaining souls are free to rest undisturbed under one of the most beautiful areas of the city, next to the Legion of Honor, a monument built to honor the American soldiers who lost their lives in the Great War, World War I

—SFgenealogy.com

SHARK ATTACK
AT BAKER BEACH

It happened one time.
In 1959.
Killed an SFSU student.
No attacks since then.

49 MILE

SCENIC DRIVE

Legion of Honor

Sutro Baths

Cliff House

Playland

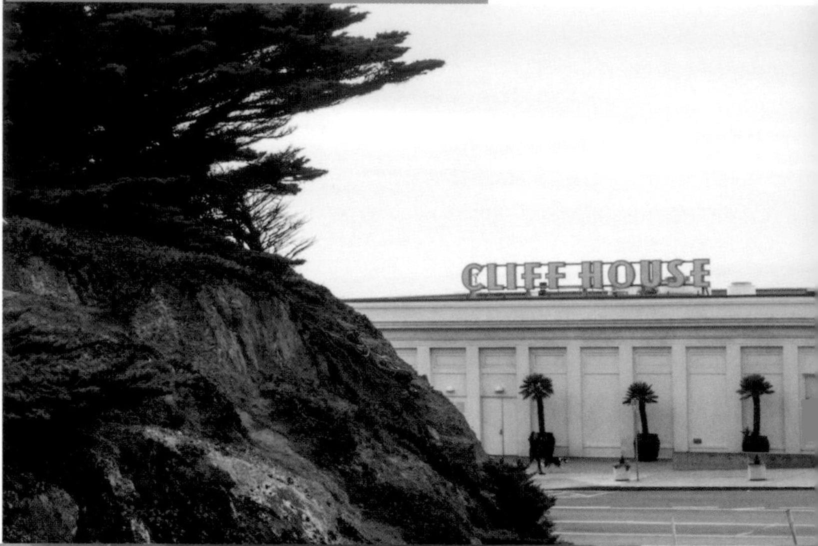

There are no bad views from Lands End.

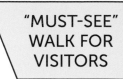
As early as the 1860s SF entrepreneurs were working to draw wealthy citizens to the outermost, rugged edge of San Francisco for shoreline recreation—the Lands End. Then in the 1880s Adolph Sutro took his Comstock silver-mining millions and let his imagination run wild. He hung a five-story, four-turreted, multispired gingerbread "Cliff House" resort over the edge of a cliff; built a mansion for himself; and created the world's largest bathhouse, complete with a passenger steam train to deliver the masses for just 5¢ a ride! And that was just the beginning of the fun.

Lands End is now in its third century of development as a recreation destination. The amusement parks have given way to history, art, and natural beauty, such as the clifftop, Lands End trails, Seal Rocks, Sutro Baths ruins, Eagle's Point labyrinth, and gorgeous ocean views.

Your walk begins on the headlands above the Golden Gate at a ¾-scale replica of the Palais de la Légion d'Honneur in Paris. You'll continue

your walk through the greens of Lincoln Golf Course, then begin a steep downhill journey back in time, first past the Sutro Baths ruins, then past the current Cliff House, and end on the beach next to the site where famous Playland-at-the-Beach entertained generations of San Franciscans. Though Playland is gone, the entire Lands End area remains SF's "playland" at the ocean. Your adventure today makes you part of this long SF tradition.

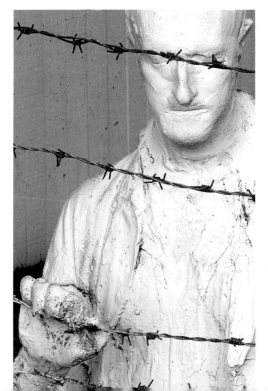

Amid the stunning natural beauty of the area stands some stark reality: the outdoor Holocaust Memorial.

Begin: El Camino Del Mar and 34th Avenue (Legion of Honor)   Hill Rating:
End: Great Highway and Fulton Street (Golden Gate Park)
Distance: ROUTE: 2.2 miles — 4,400 steps — 45 minutes
LOOP BACK: 1.7 miles — 3,400 steps — 30 minutes

3

Steep downhill

Sites you will pass on today's walk include:

MILE 15

THE RICHMOND

1. **Legion of Honor**
   100 34th Ave

2. **Holocaust Memorial** 34th Ave at El Camino Del Mar

3. *Pax Jerusalem* **Sculpture** 34th Ave, Legion of Honor parking lot

4. **Lincoln Park Golf Course**
   300 34th Ave

5. **Lands End**

DETOUR

a. **Fort Miley Reservation and VA Hospital** 4150 Clement St, or view from Lands End Trail parking lot

b. **USS San Francisco Memorial** end of Lands End Trail parking lot, left-hand side

MILE 16

6. **Sutro Baths Ruins View Point** Point Lobos Ave

DETOUR

c. **Sutro Baths ruins**

MUST-SEE

7. **Lands End Lookout and Store** 680 Point Lobos Ave

8. **Cliff House** 1090 Point Lobos Ave

9. **Playland-at-the-Beach** *GONE SF* Great Hwy between Balboa St and Fulton St

One of the few female sculptors of her time, Anna Hyatt Huntington sculpted the El Cid Campéador *bronze outside the Legion of Honor.*

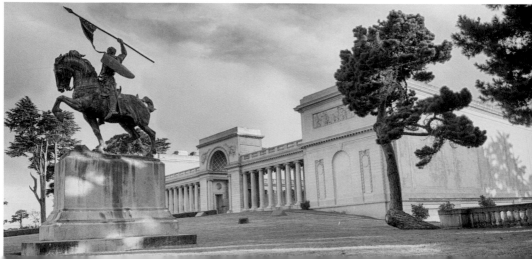

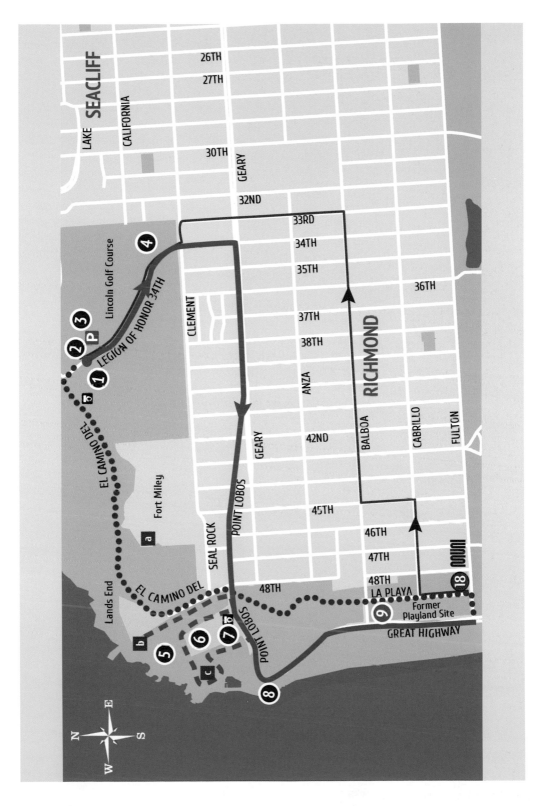

MILE 15

Begins on EL CAMINO DEL MAR at 34th Ave

THE RICHMOND

The Richmond District, along with the Sunset District and Golden Gate Park, was built on the vast, barely habitable sand dune referred to collectively as the Outside Lands. Industries that needed lots of open space, like ranches, dairies, and race-tracks, ventured "out there." The few roads that existed were built to help the farmers get their goods into San Francisco, or to bring recreation seekers to the growing amusements at Lands End. However, when the 1906 earthquake hit, the Outside Lands became a safe haven for those fleeing the rubble and fire.

At first the refugees lived in tent cities but quickly began building houses and roads. A 1913 map shows the entire area mapped for development, and by the late 1920s The Richmond was mostly built out—primarily by Irish, German, and Jewish residents. Many Russians came to the area after the upheavals of their early 19th-century revolutions and then more flooded in after the collapse of the Soviet Union in the 1990s.

In the 1950s, and especially after the lifting of the Chinese Exclusion Act in 1965, Chinese immigrants began buying homes, and now people of Chinese descent make up nearly half of the residents in the Richmond. Today, the Richmond is known for its foggy, cool weather and its extraordinary mix of cultures and languages.

1. Legion of Honor
100 34th Ave

After falling in love with the French Pavilion at the Pan Pacific Expo—a replica of the Palais de la Légion d'Honneur in Paris—Alma de Bretteville Spreckels persuaded her husband, sugar magnate Adolph Spreckels, to build and gift a replica of it to San Francisco. Opened on Armistice Day in 1924, the Legion of Honor serves as a memorial to the 3,600 Californians who died in WWI. The permanent collection spans 4,000 years of ancient and French art. Statues of Jeanne d'Arc and El Cid guard the entrance. A bronze cast of Auguste Rodin's *The Thinker* broods in the courtyard. The museum hosts international exhibits. Free the first Tuesday of the month.

2. Holocaust Memorial
34th Ave at El Camino Del Mar

Stark, disturbing. You are allowed to walk behind the barbed wire and lie down with the dead. Designed by George Segal. Dedicated in the park in 1984. Located to the left of the fountain in the Legion of Honor parking lot.

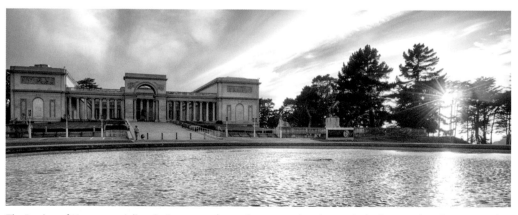

The Legion of Honor specializes in European decorative arts and sculpture, including a series of masterworks by Auguste Rodin.

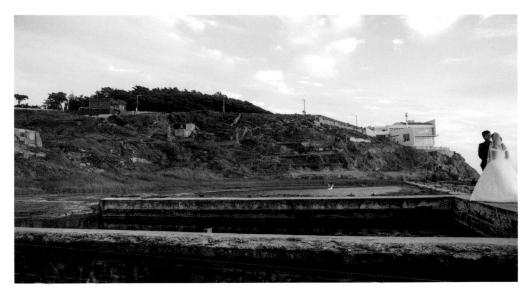

A couple has wedding pictures taken on the ruins of Sutro Baths. Photo faces south toward the Cliff House.

3. Pax Jerusalem
34th Ave, Legion of Honor parking lot

The jutting bundle of red-colored steel beams next to the fountain stands in stark urban juxtaposition to the Beaux Arts building and trees around the museum. Sculptor Mark di Suvero designed it to be twice as high as it stands now, but after outcry against the design, it was scaled down.

Head south on 34ᵗʰ out of the Park

4. Lincoln Park Golf Course 300 34th Ave

With its perch above the bay and view of Golden Gate Bridge, Lincoln Park Golf Course ranks among the most scenic urban golf courses in the world—yet its hilly terrain, strong ocean winds, and narrow cypress-lined fairways also make it challenging. This 18-hole, 5,416-yard, par-68 municipal golf course has been open to the public for over 100 years and offers discount rates for San Francisco residents with ID.

! LOOK

. . . .left through the trees over the golf course for peekaboo views of Lone Mountain College and St. Ignatius Church.

Right GEARY BLVD (west) at 42nd, bear right to join POINT LOBOS AVE

5. Lands End

Welcome to the wild, rocky, windswept, western corner of San Francisco. Many brave souls went down with their ship attempting to navigate around Lands End into the fog-strewn mouth of the Golden Gate. When the Spaniards heard the barking of the sea lions drifting up from the rocks below, they named the tip of Lands End Point Lobos, for its many *lobos marinos* ("sea wolves"). The sea lions have since relocated (from what we call Seal Rocks today) to the calmer waters of Pier 39. Trails at Lands End offer a cliff-top walk through dark cypress trees, with impressive views of the Marin Headlands, historic markers pointing out shipwrecks and old foghorns, and tempting (though slightly perilous) trailheads down to rocky wild beaches.

Spotting Wildlife

With more than 250 species of birds—including Brandt's cormorants, brown pelicans, Heermann's gulls, red-winged blackbirds, Anna's hummingbirds, and chestnut-backed chickadees—Lands End is a great place for **bird watchers**. Turn your sights to the surf and, just maybe, you might see dolphins, seals, sea lions, or a migrating whale.

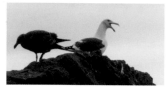

MILE 16

Begins on POINT LOBOS at Lands End Lookout building.

6. Sutro Baths Ruins View Point
Point Lobos Ave

Walk through the Lands End main parking lot or continue down Point Lobos past Louis' Restaurant to view Sutro Baths ruins. It's hard to imagine how the few decaying concrete walls sitting at the base of the cliff here once made up the largest swimming complex in the world. When former SF mayor and philanthropist Adolph Sutro's million-dollar natatorium vision was opened to the public in 1896, it boasted seven pools—one freshwater, six saltwater—ranging in temperature from icy cold to steam hot. But that wasn't all. Sutro Baths also featured a museum with Egyptian mummies, stuffed monkeys, fine art, an 8,000-seat concert hall, and more. Your 5¢ omnibus trek from the city to the Outside Lands was really worth it! Woefully, the museum burned down in 1966.

DETOUR

c. Sutro Baths Ruins

Take the dirt stairs from the parking lot, or the paved path near Louis' Restaurant (just past the Lands End Visitors Center) down and back up to the ruins.

As Sutro Baths continued to wane in popularity in the 1950s, the new owners converted the baths into an ice-skating rink. In the 1960s, developers with plans to replace the baths with a massive high-rise apartment development bought the site. When a mysterious fire destroyed all the buildings overnight in 1966 (many called it arson), the condo project fell through.

DETOUR

Go right at EL CAMINO DEL MAR to end of parking lot, and then U-turn back to main route. Or view these on the walk-back loop.

a. Fort Miley Reservation and VA Hospital
4150 Clement St

In 1885 the U.S. Army built Fort Miley as an added fortification to protect San Francisco Bay. One building and a few ruins of old battery placements are all that remain. Now it is part of the Golden Gate National Recreation Area. However, the Veterans Administration Hospital built here in 1935 remains active as a research facility, medical center, hospital, and 120-bed nursing home giving outstanding care to over 50,000 veterans a year. You can see this through the trees, to your right from the Lands End Trail parking lot (El Camino Del Mar).

b. USS San Francisco Memorial end of parking lot, left-hand side

Honored with 17 battle stars, the USS *San Francisco* is one of the most decorated ships of WWII. Her memorial, oriented toward the savage battle of Guadalcanal, which she survived, is made of actual pieces of the cruiser's shelled bridge. Located at the end of upper parking lot (EL CAMINO), on the left-hand side.

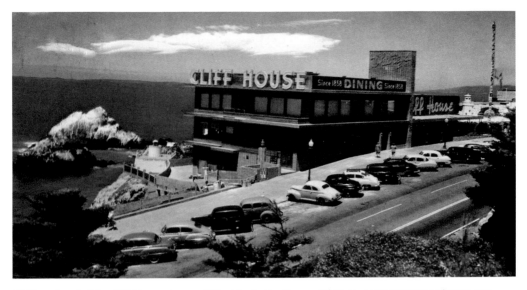

1941 postcard of the Cliff House shows off Seal Rock, the Camera Obscura, some awesome vintage cars, and, in the upper right, the world's tallest totem pole.

You can get a little taste, a virtual visit to Sutro Baths, by watching "Sutro Baths: A Forgotten Monument" and other Sutro footage on YouTube. Also, SF native and historian John Martini's outstanding book, *Sutro's Glass Palace*, is chock-full of historic photos.

! **MUST SEE**

7. Lands End Lookout and Store 680 Point Lobos Ave

This outstanding visitors center provides a (free!) fabulous and thorough overview of the area. The history displays, drawings, photos, replicas, and video loops showcase the original Yelamu Ohlone tribe inhabitants, Seal Rocks,

area wildlife, the Cliff House, Playland, Sutro Baths, Sutro mansion, and more. Plus shopping, food, and a public restroom (and hopefully many copies of this book for sale!).

· · · · · · · · · · · · · · · · · · · ·

Follow POINT LOBOS downhill as it curves around the CLIFF HOUSE and becomes GREAT HIGHWAY

· · · · · · · · · · · · · · · · · · · ·

8. Cliff House 1090 Point Lobos Ave

Over the past 160 years or so, four roadhouse/restaurant/ tourist destinations have been perched above Ocean Beach, each named the "Cliff House." The most famous incarnation would be the multistoried, turreted Victorian chateau, called the Gingerbread Palace,

built by Adolph Sutro in 1896. Alas, the dang thing keeps burning down! The most recent remodels in 2004 and interior restaurant remodel by R. H. Schaer in 2015 are exquisite—and now it has smoke alarms!

GONE SF

9. Playland-at-the-Beach, former site Great Hwy between Balboa St and Fulton St

From 1928 to 1972, 10 acres of amusement park attractions on this site across from Ocean Beach entertained generations of San Franciscans. In the 1940s and 1950s, 50,000–60,000 people came here to play every weekend. As Playland's popularity faded in the 1960s, attractions began closing. One local favorite, Laffing Sal—the giant animated cackling woman who guarded the Fun House—continued to terrify children right up until 1972 when Playland was demolished to make way for condos. The 1930s-era location of the site is outlined on your map.

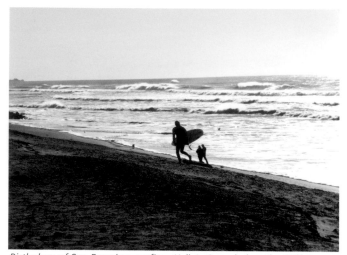

· · · · · · · · · · · · · · · ·

END on GREAT HIGHWAY at FULTON ST (beginning of Golden Gate Park)

· · · · · · · · · · · · · · · ·

Birthplace of San Francisco surfing, Kelly's Cove, below the Cliff House

In case you never made it in person, you can make a virtual visit to Playland via photos and videos at a Wix website, inspired by a Playland Facebook group (search under "PlaylandAtTheBeach"). Or pick up one of the books by local Playland expert, James R. Smith.

WALK–BACK LOOP SCOOP

Highly recommended. It begins with a steep wooden stairway but passes cool new sites. Or take the optional window-shopping loop back via Balboa Street. See details on page 95.

Playland-at-the-Beach Attractions—Where Are They Now?

A few remain in the city and can be found at:

Pier 45: Laughing Sal and the Musée Mécanique

Yerba Buena Gardens: Carousel

Cliff House: Camera Obscura

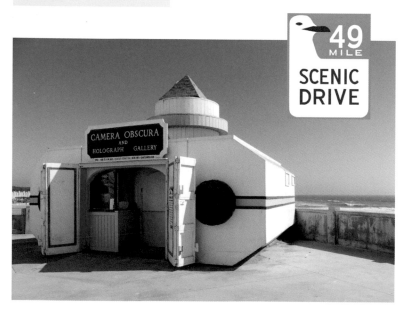

49 MILE SCENIC DRIVE

Since 1946, visitors to Playland have been lured into the kitschy camera-shaped building behind the Cliff House. Inside, a Camera Obscura based on a 15th-century design by Leonardo da Vinci produces 360 degrees of spectacular "live images" of the Seal Rocks area.

WALK 6 NEED TO KNOW

TO GET THERE
- Muni 1, 18, 38

PARKING
- Along LINCOLN BLVD
- Free 4-hour parking at the Legion of Honor parking lot

PUBLIC RESTROOMS
- Behind the Legion of Honor
- Lands End Lookout Visitors Center

TURN–BY–TURN INSTRUCTIONS
Begin: EL CAMINO DEL MAR at 34TH AVE
- Head south on 34TH AVE out of the Park
- Right GEARY BLVD (west)
- At 42ND AVE, bear Right to join POINT LOBOS AVE
- Follow POINT LOBOS AVE downhill as it curves around the CLIFF HOUSE and becomes GREAT HIGHWAY

End: GREAT HIGHWAY at FULTON ST (beginning of Golden Gate Park)

TO GET BACK
Muni
- Walk to NE corner of LA PLAYA ST and FULTON ST
- Board Muni bus 18
- Off at the Legion of Honor

Other Muni routes: 5, 31

OPTIONAL WALK-BACK LOOP DIRECTIONS
Distance: 1.7 miles, 3,400 steps, 30 minutes

Rating: 4

Option 1: The walk-back covers a few new nooks and crannies along the scenic Point Lobos and Lands End Trail you didn't see on the way down—like the ruins of Sutro's private mansion and park. If you didn't take the detour, you get a little flavor of Lands End Trail along the unpaved section of El Camino Del Mar, and a view of the USS San Francisco Memorial. The walk-back loop begins with a steep, off-road uphill stair climbs but is mild after that.

Option 2: A 30-minute Muni ride will get you all the way back to the Legion of Honor,

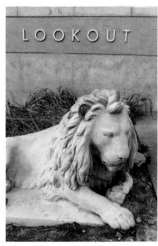

Lands End Lookout

but we suggest you hop off about halfway back at 39th Ave and Balboa to explore a cute little Outer Richmond commercial corridor. Then simply turn left at 34th Ave and follow it uphill into Lincoln Park.

Begin: GREAT HIGHWAY and FULTON ST
- Left onto FULTON ST
- Left on LA PLAYA ST
- Cross BALBOA into Sutro Heights Park
- Take DIRT TRAIL and STAIRWAY to top of park
- Where TRAIL widens (at top of hill), stay right
  ○ Continue through the park
  ○ Exit at POINT LOBOS
- Cross POINT LOBOS
- Jog right to EL CAMINO DEL MAR
- North (left) on EL CAMINO DEL MAR to the parking lot
  ○ Stay to the right
- Veer right up to DIRT TRAIL (PACIFIC COASTAL TRAIL)
- Continue on PACIFIC COASTAL TRAIL which meets back up with EL CAMINO DEL MAR
- Right at 34TH AVE

End: LEGION OF HONOR at 34TH AVE

THE DAILY CRAB

San Francisco Historical Times   Vol. 6

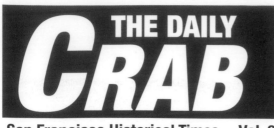

Sutro Railroad (circa 1896)

OpenSFHistory/wnp4.1055

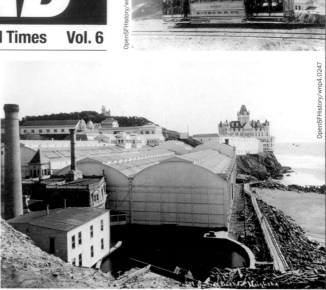

OpenSFHistory/wnp4.0247

SP RAILROAD CAN'T RAILROAD SUTRO

Adolph Sutro had an agreement with the **Ferries & Cliff House Railroad** to keep the ticket fare out to his Sutro Baths at 5¢. Just before **Sutro Baths** opened, the **Southern Pacific Railroad** bought out ferries and doubled the price to 10¢. This so angered Sutro, who had built the baths for the working people to enjoy, that he held up the opening of Sutro Baths for two years while he built a competing electric streetcar with a fare of 5¢.

Sutro Baths and Cliff House from Point Lobos (circa 1898), view south. Upper left: Streetcar depot with Sutro Heights above. Center: Sutro Baths. Upper right: Cliff House. Powerhouse and settling pond in foreground.

TRUE CONFESSIONS: TINKLE TERROR

~by Kristine

This explains a lot. Age 10: My dad took my brothers and me to Playland's Fun House. They raced ahead, but I could not find my way out of the **Fun House** maze-mirror entrance. Hopelessly lost, hopelessly in need of the bathroom, I wet my pants (last time of my life, so far). My dad finally came back and found me, led me inside. I tried to dry off in the bathroom.

The room was full of an afternoon's fun: **Giant Wooden Slide, Tumble Tube of Death, Undulating Bridge,** and the **Spinning Wheel**—you sit on a big metal disc, which spins faster and faster till you fly off.

My dad grabbed the center

Super-genius promoter **George Whitney** birthed the perfect creamy, crunchy ice cream and cookie sandwich, dipped-in-chocolate treat, **IT'S-IT**, in 1928. For four decades, you could get it at only one place: San Francisco's now-defunct **Playland-at-the-Beach**. The modern version of this San Francisco treat can now be found in flavors like mint, strawberry, and cappuccino in supermarkets and corner stores around the bay.

IT'S-IT

spot on the spinning wheel, the coveted location on the disc, thought to keep you on the disc longest. I joined the other kids around him. It spun faster and faster. Everyone else flew off,

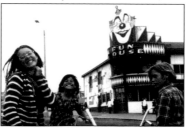

Image courtesy of Dennis O'Rorke

even my dad, but there I sat, my wet bottom keeping me glued in place.

Crowds gathered. The spinning operator stared in disbelief. I knew I had to take action. I tried a big scootch to fling myself off, but I moved only a few inches, my bottom squeaking across the disc. It took many more squeaky scootches to reach the edge.

Perhaps that is the real reason the Fun House closed. I apologize.

WAR HORROR

Guadalcanal, 1942. Screaming. Fear. Blood. Sweat. Adrenaline. Forty-five enemy shells explode as they rip through your ship. 106 of your fellow sailors die around you. Your admiral, dead. 131 wounded. You cheer as you finally sink one enemy ship and damage another... somehow your cruiser, the **USS *San Francisco***, *does not sink* and you sail away from the brutal close-quarters battle and make it back to port.

What kind of memorial could ever capture this moment? The **USS San Francisco Memorial Foundation** made a bold choice. In their words, "Our memorial ... eschews the usual symbolic folderol in favor of something far more visceral: a shell-ridden section of the *San Francisco*'s bridge. The sight of heavy gauge steel perforated like paper captures the fury and horror of that night better than any sculpture ever could."

SF HIDDEN GEM
LANDS END LABYRINTH

Along the **Lands End Coastal Trail** at **Eagle's Point** lies a hidden labyrinth overlooking the Golden Gate Bridge. **Eduardo Aguilera** created this spiritual spot for the community, and each time a vandal destroys it, Eduardo and the community that now values the labyrinth return to the sacred space and lovingly restore it. (NOTE: The uneven pathways and steps leading to the labyrinth may not be an easy trek for everyone. Follow the markers leading down to Eagle's Point Trail with care.)

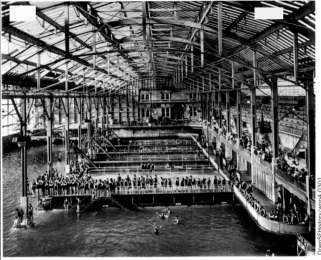

Sutro Baths. View of swimming pools looking north (circa 1910). Classic view that became a poster.

"NEGROES CLAIM CIVIL RIGHTS"

In 1897, an SF newspaper reported the story of **Mr. John Harris**, "a colored man" who attempted to buy a ticket to go swimming at **Sutro Baths**. Mr. Harris was refused entrance to the pools and subsequently filed a lawsuit, which became an early test case for a new California civil rights law called the **Dibble Bill**. The new law, which had gone into effect three months earlier (April 1897), declared that "no railway, hotels, restaurants, barber-shops, bathhouses and other like institutions licensed to serve the public shall discriminate against any well behaved citizen, no matter what his color."

The superintendent of Sutro Baths attempted to clarify company policy saying, "Negroes, so long as they are sober and well behaved, are allowed to enter the baths as spectators, but are not

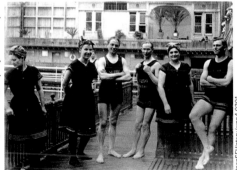

Sutro Baths, men and women bathers (1906)

permitted to go in the water. It is not a matter of personal feeling with us but of business necessity. It would ruin our baths here because the white people would refuse to use them if the Negroes were allowed equal privileges in that way."

The law was upheld and Mr. Harris was awarded the minimum penalty allowed by law.

—Woody LaBounty, Outsidelands.org

49 MILE SCENIC DRIVE

Ocean Beach
Great Highway
SF Zoo

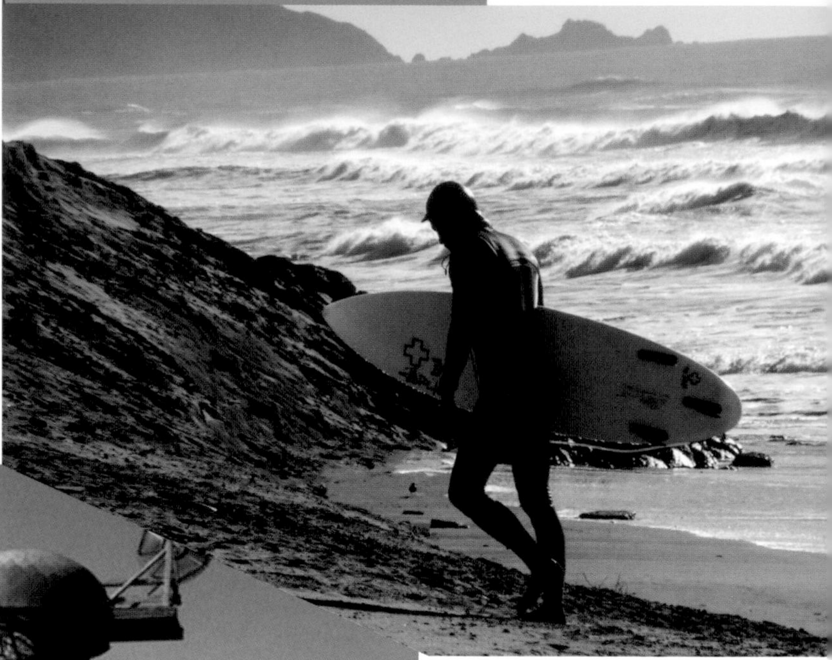

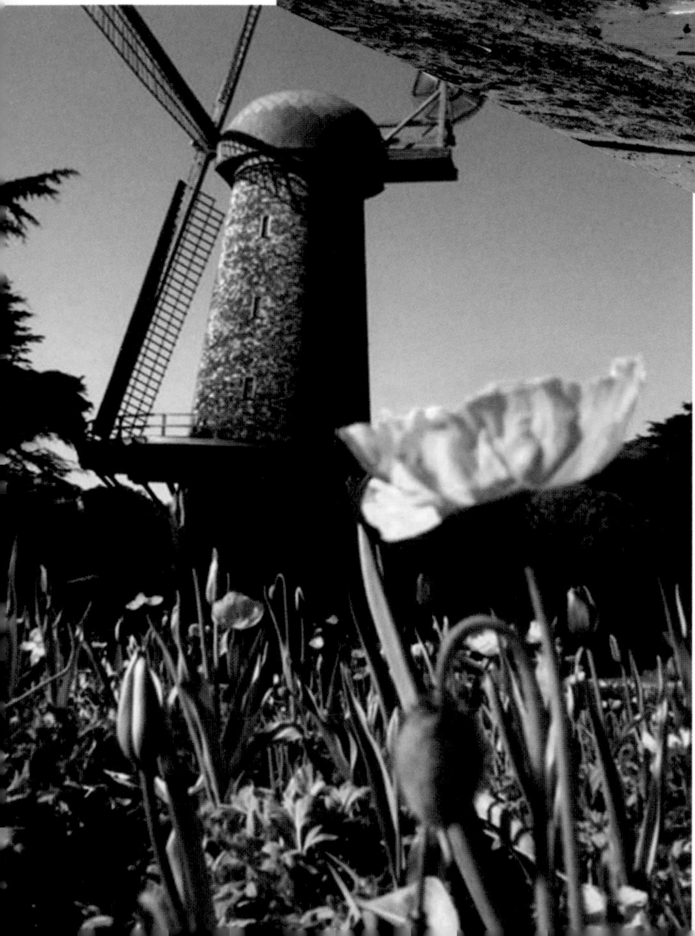

Ocean Beach surfer and Golden Gate Park's Dutch Windmill

Check the weather before you go!

This walk can be a gorgeous 80° beach day stroll in the surf, waving at dolphins, watching the surfers or a bone-chillingly cold day with punishing winds sandblasting off the top layer of your skin. Average temperature: 50°–60°. (That's why this is one of the few beach towns where it's actually cheaper to live right on the ocean.) Late summer and early fall tend to be warmer. The wind picks up around 3 p.m. Wear layers.

Regardless of the weather, Ocean Beach is powerful, it's romantic, it's so San Francisco.

After a little detour in Golden Gate Park, Walk 7 lets you choose to stroll along the beach itself on the hard-packed sand close to the surf, or take the jogging path that runs along the Great Highway. If you take the jogging path, glance away from the beach occasionally toward the avenue below and you may catch some interesting house designs and paint styles along La Playa Street. ("Ooo, look at that house designed to look like a boat." "Mondrian-inspired paint job—nice." "Could that be an old earthquake shack?" "Is that handsome surfer stripping completely out of his wet suit? My, my.")

As you walk past San Francisco Zoo at the very end of the walk, peek through the fence. What do you see? Kangaroos? And if you listen for a moment, you may hear some wild beasts. Or better yet, detour over to the zoo's front entrance—to see some wild animals and the remnants of a two-and-a half-football-fields-long outdoor swimming pool.

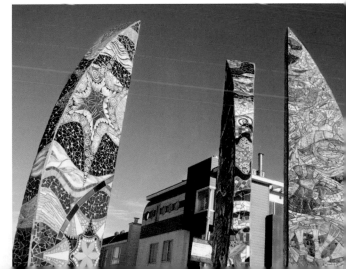

Roundabout street art at Taraval and 48th

Begin:	Great Highway and Fulton Street (north edge of Golden Gate Park)
End:	Skyline Boulevard and Lake Merced Boulevard (Lake Merced)
Distance:	ROUTE: 3.25 miles — 6,500 steps — 1 hour
	LOOP BACK: 3.25 miles — 6,500 steps — 1 hour

Hill Rating: **1**

Sites you will pass on today's walk include:

MILE 17
1. **Golden Gate Park**
   Great Hwy between Fulton St and Lincoln Way

   DETOUR

2. **Dutch Windmill**
   1691 JFK Blvd

3. **Beach Chalet**
   1000 Great Hwy

4. **Murphy Windmill**
   MLK Blvd, off Lincoln Way

5. **Ocean Beach**

MILE 18
6. **Surf's Up!**

7. **Java Beach**
   1396 La Playa St (Judah St)

8. **Former Breakers Carriage House**
   1536–1540 La Playa St (Kirkham St)

9. **Former Carville Home**
   1632 Great Highway (past Lawton St)

MILE 19
10. **The Great Highway**

11. **Former Chickery Restaurant** Vicente St at Great Hwy

MILE 20
12. **Westside Pump Station** 3000 & 3500 Great Hwy

13. **San Francisco Zoo**

   DETOUR

a. **Parking Lot and Zoo Entrance**

14. **Doggie Diner Head**
   Sloat Blvd median at 45th Ave

NOTE: Lake Merced, the designated end of this walk, is just below your map at the intersection of Lake Merced Blvd and Skyline Blvd, but if you want to stop at the end of the zoo parking lot and turn around, you are welcome to do so.

On Walk-Back Loop
b. **United Irish Cultural Center of San Francisco**
   2700 45th Ave at Wawona St

c. **Robert's at the Beach Motel**
   GONE SF
   Sloat Blvd at 46th Ave

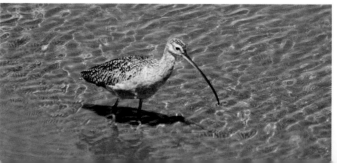

Our native "candlestick bird" (long-billed curlew) inspired the naming of Candlestick Point and subsequently Candlestick Park stadium.

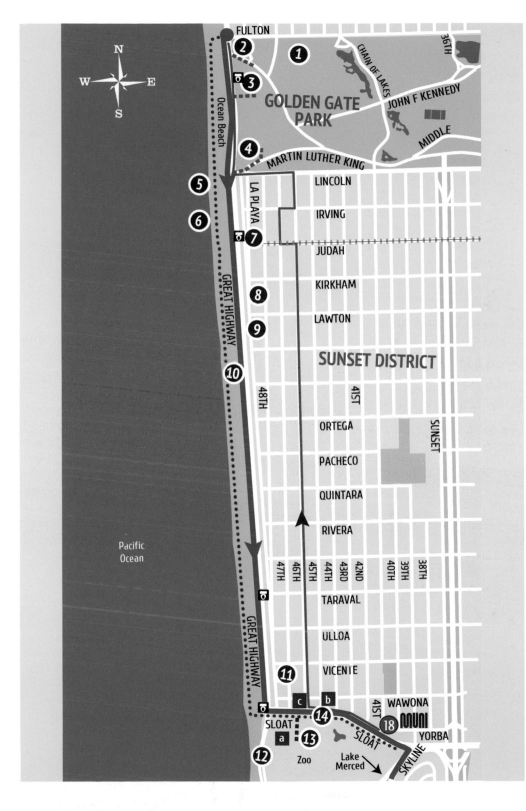

MILE 17

Begins on GREAT HIGHWAY
at FULTON ST

Before You Begin:
- Bob Wise has been building surfboards at Ocean Beach since 1968. You can visit Wise Surfboards on the site of the defunct Playland: 800 Great Highway.
- **Picnic anyone?** Safeway is located one block up Fulton between La Playa and 48th.

....

Continuing from Walk 6, head south on GREAT HIGHWAY

....

15. Golden Gate Park

Three miles long by half a mile wide, Golden Gate Park ends

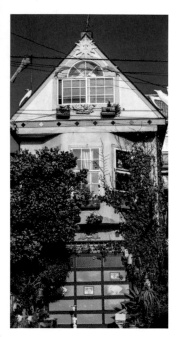

here at the beach and divides the Richmond and Sunset Districts. (GG Park is detailed in Walks 10 and 11.)

DETOUR

> At FULTON, cross to the park side of GREAT HIGHWAY

> Take first Left onto JOHN F KENNEDY

> Admire the Dutch Windmill on your left

> Return to GREAT HIGHWAY and continue south

16. Dutch Windmill First left off Great Hwy into the park on JFK Dr

To save the city from the exorbitant water fees charged by the Spring Valley Water Company in the city's early years, some civic-minded San Franciscans donated Queen Wilhelmina's Windmill, also called Dutch Windmill, to the city in 1903. The windmill allowed the city to irrigate the western end of the park for free by using free wind power to pump 30,000 gallons of water a day from free underground aquifers.

It was so successful a second windmill began pumping free water in 1908. This windmill was donated by Samuel G.

Murphy, president of First National Bank, as "partial payment for the pleasures derived during many years' visits to the park."

But for some reason, in 1913 the city decided to install motorized pumps run by electricity purchased from the power company instead. Neglected, the windmills fell into ruin. Fortunately, beginning in 1964 some fabulous San Franciscans (led originally by Eleanor Rossi Crabtree) stepped in and began raising funds to restore them. The Dutch Windmill came back to life in 1981 and the Murphy Windmill in 2011. Though they no longer pump water, the sails turn and they look magnificent.

In 1980 the Netherlands donated the Queen Wilhelmina Tulip Garden, along with the thousands of tulips and Icelandic poppies in it, which bloom annually throughout March and April under the Dutch Windmill. The garden blooms with other types of flowers the rest of the year.

❗ NICE STOP

....

Left to the Beach Chalet

Return to GREAT HIGHWAY and continue south

....

17. Beach Chalet
1000 Great Hwy

Delightful restaurant, brewery, pet-friendly lawn area with Adirondack chairs, and visitors center—complete with a model of Golden Gate Park, original Depression-era murals of San Francisco by Lucien Labaudt—and public restrooms. Built in 1925 as a bathhouse for visitors to Ocean Beach, later it housed soldiers in WWII and finally served as a club for veterans before closing in 1981. After a badly needed renovation, it reopened in 1996.

18. Murphy Windmill
at the end of the park turn left on Lincoln Way, then left on MLK

See page 102 for a description.

• • • • • • • • • • • • • • • • • •

Left at LINCOLN BLVD (at the end of the park)

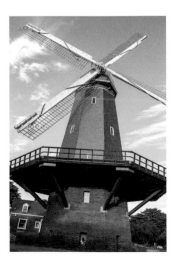

Take first left at MARTIN LUTHER KING DR

Stare up at the Murphy Windmill on your left

Return to GREAT HIGHWAY and continue south

Or cross GREAT HIGHWAY down to Ocean Beach to walk there

• • • • • • • • • • • • • • • • • •

19. Ocean Beach at the end of the park cross Great Hwy, walk down to the beach

Our wild, gorgeous six-mile stretch of sand and sea has long been a city playground. It all happens here: fire pits blazing at night, lots of four-legged scampering at the Saturday little dog walk, kites flying, sand castle competitions, wetsuit-clad surfers, cargo ships and sailboats cruising by, views of the Farallon Islands, even dolphin sightings. Occasionally you'll even see some brave souls playing in the icy water! WARNING: Owing to riptides, swimming is not recommended.

• • • • • • • • • • • • • • • • • •

Continue on GREAT HIGHWAY (or Ocean Beach) to SLOAT BLVD

• • • • • • • • • • • • • • • • • •

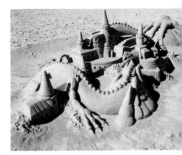

LEAParts.com's annual giant sand sculpture contest raises funds to support arts programs for Bay Area students.

MILE 18
Begins on GREAT HIGHWAY at LAWTON ST

20. Surf's Up!

SurfingCal.com sums up Ocean Beach surfing as "Miles of beach break and fantastic sandbars on the good days, miles of brutal swells and frustration on bad days." Kelly's Cove, North Ocean Beach, and South Ocean Beach have long been among the most popular, and difficult, surf spots in Northern California. In fact it was the icy waters of Ocean Beach that inspired famed surf innovator Jack O'Neill to invent the neoprene wetsuit in the 1950s. O'Neill Surf Shop, formerly on Great Highway, was one of the first in California, but in 1959 Jack permanently moved his surfing and shop to the warmer climes of Santa Cruz.

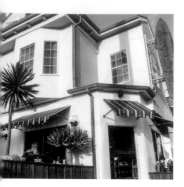

21. Java Beach, So Cool
1396 La Playa St
(Judah St)

Some say the day Patrick and Buffy Maguire opened Java Beach Café on Judah at La Playa in 1993, the Sunset started turning just a little bit hip. Is it the beer, comedy, and music in the evenings? Or the awesome bagels and coffee on a cold morning? Stop by, grab a snack, take in the neighborhood atmosphere, and decide for yourself.

22. Former Breakers Carriage House
1536-1540 La Playa

According to Outsidelands. org, the flat stuccoed facade of 1536 La Playa and the smaller 1540 La Playa hide its past as a former roadhouse (The Breakers) and carriage house.

23. Former Carville Home 1632 Great Hwy (past Lawton St)

The unimposing two-story house behind the fence at 1632 Great Highway looks pretty normal from the outside. But like a lot of things in San Francisco, this house is not what it seems. The second story is built of two old cable cars joined together and also has a side room made from an old San Francisco horsecar. The house is the last survivor of Carville-by-the-Sea, a long-gone, oceanside, neighborhood cobbled together from old streetcars.

Drag Race

Teens loved drag racing along the Great Highway in the 1950s and 1960s, but joy riders on the scenic road have been a nuisance since the early 1900s. So much so that in 1912 the city's Police Commission responded by forming a 30-officer motorcycle squad to round up miscreants in Golden Gate Park and along Ocean Beach. Now that alternate, official racetracks have been built around the bay the drag racers seem to have moved on.

MILE 19

Begins on GREAT HIGHWAY at SANTIAGO ST

24. Great Highway

Even before the 3.5-mile stretch of unpaved road connecting the Cliff House and Sloat Boulevard was officially named the Great Highway in 1874, the wind was blowing mounds of sand over the road and riders.

Since the 1930s different government agencies have attempted to control the traveling dunes that regularly block the road. They have tried everything from building embankments and wind breaks to planting native plants. Mother Nature is winning the battle.

In 2012 the SF Department of Public Works reported that it had been spending about $300,000 a year to keep the road clear. The Ocean Beach Master Plan is the latest interagency effort working to develop a long-term vision for Ocean Beach. Nonetheless, on a sunny day, it's still the most majestic walk in the city.

25. Former Chickery Restaurant
2600 Great Hwy

In the 1920s, the big brick building on the corner of Vicente and Great Highway sold lip-smacking, 50¢ roasted chicken dinners.

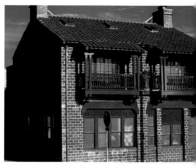

"Is that roasted chicken I smell?"

MILE 20

Begins on GREAT HIGHWAY at SLOAT BLVD

. . . .

Cross to southeast corner (zoo side) of SLOAT BLVD

NOTE: Since there is no pedestrian sidewalk or trail here, the 49 mile walk does not follow the official driving route and signs, which direct you to continue on the Great Highway as it curves around the zoo.

LEFT (east) on SLOAT

. . . .

26. Westside Pump Station 3000 Great Hwy

This important part of the San Francisco sewer system stands on much of the area around and below the former Fleishhacker Pool. The Westside station pumps into the Oceanside Water Pollution Control Plant located farther down on the Great Highway. Seventy percent of its 12 acres are located underground.

DETOUR

> Take entrance path on your right.

> Follow sidewalk to zoo entrance.

> Return the way you came.

> Turn right (east) onto SLOAT BLVD to rejoin route.

a. Parking Lot and Zoo Entrance

The zoo parking lot covers the approximate space of the former Fleishhacker Pool, a giant outdoor pool, approximately the length of two and a half football fields that could hold up to 10,000 swimmers. The framing that went around the original entrance to the Fleishhacker Pool stands west of the parking lot. Zoo entrance: You are allowed to go into the gift store and are welcome to take a peek at any animals close by the front of the zoo.

50,000 People, 1,014 Musicians—That's a Beach Party

Proclaimed the "finest stretch of highway ever constructed," the Ocean Beach Great Highway Esplanade opened to great fanfare in 1929. It cost $1 million and featured an equestrian ramp down to the beach, traffic signals, modern electroliers (street lamps), and underpasses to the beach at Fulton Street, Judah Street, Taraval Street, Sloat Boulevard, and the Beach Chalet. To maintain the landscaping, the city installed the most modern and largest sprinkling system in the world: a 30,000-foot sprinkling system operated in 150-foot separate valve sections each lined with spray nozzles every two feet.

27. San Francisco Zoo

The SF Zoo is the birthplace of Koko the gorilla (1971); a bald eagle named after comedian Stephen Colbert (2006); a baby gorilla (2013) named Kabibe (Swahili for

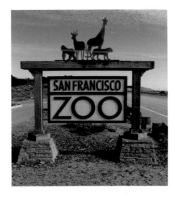

And the award for "2014 Best S.F. History Lesson in One Minute" goes to the Western Neighborhoods Project—as voted by *SF Weekly*. This nonprofit has been gathering stories, images, and videos of the western portion of San Francisco since 1999. The site boasts approximately 80-minute-long videos—mostly by David Gallagher and Woody LaBounty— each covering a small, cool, often unknown snippet of SF history. Enjoy at Outsidelands.org.

"little lady"); and a lion cub born in 2015. Originally named the Fleishhacker Zoo after its founder, banker, and San Francisco Parks Commission president Herbert Fleishhacker, it was built in the 1930s and 1940s with funds from the Depression-era Works Progress Administration (WPA). In 1997 a $48 million Zoo Bond plus $25 million in private donations funded a complete overhaul. Though Monkey Island, Storyland, and the big black locomotive (that many older San Franciscans remember) disappeared with the remodel, today our SF Zoo has been transformed into a modern conservation zoo with over 1,000 exotic, endangered, and rescued animals and majestic, peaceful gardens full of native and foreign plants. Open 365 days a year.

· · · · · · · · · · · · · · · · · ·

Continue on SLOAT BLVD, but feel free to walk next to the zoo fence as it curves around zoo

· · · · · · · · · · · · · · · · · ·

28. Doggie Diner Head
Sloat Blvd median across from Java Beach

Once upon a time, fast-food eaters throughout the Bay Area were welcomed to the popular (unionized) Doggie Diner restaurants by a seven-foot-tall rotating fiberglass head of a wide-eyed, grinning dachshund, wearing a bow tie and a chef's hat. Most

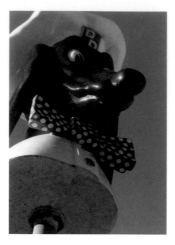

heads were taken down and lost when the chain closed in 1996. Fortunately, Diana Scott and Joel Schechter of the Ocean Beach Historical Society worked to save this iconic doggie head for posterity. *Thank you!*

(To save more Doggie Diner heads visit DoggieDiner.com)

· · · · · · · · · · · · · · · · · ·

RIGHT on SKYLINE BLVD

END at Lake Merced

SKYLINE BLVD and LAKE MERCED BLVD (a multi-street intersection right across from the lake)

· · · · · · · · · · · · · · · · · ·

WALK–BACK LOOP SCOOP

To continue the route around lake Merced, flip over to Walk 8 for directions. Or, save that four-mile walk for another day and head back down Sloat for a bite to eat before walking back to the beginning of the

route via Ocean Beach. On your way back down Sloat you will pass:

b. United Irish Cultural Center of San Francisco 2700 45th Ave at Wawona St

Built entirely by volunteer labor and community contributions in 1975, this Irish social center and restaurant continues the work of its predecessors such as the Knights of the Red Branch (Clan na Gael). If it's a cold day you can stop by for a nice Guinness stew there.

GONE SF

c. Roberts-at-the-Beach Motel site Sloat Blvd at 46th St

Once billing itself as the "Most Unusual Place in the West," Roberts-at-the-Beach Seabreeze Resort had many incarnations between 1897 and 2015. For example: The popular roadhouse tried unsuccessfully to skirt prohibition in the 1920s. In the 1930s one owner bet Bay Meadows Racetrack that his horse "Blackie" could swim the Golden Gate channel—which he did in a brisk 23 minutes. In the 1960s the owner of the Condor Club, where Carol Doda was dancing topless, tried to buy it, but the sale was stopped by neighborhood outrage and the fear that a strip club might move in. In recent years it had been a basic family-friendly motel. Torn down in 2015.

WALK 7 NEED TO KNOW

TO GET THERE
Muni 5, 18, 31

PARKING
- Non-metered street parking
- Non-metered Ocean Beach parking lots
- Balboa St near the surf shop or across from Beach Chalet
- On JFK, near the Dutch windmill

PUBLIC RESTROOMS
- Beach Chalet
- Judah at Great Highway
- Taraval at Great Highway
- Sloat at Great Highway

TURN–BY–TURN INSTRUCTIONS
Begin: GREAT HIGHWAY and FULTON ST
- Continuing from Walk 6, head south on GREAT HIGHWAY
- DETOUR: Golden Gate Park
  - At FULTON ST, cross to the park side of GREAT HIGHWAY
  - Take first left onto JOHN F KENNEDY DR
  - Admire the Dutch Windmill on your left
- Return to GREAT HIGHWAY and continue south
- Left to the Beach Chalet
- Return to GREAT HIGHWAY and continue south

- Left at LINCOLN BLVD (at the end of the park)
- Take first left at MARTIN LUTHER KING DR
- Stare up at the Murphy Windmill on your left
- Return to GREAT HIGHWAY and continue south
- Or cross GREAT HIGHWAY down to Ocean Beach to walk there
- Continue on GREAT HIGHWAY (or Ocean Beach) to SLOAT BLVD
- Cross to southeast corner (zoo side) of SLOAT BLVD
  - NOTE: Since there is no pedestrian sidewalk or trail here, the 49 mile walk does not follow the official driving route and signs, which direct you to continue on the Great Highway as it curves around the zoo.
- Left (east) on SLOAT BLVD
- DETOUR to SF Zoo
  - Take entrance path on your right
  - Follow sidewalk to zoo entrance
  - Return the way you came
  - Turn right (east) onto SLOAT BLVD to rejoin route
- Continue on SLOAT BLVD, but feel free to walk next to the zoo fence as it curves around zoo
- Right on SKYLINE BLVD

- End: SKYLINE BLVD and LAKE MERCED BLVD (a multi-street intersection right across from the lake)

HOW TO GET BACK
Muni
- Board bus 18 on north side of Sloat Blvd at 41st Ave (toward Legion of Honor)
- Get off at Fulton St and La Playa St

Other Muni routes: 23, 29, L at 46th Ave & Sloat Blvd, N on Judah St, L at Wawona St and 46th Ave

OPTIONAL WALK-BACK LOOP DIRECTIONS
Distance: 3.25 miles, 6,500 steps, 1 hour

Rating:

Begin: U-turn back down SKYLINE BLVD
- Left on SLOAT BLVD
  - Cross street at 45th AVE, continue on SLOAT BLVD
- Right on GREAT HIGHWAY
  - or if taking beach back, cross GREAT HIGHWAY to the beach
  - Right on Ocean Beach
- Walk past GOLDEN GATE PARK to the NW edge
- Turn right on FULTON ST
  - or if on beach, cross GREAT HIGHWAY at FULTON ST
- End: FULTON ST and GREAT HIGHWAY

THE DAILY CRAB

San Francisco Historical Times   Vol. 7

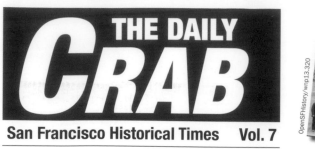

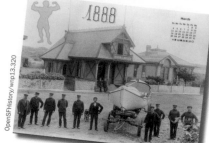

OpenSFHistory/wnp.13.320

BARKING "WATCH DOG" SEAL

The *Gjøa*, the ship in which the Norwegian heroic explorer **Roald Amundsen** launched his world-famous arctic expedition, was retired here at the edge of Golden Gate Park in 1909. A guard, a fence, and a barking-seal watchdog were not enough to keep souvenir hunters and vandals away. (Yes, a seal. They put a seal in a tank to bark when strangers approached.) Within a few years, however, interest in the ship dwindled, the ocean air took its toll, and by the 1970s the ship was mostly used as an overnight camp for LSD-dropping hippies. In 1972 the Norwegians took her back. We hear she is doing well.

— Woody LaBounty, Outsidelands.org

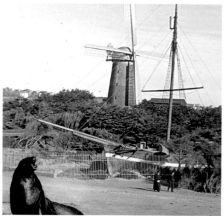

OpenSFHistory/wnp4.1136

Golden Gate Park, Dutch Windmill, and ship Gjoa. Inset: barking seal

HOT 'N' HUNKY CALENDAR: 1888

Nearly 100 ships have wrecked on the dangerous shoreline around **Lands End** and **Ocean Beach** over the past 150 years. In 1871, the federal government created the **United States Life-Saving Service** and built two stations for San Francisco along Ocean Beach (real SF crew pictured on photoshopped calendar, above). Crews launched themselves into treacherous waves in 36-foot lifeboats, used cannons to shoot rescue lines to foundering boats, and regularly risked their lives to save others.

In 1915, the U.S. Life-Saving Service merged with the Revenue Cutter Service to create the **United States Coast Guard**.

We're still waiting for the calendar to come out!

IRISH–MEXICAN HISTORIA DE AMOR

Driven by a desire to own their own land, a few thousand Irish immigrants headed to the "Mexican West" in the early 19th century.

They found a friendly welcome from fellow-Catholic Mexicans. They learned to speak Spanish and some were even given land grants in California by the Mexican government, especially in Marin County, which was nicknamed Little Ireland.

Tens of thousands more came for gold, and by 1880, the Irish made up one-third of San Francisco's population.

Groups despised on the East Coast, such as the Irish, Jews, East Europeans, and even Mormons, were fully accepted in San Francisco society. San Francisco street names, like **McCoppin, Brannan, O'Shaughnessy, Geary, O'Farrell, Broderick, Haight,** and **Phelan,** have immortalized many of the early Irish who became prominent in politics, business, and city life.

Unfortunately, as the U.S. took ownership of California in the Mexican-American War and hundreds of thousands of people from around the world flooded into San Francisco competing for gold and then jobs, relations between the Mexicans and the Anglos (including the Irish) deteriorated rapidly. For the next century most of San Francisco society defined "native" as "white" and "foreign" as "non-white." Fortunately, racial tensions have been thawing for the last half-century and groups like the **San Francisco Irish–Mexican Association** flourish today.

POOL PARADISE PLUNGE

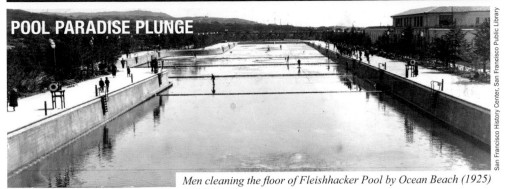

Men cleaning the floor of Fleishhacker Pool by Ocean Beach (1925)

Upon its completion in 1925, **Fleishhacker Pool** was the largest heated outdoor swimming pool in the world, boasting a tank 1,000 feet long by 160 feet wide in the center by 100 feet wide at the ends. It was filled with 6.5 million gallons of heated seawater and patrolled by up to 24 lifeguards, some in rowboats.

Your 25¢ admission, 15¢ for swimmers under age 12, purchased use of the grounds, including a tree-sheltered beach, large dressing room with showers, and cafeteria, plus the loan of a bathing suit and large towel, sterilized between uses. Child care cost extra.

Though the water was heated to 72°, the average ambient temperature was 60°, and attendance soon fell. It limped along for decades, until a storm dealt it the final blow, closing the pool in 1971. It was demolished in 2000.

The pool was a gift from Park Commissioner **Herbert Fleishhacker**, also the arts commissioner (responsible for Coit Tower on Walk 2) and a philanthropist who donated the land for the SF Zoo.

GHOST RIDER

On August 12, 1912, **George Haviland Barron,** former curator of the **de Young Museum** in Golden Gate Park, gave this eyewitness account and warning:

"*Should you find yourself alone in the park at midnight and out of the fog bursts a large black stallion galloping at full speed bearing a young woman wearing a straw hat with an expression of sheer terror on her face... you've seen the ghost of the horse and rider who were*

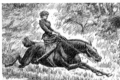

found drowned at Ocean Beach in the 1880s. I saw it too."

If you see it, try checking the sand in front of the Beach Chalet in the morning for horse prints heading into the ocean.

In the mid-1890s, San Francisco transit companies started selling surplus horse-pulled cars and cable cars to the public—$20 with seats intact, $10 without. These obsolete public transportation shells were soon turned into bars, restaurants, shoe repair shops, playhouses, laundries, artists' studios, and even houseboats. A bohemian settlement erupted at **Ocean Beach** as written by...ers, judges, and lady bicyclists arranged, combined, and even stacked old transit cars to create **"Carville-by-the-Sea."**

—*Carville-by-the-Sea,* by Woody LaBounty

CABLE CAR CONDOS

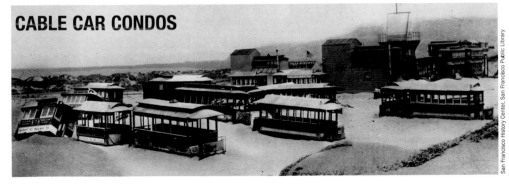

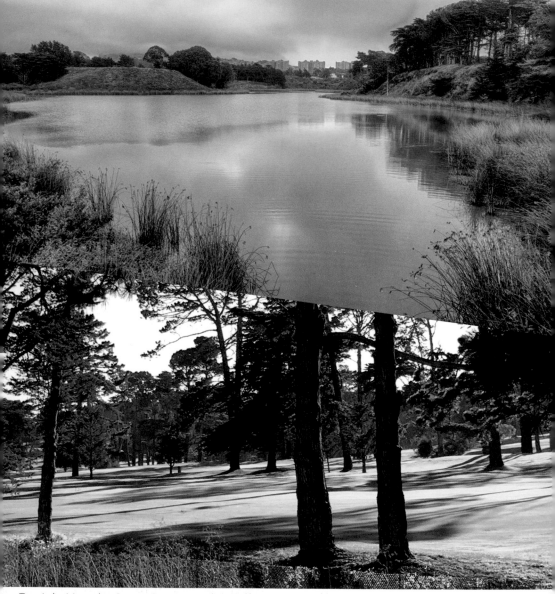

Top: Lake Merced at Sunset. Bottom: Harding Golf course. PHOTO BY SCOTT WALTON

Many people are surprised to learn that Lake Merced is *not* man-made; it's a natural freshwater lake! In fact, the abundant natural resources supported the native Ohlone people's village here for centuries. Be sure to look for the tule reeds along the shoreline. The Ohlone used tule to build houses and boats. (HINT: You can see a re-creation of a tule boat at the Maritime National Park Visitor Center on Walk 3, and a tule hut in Mission Dolores on Walk 14)

Lake Merced remained San Francisco's main source of freshwater for nearly 50 years. Today it's a source of fresh-air recreation—with a rowing club, boathouse, recreational fishing, picnic areas, and cafés surrounded by three golf clubs and a 4.5-mile walking/jogging/biking loop. The official 49 mile route covers 3.8 miles of its circumference, but this walk navigates the entire loop. Take your time. Pause and notice the wildlife and plant life around you.

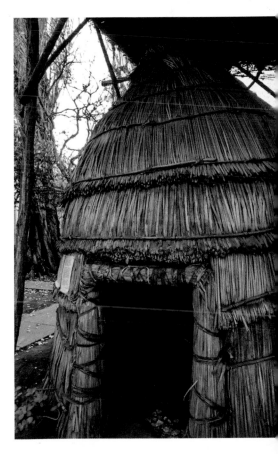

Ohlone people lived along Lake Merced in tule reed huts (see this replica inside Mission Dolores on Walk #14)

Begin:	Skyline Boulevard at Lake Merced Boulevard (Lake Merced)	Hill Rating:
End:	Sunset Boulevard at Lake Merced Boulevard	
Distance:	ROUTE: 4.5 miles — 9,000 steps — 1:30 hour	2
	LOOP BACK: none	

Sites you will pass on today's walk include:

MILE 21

1. **Lake Merced**
   Skyline Blvd, John Muir Dr, and Lake Merced Blvd

2. **Rowing Clubs**
   1 Harding Rd

a. **Fort Funston**
   Fort Funston Rd

MILE 22

3. **San Francisco Police Pistol Range**
   700 John Muir Dr

4. **Former Pacific Rod and Gun Club**
   GONE SF

5. **Lakewood Apartments**
   515 John Muir Dr

b. **Fishing Pier and Bridge**

MILE 23

> **DETOUR**
c. **Broderick-Terry Duel Site** 1100 Lake Merced Blvd

6. **The Olympic Club**
   599 Skyline Blvd

7. **San Francisco Golf Club** 1310 Junipero Serra Blvd

8. **TPC Harding Park Golf Course**
   99 Harding Rd

9. *Penguin's Prayer* **Sculpture** Lake Merced Blvd

MILE 24

10. **San Francisco State University (SFSU)**
    1600 Holloway Ave

11. **Lowell High School**
    1101 Eucalyptus Dr

d. **Captain Juan Bautista de Anza Statue** parking lot off Lake Merced Blvd

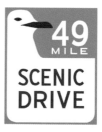

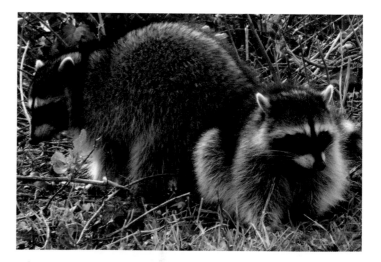

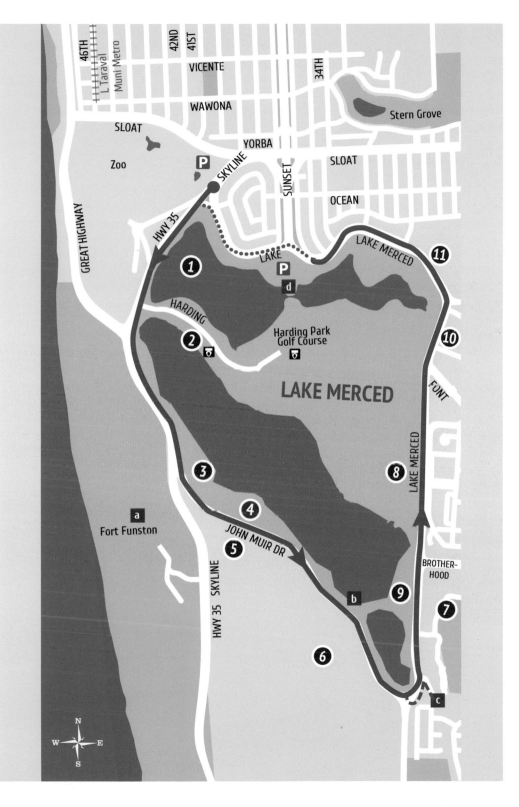

MILE 21

Begins on SKYLINE BLVD at
LAKE MERCED BLVD

• • • • • • • • • • • • • • • • •

South on SKYLINE BLVD on lake side of street

• • • • • • • • • • • • • • • • •

1. Lake Merced Skyline Blvd, John Muir Dr, and Lake Merced Blvd

When the Spanish arrived in 1774, they found a freshwater lake teeming with fish, surrounded by oak trees, Ohlone natives, and grizzly bears. They named the lake Laguna de Nuestra Señora de la Merced (Lake of Our Lady of Mercy).

An underground spring feeds Lake Merced, but early surveys show that at one time it had an outlet to the ocean, thus it contains fish that are adapted to both saltwater and freshwater. Watch for the large concrete marker detailing the ecology of Lake Merced along Mile 24 just past the golf course. Today fishing is limited to designated areas (not along the shoreline), and you must acquire a daily permit.

2. Rowing Clubs
1 Harding Rd

Three rowing clubs use Lake Merced. Thanks to many generous donations, Lake Merced now has a new state-of-the-art dock to replace the old rotting wooden one.

• **Pacific Rowing Club:** Highly competitive junior rowing program recruits high-school-age boys and girls and welcomes skilled adults who want to help. Since 1980.

• **San Francisco Rowing Club:** This club offers state-of-the-art equipment for beginners and elite racers alike. Since 1984.

• **Dolphin Club:** The main clubhouse is on Walk 3, but the club maintains a boathouse here for its nationally and internationally recognized rowers as well as recreational rowers. Since 1877.

DSE Motto: "Start Slowly and Taper Off"
The oldest and largest running club in the city, the all-volunteer Dolphin South End Running club proudly offers low-key, low-cost, weekly timed runs that welcome every race, age, and skill level! A typical run may include a 12-year-old girl toeing the starting line, next to a 75-year-old man, standing next to a seasoned athlete—and all three may beat your time. But really, just run your own pace and have fun. They run weekly races around Lake Merced in the summer.

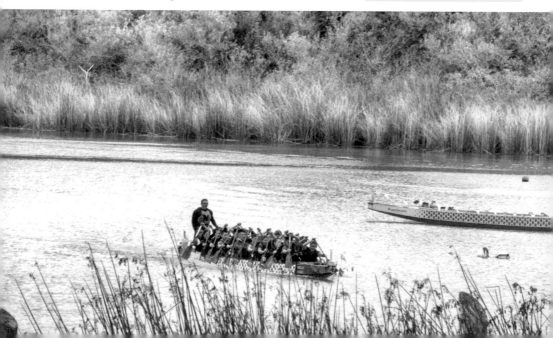

(NOTE: on Walk 3 you pass the clubhouse of two DSE founding clubs: the South End Rowing Club and the Dolphin Swim Club. The third DSE founding club, San Francisco Rowing Club, meets at Lake Merced.)

a. Fort Funston
Fort Funston Rd

All the land you see on the right side of Skyline is Fort Funston. Named after the army commander who patrolled the streets after the 1906 earthquake, this military reservation was deactivated after World War I, then reactivated during World War II, then declared surplus and given to the city of San Francisco. Ruins of gun batteries remain (as well as an underground Nike missile silo, which we assume is empty). Today, as part of the GGNRA, these ocean cliffs form an awesome off-leash dog park (greatly needed and fiercely protected by dogowners) and a launching ground for hang gliders.

MILE 22

Begins on SKYLINE BLVD at JOHN MUIR DR

· · · · · · · · · · · · · · · · · ·

Follow sidewalk left, street turns into JOHN MUIR DR as it heads around the lake

· · · · · · · · · · · · · · · · · ·

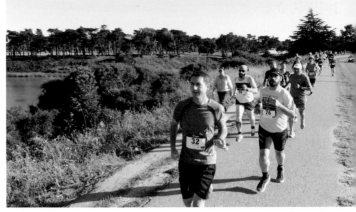

Like these Dolphin South End runners, people love to run, walk, and perambulate around the lake's 4.4-mile circumference.

3. San Francisco Police Pistol Range
700 John John Muir Dr

The pistol range provides training "so that sworn members of the San Francisco Police Department are proficient and qualified in the proper use of firearms."

—sf-police.org

GONE SF
4. Pacific Rod and Gun Club

In 2015 the city closed this unusual club that had been in operation on Lake Merced since 1934. Its 10 acres next to the police shooting range offered the only Olympic skeet field and training facility within 40 miles and the last facility of its kind in a major metropolitan area. Over the course of 80 years this all-volunteer, non-profit club taught thousands of people trap and skeet shooting, shotgun safety, and

training for hunting licenses. It's sad to see old SF places disappear, but it's also good that the city is cleaning up the toxic residue left over from the early days when the club used lead ammunition.

NOTE: The 49 Mile Walk authors considered renting the club's funky, kitschy (inexpensive) clubhouse for their wedding reception, until they realized gun practice would be taking place at the same time. Eh, not the best soundtrack for a wedding dance.

5. Lakewood Apartments
515 John Muir Dr

Across the street on your right, this seven-story, 722-unit apartment complex with tons of on-site amenities has been offering "resort-style" living since 1974. 510-square-foot studios begin at $2,300 a month.

b. Fishing Pier and Bridge

About two miles into the walk, just before the parking lot in front of the bridge that crosses the lake, is a path through the bushes that leads out to a small fishing pier. Shore fishing is allowed one hour before sunrise to one hour after sunset. California State Fishing License required.

MILE 23

Begins on LAKE MERCED BLVD at JOHN MUIR DR

• • • • • • • • • • • • • • • • •

Follow sidewalk left, street turns into LAKE MERCED BLVD as it heads around the lake (or take the detour)

• • • • • • • • • • • • • • • • •

c. Broderick–Terry Duel Siter
1100 Lake Merced Blvd

This site marks where the "last notable duel" in the U.S. took place. On September 13, 1859, former California Supreme Court justice David S. Terry, a pro-slavery proponent, shot California United States senator David C. Broderick, an abolitionist. (On Walk 3 the 49 mile route passes near the house in which the loser died three days after the duel.)

THREE GOLF COURSES

Private Courses:

6. The Olympic Club
599 Skyline Blvd

The Olympic Club hosted the U.S. Open in 2012. Webb Simpson crowned (+1), with Tiger Woods (+7). The club has two 18-hole, 71-par courses and one 9-hole, par-3 course on the bluffs over the Pacific Ocean. (The 49 mile route also passes the Olympic Club's downtown clubhouse on Post Street in Walk 2.)

7. San Francisco Golf Club 1310 Junipero Serra Blvd

Rated no. 27 in the country, the San Francisco Golf Club is old money, conservative, and proud that they denied membership to early Internet millionaires. 18 hole, 71 par.

Municipal Course:

8. TPC Harding Park
99 Harding Rd

Formerly **Harding Park Golf Club**, this 18-hole, 72-par course opened in 1925 and struggled after the 1960s. Then, after much public debate, the PGA Tour took over running the club in 2010 and today she is once again hosting major tournaments.

9. *Penguin's Prayer Sculpture* Lake Merced Blvd

Why is there a penguin statue here, you ask? Two reasons: (1) *Penguin's Prayer* was originally made for the Golden Gate International Exposition of 1939 and (2) It was sculpted by popular SF artist/icon Benny Bufano (1890–1970) in his signature rounded style.

DETOUR

> At the bottom of the lake, as JOHN MUIR DR becomes LAKE MERCED BLVD, cross over to the median and cross LAKE MERCED BLVD at the light.

> Turn left. You'll quickly run out of sidewalk, but walk along the grass just around the bend to the first street. You'll see a sign for the Broderick–Terry Duel.

> Take first right to Lake Merced Hill (private club). Again, there is no sidewalk walk on the road.

> Pass the tennis courts on your right.

> At the dead-end roundabout (stairs to your left), head into the woods and you'll see the landmark plaque.

> Pass through the opening in the chain-link fence.

> A short walk away, you will see two granite shafts, one marked Terry, the other Broderick.

> Reenact the duel.

> Return the way you came back to the route.

Bufano's five-foot stature belied his outsized personality and skill. For example, he claimed to have cut off his trigger finger and then mailed it to President Wilson as a pacifist act of protest. (You'll pass another Bufano on Walk 12).

Search YouTube for "Benny Bufano Sculptures of San Francisco" to see his many other penguins and bears and sculptures of the Madonna and Saint Francis placed throughout the city.

MILE 24

Begins on LAKE MERCED BLVD at FONT ST

10. San Francisco State University (SFSU)
1600 Holloway Ave

Once you pass Font Street the tall apartment buildings across the street on your right are SFSU dorms. It opened as a teacher training college for women in 1899, called San Francisco State Normal School. Today SFSU is one of 23 California State University campuses, which serve nearly 437,000 students statewide. About 30,000 attend SFSU. *Go, Gators!*

Born in SF in 1946, actor Danny Glover grew up in the Haight (Walk 11), attended George Washington High School in the Richmond (Walk 10) and SF State (Walk 8), and saw Jimi Hendrix at Marx Meadow (Walk 10).

11. Lowell High School
1101 Eucalyptus Dr

Past Winston, the stadium across the road on your right is Lowell's football field. Founded in 1856 in San Francisco, Lowell is the oldest public high school west of the Mississippi. Admission to Lowell is competitive, merit based, and tuition free. In *U.S. News & World Report*'s "Best High Schools in America for 2015," Lowell ranked the second highest for schools with over 2,000 students. And there's more—Lowell students participate in over 100 active clubs and service organizations, 32 athletic teams, a large Visual and Performing Arts Department, and a World Language Department of nine languages. *Yay, public schools!*

END on SUNSET BLVD at LAKE MERCED BLVD

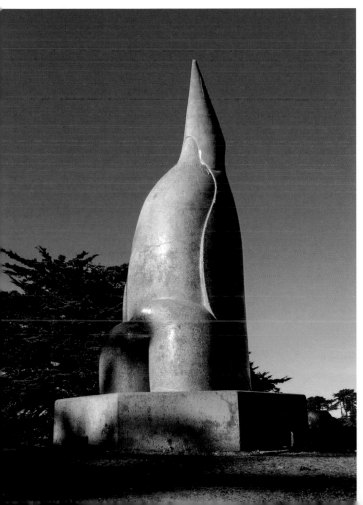

Penguin's Prayer, by Benny Bufano

ON WALK–BACK LOOP

d. Captain Juan Bautista de Anza Statue parking lot off Lake Merced Blvd

At the southern end of the parking lot at the top of Lake Merced stands an 8,000-pound, 11.5-foot-tall bronze equestrian statue of Captain Juan Bautista de Anza, founder of the city San Francisco in 1776. Artist: Julian Martinez.

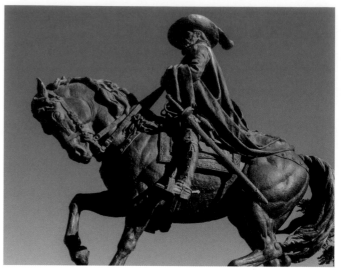

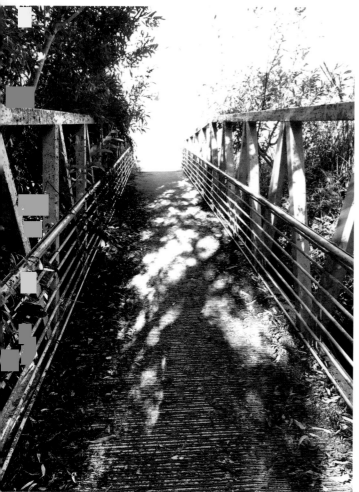

Just down the pathway south of the de Anza statue you can take a pedestrian bridge across the lake to the heart of the golf course. BRIDGE PHOTO: SCOTT WALTON

WALK 8 NEED TO KNOW

TO GET THERE
Muni 18, 23, 29

PARKING
Non-metered street parking and free parking lots. Parking in the Lake Merced lot at the top (north end) of the lake at the end of Sunset Blvd is recommended.

PUBLIC RESTROOMS
- Lake Merced Boat House 1 Harding
- Harding Park Golf Course 99 Harding

TURN–BY–TURN INSTRUCTIONS
Begin: SKYLINE BLVD at LAKE MERCED BLVD

- South on SKYLINE BLVD on lake side of street

- Follow sidewalk left, which turns into JOHN MUIR DR as it heads around the lake
- Follow JOHN MUIR DR, which turns left (north) onto LAKE MERCED BLVD
- Continue around the lake on LAKE MERCED BLVD

End: SUNSET BLVD at LAKE MERCED BLVD

TO GET BACK
- Board Muni bus 18 at NW corner FONT ST and LAKE MERCED BLVD
- Get off at SKYLINE BLVD & and SLOAT BLVD

Other transit routes:

- Muni 17, 18, 29
- SamTrans 122

OPTIONAL WALK-BACK LOOP DIRECTIONS

Rating:

Since the walk is a near loop around the lake, the walk-back is just walking back to your car.

Begin: SUNSET BLVD and LAKE MERCED BLVD

- Continue on LAKE MERCED BLVD to SKYLINE BLVD

End. LAKE MERCED BLVD at SKYLINE BLVD

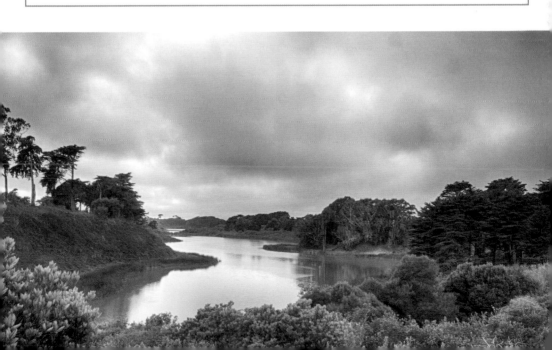

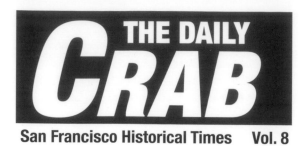

THE DAILY CRAB

San Francisco Historical Times   Vol. 8

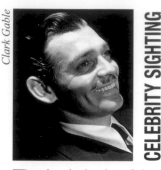

Dastardly Discourteous Duel Debacle

D uring the heyday of skeet shooting, 1946–1957, Hollywood actors who shot at the **Pacific Rod and Gun Club** included **Clark Gable, Ernest Hemingway, Greer Garson, Rex Harrison,** and **Barbara Stanwyck**.

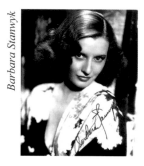

1859 **Chief Justice David Terry**, a known brawler, was well practiced with the Belgian .58 caliber pistols chosen for the duel with **U.S. senator David Broderick**. Broderick, unaccustomed to dueling, did not know about the hair-trigger mechanism of the pistols and, as the duel began, his gun discharged prematurely into the dirt. Terry declined to give a "gentleman's offer" for Broderick to reload, so Broderick bravely stood up full frame, making himself an easy target for Terry's fatal shot. Some called it murder.

Though he was acquitted in court, Terry's behavior generated so much hatred he felt compelled to retire to (gasp) Stockton.

As Broderick, an abolitionist, lay dying he said, "They killed me because I was opposed to the extension of slavery." He was hailed as a martyr in the antislavery cause and his funeral at Lone Mountain had one of the largest turnouts in city history.

HUT, HUT, FORE!

J ohn Madden, Super Bowl–winning coach of the **Oakland Raiders** and popular football commentator, grew up in **Daly City** within walking distance of the **Lake Merced** area golf courses. He worked as a caddy at the **San Francisco Golf Club** and in his autobiography admits to sneaking into the golf clubs often to play with his friends.

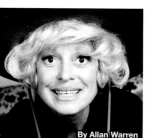

By Allan Warren

Hello, Dolly!

C arol Channing, Golden Globe–winning actress, co-median, singer, and graduate of **Lowell High School** class of 1938, surprised her classmates with a cameo appearance at their 1988 50th-year reunion.

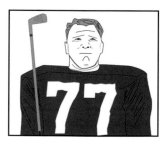

MURDER AND MOURNING

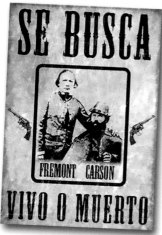

In 1837, Yerba Buena's first alcalde (aka San Francisco's first mayor), **Francisco de Haro**, bought **Lake Merced** for 100 head of cattle and $25. In 1846, during the Mexican-American War, U.S. Army captain **John Fremont** proclaimed himself the U.S. commander of California and ordered frontiersman **Kit Carson** to execute Mayor de Haro's 19-year-old twin sons. Many called it murder. (Read more about this story in Walk 15.) A despondent de Haro spent the remaining years of his life rambling around his hacienda on the southern end of Lake Merced before his death in 1849. You can see de Haro's tombstone in the Mission Dolores cemetery on Walk 14.

"Little Boxes on the Hillside..."

Malvina Reynolds wrote and sang "Little Boxes" in 1962 to satirize **Henry Doelger**'s tract-home development of "ticky-tacky" identical-looking houses at Westlake, located south of Lake Merced. ("Little Boxes" became the theme song of Showtime's *Weeds*.)

H₂O HOGS SOCK IT TO SF

Early San Francisco relied on freshwater **Lake Merced** as her main water supply. In 1868, the moguls of the **Spring Valley Water Company** (SVW) bought water rights to the lake and the surrounding watershed and began capitalizing on their powerful private monopoly over the city's water supply. They charged exorbitant rates and used eminent domain to grab up land around the bay for their own aggrandizement.

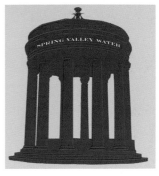

Various reformers tried to break the monopoly, especially when SVW announced it would no longer provide water for the growing needs of Golden Gate Park, but SVW's influence and bribes to city supervisors squelched those efforts.

It took the 1906 earthquake to bring SVW down. As the city was burning to the ground, SVW's inadequate fire hydrants and water systems delivered only a trickle of mud. The resulting civic outcry gave reformist **Mayor James Phelan** a chance to take action. In 1908, when the city approved construction of the **O'Shaughnessy Dam**, creating the **Hetch Hetchy Reservoir** in the Sierra Nevada range, the city finally gained municipal control of her water.

—FoundSF.org

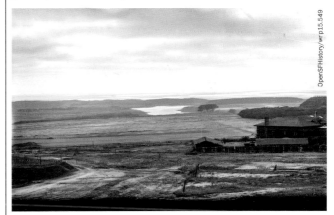

View west toward the Pacific Ocean: Ingleside Golf Course clubhouse to the right with Lake Merced in the distance (1915)

HEROES OF THE LAKE

Just a few decades ago, we nearly lost Lake Merced through excessive pumping and poor development planning—but thanks to the work of **CalTrout**, the **Lake Merced Task Force**, the **Friends of Lake Merced**, and many volunteers, the lake is rebounding wonderfully. *Thank you!*

BONUS CHAPTER

MAKING SAN FRANCISCO A WALKER'S PARADISE

Some thoughts from the SF pedestrian advocacy group Walk San Francisco

By Natalie Burdick, Outreach Director of Walk San Francisco

With over three-dozen parks packed into 49 square miles, it takes mere minutes to walk to green, open space in San Francisco.

Golden Gate Park, while not quite as well known as its East Coast counterpart, is actually 20% larger than New York's Central Park. The hilly terrain of the city's streets and parks grace visitors and residents alike with breathtaking views of the Pacific Ocean, the San Francisco Bay, across to the Marin Headlands, and all the way to the Contra Costa Hills—not to mention the city's own ever-changing, fog-wrapped skyline.

There is also much to see between the 48 (named) hills, which dot the city's scant seven by seven miles. The rich patchwork of intimately-scaled and distinct neighborhoods and the unique Victorian and Edwardian architecture—all influenced by San Francisco's turbulent economic, geologic, and social history—ensure there's no end to a walker's delight.

Google "walk san francisco" and page after endless page of walks are returned—pick from your choice of historic, cultural, or nature focused. There are walks about chocolate, beer, art, and niche interests from hidden stairways to ghost hunts—there's even an annual, all-day urban trek that stretches 12 to 14 miles across at least 10 of the city's hills each September called Peak2Peak.

> About 250,000 people a day walk on Market Street, SF's main boulevard, which stretches from the Ferry Building to Twin Peaks.

It's thrilling to see the latest entry to that list—San Francisco's 49 Mile Scenic Drive reborn as a 49 Mile Scenic Walk. In fact, with its mild climate, compact geography, and second-highest-ranked transit access in the U.S., San Francisco has been the obvious choice for many new walking adventures:

- San Francisco was the first American city to host Walk to Work Day.

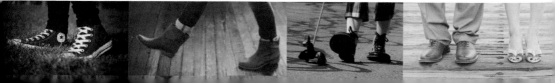

- San Francisco was the first to implement Sunday Streets. One weekend a month, the city closes a different neighborhood corridor to traffic and welcomes tens of thousands of pedestrians to walk the streets (April to October).
- San Francisco innovated the "parklet," which extends the sidewalk over (former) parking spots, to create open spaces with art or benches where people can stop, sit, and relax. (San Francisco has over 40 parklets, the most of any U.S. city.)

So, Why Is THIS Tragedy Four Times More Likely to Happen in San Francisco?

Indeed, the shining city on the hill seems to be a walker's paradise. Which is why many people are surprised when they learn that in San Francisco, at least three people a day are hit by cars while they walk. Annually, 30 people are killed and over 200 suffer serious, life-changing injuries. San Francisco is literally California's most dangerous city for pedestrians, where they make up an unprecedented 60% of all car crash fatalities—a number, which is over four times the national average of around 12%.

What accounts for such a disproportionate number of injuries and deaths? And more importantly, is there anything that can be done to make the city's streets safe for people walking here?

> San Francisco is redesigning the 6% of streets where more than 60% of pedestrian crashes occur.

The 6% Solution

The good news for San Francisco: only 6% of its streets account for more than 60% of the total crashes involving those who walk. As part of a Pedestrian Strategy released by the Mayor's Office in 2013, these high-injury corridors and intersections were identified using years of collected data from the San Francisco Police Department and the Department of Public Health. The city has detailed information on both the most common locations for injuries and deaths and the top illegal driving behaviors that lead to these collisions.

A quick look at the list of the most dangerous corridors, including Geary Boulevard, Sunset Boulevard, Mission Street, 19th Avenue, Polk Street, and streets that cross Market, like 6th and 8th, shows that most crashes involving pedestrians happen on wide arterials and/or fast, one-way streets.

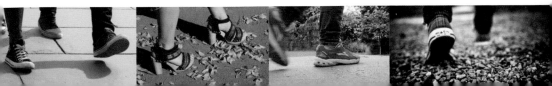

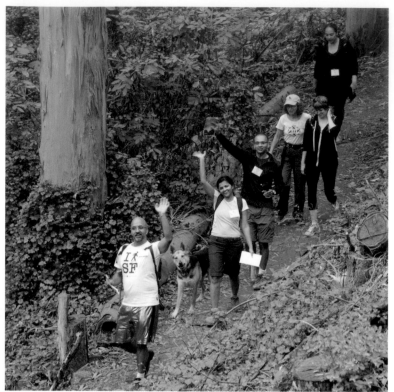

Sign up at WalkSF.org to join Peak2Peak hikers like these on an annual 12-mile, all-day, urban trek across 10 of the city's hills.
Photo: Robin Allen, ROBINALLENPHOTO.COM

Vision Zero

In 2014, a coalition of community groups, led by the pedestrian advocacy nonprofit Walk SF, launched Vision Zero with a goal to eliminate *all* traffic-related deaths in ten years. The effort would require the city to commit to funding and implementing targeted engineering, enforcement, and education solutions to bring to zero the number of motorist, bicyclist, and pedestrian deaths. While it's an aggressive goal, it is a realistic one.

Sweden, where Vision Zero originated, has clearly demonstrated success in bringing down road fatalities, even as overall car ownership and driving has increased. In the U.S., cities like New York, Chicago, and even Los Angelese have also adopted Vision Zero.

Vision Zero SF—a goal to eliminate *all* traffic-related deaths in SF by 2024

With speed being the key factor in safety, particularly for the most vulnerable road users—seniors and

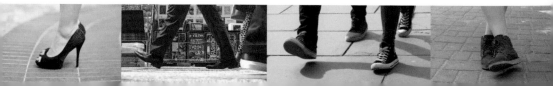

children—there are proven interventions. Increased enforcement for illegal driving behaviors like speeding, not stopping at lights and stop signs, making improper turns, and not yielding to people in crosswalks helps tremendously, but the most important and effective changes involve street designs, which prioritize safety and enjoyment over vehicle volumes and speed.

In a dense, urban environment like San Francisco, solutions that can result in dramatic increases in safety, include:

- countdown signals for pedestrians
- sidewalk extensions at intersections called "bulb-outs"
- well-marked crosswalks
- lower speed limits (Walk SF led and won an effort to make San Francisco the first major city in the state to adopt slower 15 mph limits around schools in 2012)
- retimed signals for safer traffic flow
- turn restrictions on red lights
- road diets (e.g., converting a fourth traffic lane to a bicycle lane)

Moreover, traffic-calming solutions like these can be augmented by the addition of crossing islands (medians), parklets, and planting greenery on sidewalks and medians, which all work together to slow drivers down and reinforce the idea that roads are shared by motorists, bicyclists, and people walking.

Walk, Enjoy, Relax

As the city works toward implementing Vision Zero, visitors and residents alike will be able to continue enjoying a bounty of scenic views, a treasure trove of hidden gems discoverable only from a walker's perspective, all the tremendous benefits to one's health and the environment that come from travel by foot—*and* they will be able to do so without the added risk of having to navigate fast, unsafe streets.

By realizing Vision Zero, San Francisco will be a veritable walker's paradise.

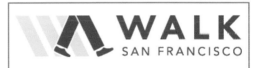

San Francisco's pedestrian advocacy organization, Walk San Francisco, and its members are making San Francisco a more **livable, walkable city** by reclaiming streets as safe, shared public space for everyone to enjoy. Join Us! WalkSF.org.

49 MILE
MILE

SCENIC DRIVE

Sunset Boulevard to

Golden Gate Park

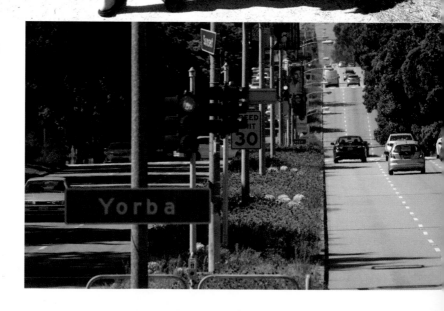

A young couple takes an amble down the tree-lined path along Sunset Boulevard.

If you're looking for a flat, easy stroll, this is it. On this long, straight stretch down the entire length of Sunset Boulevard the historic 49 mile route takes you across the Outer Sunset District and gives you a taste of life in "the Avenues" (so called because 46 of the north—south-running streets are numbered avenues).

The key on this walk: Ignore the traffic, take in the plants and birds, smell the salt air, and look westward at intersections for some surprising glimpses of the ocean. Also watch for the new, tiered rain gardens being built along the boulevard.

Of note: Even though you can see some beautiful sunsets from here, the name Sunset was a marketing gimmick meant to distract people from the area's reputation as the foggiest neighborhood in the city. Dress accordingly.

Then, if you're up for a little adventure after three miles of residential calm, take a stroll west down Judah Street's funky restaurant/business corridor, for a hidden SF neighborhood experience.

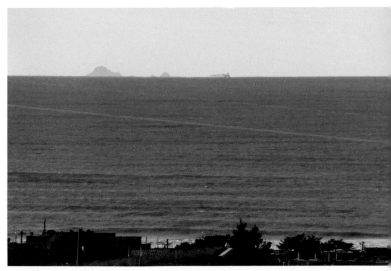

On a clear day you can see the Farallon Islands.

Begin: Sunset Boulevard at Lake Merced Boulevard
End: Sunset Boulevard and Martin Luther King Jr. Drive
            (Golden Gate Park)
Distance: ROUTE: 2.5 miles — 5,000 steps — 50 minutes
            LOOP BACK: none

Hill Rating: 2

Sites you will pass on today's walk include:

MILE 25

OUTER SUNSET

1. **Sunset Boulevard**

2. **Sloat Boulevard**

3. **Yorba Street**

MILE 26

4. **St. Ignatius College Preparatory**
   2001 37th Ave

5. **"Doelger City"**
   Kirkham St to
   Ortega St

MILE 27

a. **Polly Ann Ice Cream Parlor**
   3138 Noriega St
   at 39th Ave

6. **Audley and Josephine Cole Home** 1598 36th Ave

7. **Holy Name of Jesus**
   1555 39th Ave at
   Lawton St

b. **Judah Street Corridor**

NOTE: If you want to avoid the noise of Sunset Blvd's six-lane thoroughfare, feel free to go one block east or west to walk down a parallel residential avenue (36th or 37th Ave). Likewise, if you are using a wheelchair or pushing a stroller you may want to swing up to the Avenues' paved streets to avoid the dirt paths in those sections. The west side of Sunset is paved with concrete while the east side is often graveled.

Hop on the westbound N-Judah at the end of your walk to explore the 44th–48th Avenue corridor of funky shops and eateries.

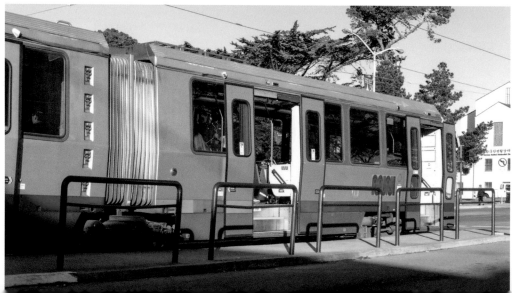

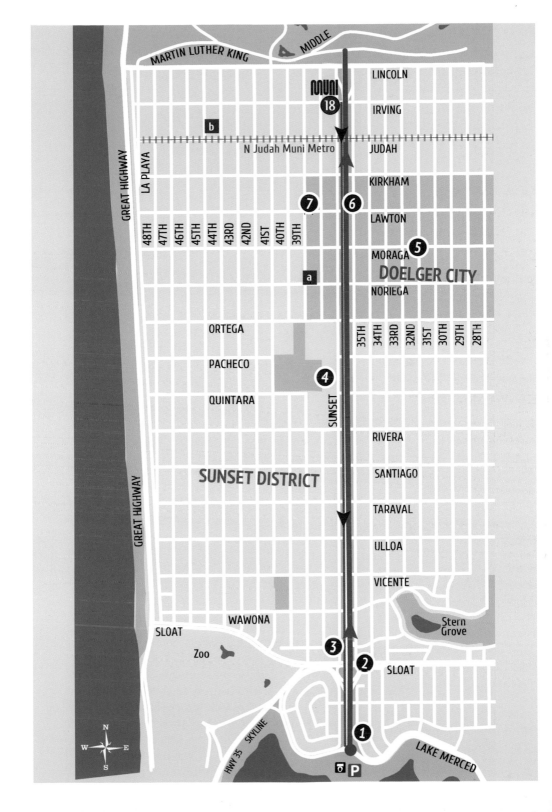

MILE 25

Begins on SUNSET BLVD at
LAKE MERCED BLVD

· · · · · · · · · · · · · · · · · · · ·

Walk north on
SUNSET BLVD into
GOLDEN GATE PARK

· · · · · · · · · · · · · · · · · · · ·

OUTER SUNSET:
HIP BY THE BEACH?

Many who've lived in the Outer
Sunset say this fog-shrouded
neighborhood of modest
stucco family homes feels miles
away from the fast-paced
urban city center. But a 2013
SF Examiner article made this
bold claim: The Sunset has
"made it to the high standards
of San Francisco hipdom."
What?! Yes, apparently as
the affordable real estate,
public transportation, and
quiet neighborhoods began
drawing "quirky locals" from
the rest of town, businesses
sprang up to meet the new
needs—like a tattoo parlor,
vegan juice bar, pizza parlors,
coffee shops, corner stores,
bakery, a co-op nursery school,
and more. The new residents
seem quite happy to support
longtime Sunset residents'
historic opposition to big retail
chains. Together in 2003 and
2004 they "gathered 5,000
signatures and withstood a
marathon City Hall hearing
to block a Starbucks coffee
shop from pushing out a local
coffee shop." Can you really
be hip without a Starbucks? In
the Sunset you can!—"*Outer*

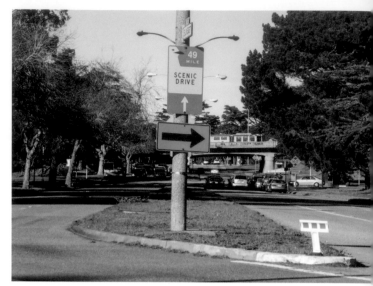

Sunset: Hip by the Beach," SF
Examiner, 2013

1. Sunset Boulevard

Built amid the sand dunes
in 1931, this thoroughfare
was meant to move a lot of
traffic quickly between Sloat
Boulevard and Golden Gate
Park. Sunset Boulevard divides
the Outer Sunset from the rest
of the Sunset District, namely,
Parkside, West Portal, and the
Inner Sunset.

2. Sloat Boulevard

Sloat Boulevard is the widest
street in SF and, coincidentally,
begins a few miles north at St.
Francis Circle, which has the
longest traffic light in the city.

3. Yorba Street

The street was originally set
to be named Xavier Street,
to fit with the alphabetized
street-naming convention for
east–west-running streets,
but planners deemed the
name Xavier too difficult to
pronounce so it was changed
to Yorba.

Be Careful

Unfortunately Sunset Boulevard's car-focused design invites
freeway-like habits from many of its 35,000 daily vehicle
drivers, making it one of the most dangerous streets in SF
for pedestrians. After cars struck 44 pedestrians in a six-year
period, the city began efforts to make it safer, such as adding
a new stoplight, reducing the speed limit, and giving out
more traffic citations. The actions are part of Vision Zero— a
civic and community goal to eliminate all traffic deaths in San
Francisco by 2024 (see page 122).

MILE 26

Begins on SUNSET BLVD at TARAVAL ST

4. St. Ignatius College Preparatory
2001 37th Ave

This Jesuit school has been in the city since 1855. Typically, 100% of its graduating students go on to college. In keeping with its spiritual origins, the school requires each student to perform 100 hours of service per year—many students serve more hours. Nearly a quarter of the school's 14,000+ students receive aid to cover the $18,350 annual tuition.

St. Ignatius and Sacred Heart have been butting heads on the athletic field since 1893, giving them the oldest high school football rivalry west of the Rockies and the oldest Catholic school football rivalry in the United States.

! LOOK westward at Ortega Street

Stop a moment and look west for a great view of the Pacific Ocean and possibly even the Farallon Islands (on a clear day). Great photo opportunity.

5. "Doelger City": Cookie Cutter Houses Ortega St to Kirkham St

Henry Doelger, the best-known developer of houses in the Sunset District, specialized at mass-producing houses on little lots. He studied and implemented Henry Ford's factory techniques to home building. By the late 1930s he was churning out two complete houses a day, building over 24,000 homes in his lifetime. The tracts he built from 27th to 39th Avenues between Ortega and Kirkham Streets were known as Doelger City. People accustomed to the details of Victorian and Edwardian buildings scoffed at the "cookie-cutter" way these houses were built, but the houses were not only affordable to people who could not have otherwise owned a home, they were well built and have stood the test of time.

In that spirit, a number of new multiunit buildings are being proposed along the Sunset corridor in response to SF's current housing shortage

Sewage Spillover Solved with Rain Gardens
What happens when inches and inches of storm water fall on paved city streets, sidewalks, and driveways? The water surges into the sewer—overwhelming the system and flooding neighborhood streets. With input from residents, the SF Public Utilities Commission wants to turn Sunset Boulevard into a greenway to help solve that problem. The innovative green infrastructure technologies the commission is evaluating include tiered rain gardens to capture storm water and allow it to soak into the landscape. Construction on Sunset should be well under way or completed by the time you walk it.

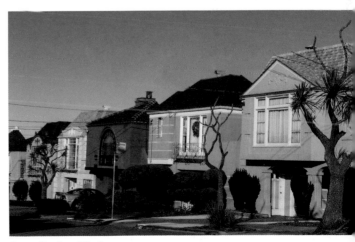
Some Doelger City homes

MILE 27

Begins on SUNSET BLVD at NORIEGA ST

a. Polly Ann Ice Cream Parlor 3138 Noriega St at 39th Ave

OPTIONAL: Head two blocks toward the ocean. Opened in 1955, today this neighborhood ice cream parlor serves up to 50 of its 500 flavors at a time. If you're having trouble picking a flavor, you can spin the flavor wheel to help you decide. Charlie Wu, the owner since 1985, learned to make ice cream in the Cornell University food science program—where many ice cream executives

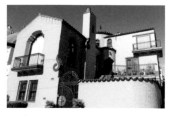

Look east at Lawton to see the Cole family's Rousseau home.

(including those from Ben & Jerry's and Baskin-Robbins) learn the science of ice cream. Charlie was the first Asian in the program.

6. Audley and Josephine Cole Home
1598 36th Av e at Lawton St

Two unsung heroes in the fight for civil rights, Audley Cole, the first black Muni driver (1940) and his wife, Josephine, who became the first black schoolteacher in the San Francisco public school system (1944), purchased an Oliver Rousseau home in the nearly all-white Sunset District in 1957. An outstanding educator, Josephine received numerous awards during and after her distinguished career and used her home as a student gathering place, inviting notable guests such as singer Josephine Baker and

actor Vincent Price. In 1992, SF City College named the southeast campus library after her.
—*Stories in the Sand: San Francisco's Sunset District, 1847-1964*, by Lorri Ungaretti

7. Holy Name of Jesus
1555 39th Av

As you pass Lawton, look left down the street at the large church. In 1925, a young Father Richard Ryan (originally from County Cork, Ireland) was assigned to serve the 125 families in San Francisco's Sunset District. Together they built the Holy Name of Jesus Catholic Parish. As the Sunset's population grew so did church attendance. Holy Name could count 560 men from the parish who had gone to serve their country in WW II. The Sunset housing boom that greeted the GIs on their return brought in even more families. The church grew and changed with

---

Rousseau-Style Homes

Sunset between 33rd and 36th Avenues from Kirkham to Lawton Streets is home to the city's largest cluster of Rousseau-style homes—those storybook houses dressed in pastels that blend fanciful turrets with practical garage bases. The late developer Oliver Rousseau built these fairy-tale-conjuring yet modest homes for the working and middle classes in the 1930s for people who were priced out of places like Forest Hill and St. Francis Wood. Mediterranean archways or ornate medallions adorn the facades, and the interiors are at once formulaic and romantic, mixing vaulted ceilings and interior patios with sunken living rooms—as though a ranch house had signed up for castle lessons.

In the 1920s, neighborhood-based, racial covenants—discriminatory practices legally prohibiting the sale of property to African Americans, Asians, Jews, and other specified non-Caucasian groups—became widespread throughout the country. San Francisco was slow to adapt these covenants. However, by the late '30s, most developers, including the biggest developer, Henry Doelger, had added these covenants. Rousseau homes *did not* have covenants. In 1948 the U.S. Supreme Court ruled the practice unconstitutional.

—SFCurbed.com and the SF Planning Department

the changing neighborhood over the decades, and today the largest group serving the parish is the Fil-Am Club of Holy Name. In the spirit of *bayanihan* (Tagalog for "a sense of community), the club started accepting non-Filipino members back in 2006.

· · · · · · · · · · · · · · · · · ·

END on MARTIN LUTHER KING JR DRIVE

· · · · · · · · · · · · · · · · · ·

WALK-BACK LOOP SCOOP

Take the bus back.

However, if you want a real SF adventure after your three-mile stroll through this residential neighborhood, hop on a bus and head west down Judah Street. HiddenSF.com calls it a hidden gem that SF residents, let alone tourists, rarely get out to see. The **Mollusk Surf Shop** (46th), many coffee shops, 44th Ave's **Other Avenues Natural Food Coop** (worker owned since 1974), and cute stores, such as **The Last Straw** jewelry store (47th) give it a "little Santa Cruz" vibe. The surprise is the quality of the restaurants. Their attitude seems to be "We better have really great food if we expect people to drive clear across town for it." And the Yelp reviews show it's working—you may not get into restaurants like **Pisces** (39th) or **Thanh Long** (43rd) without reservations. Expect a wait for brunch at **Outerlands** (39th).

Did the FHA Create the Middle Class?

A typical home purchase in the 1920s required a minimum 30% down payment, plus refinancing every 5 to 10 years. This not only priced working folks out of the market, it meant foreclosures often occurred because owners could not secure financing to renew. When the Great Depression hit in the 1930s the country faced an alarming drop in home construction and a rise in foreclosures. To revive the moribund housing industry, the federal government created the Home Owners' Loan Corporation (HOLC) in 1933 and the Federal Housing Administration (FHA) in 1934.

HOLC pioneered the concept of a long-term, fully amortized mortgage and the FHA insured long-term mortgage loans making it less risky for banks and homeowners to finance mortgages. With low 10% down payments and affordable 30-year fixed payment plans, anyone with a steady job could afford to purchase a home, building both equity and security for themselves and their children.

The construction industry boomed and so did home ownership, which grew from 44% of American families in 1934 to 63% in 1972.

If it's true that sustainable homeownership is the "gateway to the middle class," the Feds got one right on this one! *Thanks, U.S. government!* —SF-Planning.org

NEED TO KNOW

TO GET THERE
- Muni 17, 18, 29
- SamTrans 122

PARKING
Free street parking

PUBLIC RESTROOMS
- Lake Merced parking lot (near Sunset)
- Golden Gate Park (see Walk 10)

TURN-BY-TURN INSTRUCTIONS
Begin: SUNSET BLVD at LAKE MERCED BLVD

- Walk north SUNSET BLVD into GOLDEN GATE PARK

End: MARTIN LUTHER KING JR DRIVE

TO GET BACK
Muni
- Board bus 29 at SW corner of SUNSET BLVD and IRVING
- Get off at WINSTON DR and LAKE MERCED BLVD

Other Muni routes: N at Judah

NO WALK-BACK LOOP— TAKE THE BUS

THE DAILY CRAB

San Francisco Historical Times   Vol. 9

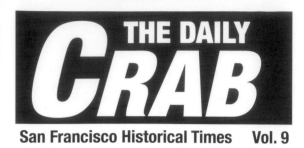

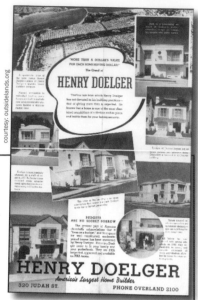

courtesy: outsidelands.org

"MORE THAN A DOLLAR'S VALUE FOR EACH HOMEOWNING DOLLAR"

The Creed of

HENRY DOELGER

HENRY DOELGER
America's Largest Home Builder

320 JUDAH ST.   PHONE OVERLAND 2100

SANDLOT SUCCESS

Before the 1906 earthquake, the area south of Golden Gate Park (today's Sunset District) was a vast area of scrub grass and sand dunes sparsely populated, save a few farms, a few criminals hiding in makeshift shacks, and two dynamite plants (that exploded occasionally). A Hollywood motion picture company once shot desert scenes here. The completion of Golden Gate Park in the 1880s, the earthquake

In 1941, the FHA helped aspiring San Francisco homeowners buy $5,560 Doelger tract homes for $560 down, $37.50 month.

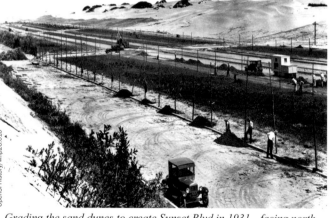

OpenSFHistory/wnp26.010

Grading the sand dunes to create Sunset Blvd in 1931—facing north

of 1906, and the boring of the Twin Peaks tunnel in 1917 each prompted waves of housing development here. More robust development in the 1930s and finally tract homes built for the post-WWII "baby boom" families in the 1950s created the Sunset neighborhood we know today. It's the largest, most populated neighborhood in the city.

"SPANISH TOWN" REVOLT

When the city first laid out the streets of the Outside Lands, planners simply numbered the north–south-running streets 1st to 49th Avenue, and lettered the east–west streets A to Z.

In a post-earthquake attempt to correct the confusing street naming conventions across the city, the Board of Supervisors created a commission to clean it all up. They suggested renaming all the north–south avenues in the Rich-mond and Sunset in alphabetical order after Spanish historical fig-ures, Arguello, Borca, to Zamo-rano on 26th Avenue, and then start again with Spanish saints.

The Richmond and Sun-set community organizations claimed this would cause them to be mocked as a "Spanish Town" and threw a fit. So, the numbered avenues remained, with the com-promise of Arguello for 1st and La Playa (which means "beach")

for 49th Avenue. In the renam-ing of the east–west A–Z streets, the Richmond residents on the north side of the park had only three streets to name, so they were willing to have Anza, Bal-boa, and Cabrillo, but the Sunset community wanted some streets named after "American heroes, dammit!" Thus, Irving, Judah, Kirkham, and Lawton break the pattern of Spanish east–west street names in the Sunset.

—source: John Freeman, *Encyclopedia of San Francisco*

PINOY POWER

Did Filipinos land in America before the Pilgrims' 1620 arrival? *Yes.* As a colony of Spain, the Philippines supplied sailors for Spanish worldwide explorations, which included Filipino sailors landing in Marin County on November 1595 as part of the crew of the galleon *San Agustin*.

San Francisco has long played a role in the history of Filipinos. San Franciscans were recruited to fight in the 1898 **Spanish-American War** in the Philippines. When Spain surrendered, it gave sovereignty over the Philippines to the U.S. The Filipinos, who had been fighting a war of independence against the Spaniards, kept fighting for independence, which led to the very short **Philippine-American War**.

Many American troops, reflecting the prevailing attitudes about white racial superiority of the era, derisively called it "another Indian war." In fact, U.S. African American troops fighting in the Philippines (the **Buffalo Soldiers** stationed at the Presidio) were so incensed by the extreme racism directed against

Filipinos, some even joined the Filipino rebels to fight against U.S. imperialism. The rebels lost.

Later, Filipinos were American allies in World War II, and over the last 100 years, hundreds of thousands of Filipino American families have become integral to life in San Francisco. In fact, the highest concentration of Filipinos outside the Philippines is in Daly City. *Mabuhay!*
— James Sobredo, CSUS.edu

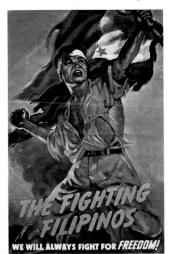

Photo: courtesy of a private collector

San Francisco's official Soap Box Derby racecourse ran down Sunset Boulevard between Ulloa and Wawona.

SUNSET BLVD SOAP BOX DERBY

The first soapbox derby race took place in Ohio in 1933. When the second-place winner was announced, the crowd gasped as the driver took off his hat and out flowed long hair, revealing he was a she, **Alice Johnson.** After two more girls competed in a 1934 race, the newly formed **All-American Soap Box Derby** organization officially banned all girls from racing.

In 1937, the **San Francisco Chronicle** and **Chevrolet** brought the Soap Box Derby to San Francisco. The racecourse ran down Sunset Boulevard between Ulloa and Wawona. The *SF Chronicle* described Sunset Boulevard as a "lovely, peaceful parkway drive in the Sunset district that is seldom used even on Sunday."

San Francisco boys have placed, though not won, in five Derby finals. The Derby left the city in the 1960s.

Girls were allowed (back) into the Soap Box Derby in 1971 and, in 1975, an 11-year-old girl from Pennsylvania won.
— Outsidelands.org, by Lorri Ungaretti

"LITTLE CHINATOWNS"

As in much of the city, the Sunset has transformed from a predominantly Irish neighborhood to a wonderfully diverse community including about 50% Asian American residents. Several informal "little Chinatown" commercial areas thrive around 19th Avenue on the district's main corridors: Irving, Noriega, and Taraval.

A U.S. military propaganda poster depicts World War II Philippine guerrilla fighters, who ambushed occupying Japanese forces and provided valuable behind-the-lines intelligence reports to Allied strategists.

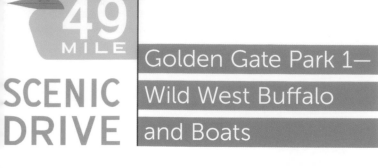

49 MILE

SCENIC DRIVE

Golden Gate Park 1—
Wild West Buffalo
and Boats

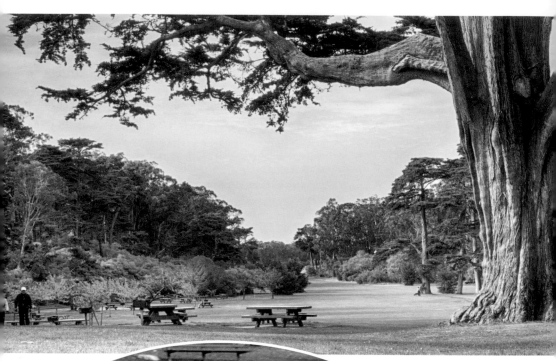

Enjoy a picnic at Lindley Meadow and then cross JFK Drive to watch the boat races at Spreckels Lake.

When the creator of New York's Central Park, Frederick Law Olmsted, was invited to build Golden Gate Park in the 1860s, he took a good look at the three-mile-long stretch of treeless sand and scrub extending to the ocean, declared the task impossible, and turned down the job. So 24-year-old William Hammond Hall, and later his assistant, John McLaren, stepped in to show New York how San Francisco does "the impossible." Yo!

Your exploration today begins in the wild western end of Hall and McLaren's 1,017-acre woodland miracle—and will lead you on a jaunt past buffalo, model boats, grassy meadows, 1906 quake remnants, and old hippie haunts. Put some flowers in your hair and relax into this easy-flowing, tree-lined amble. We also recommend you take your adventure off-road on the detour past the fly-casting pools, police department horse stables, and polo fields. There are plenty of spots to enjoy a picnic on the way, or you can end with a cup of tea at the Japanese Tea Garden, or a stroll through the Botanical Gardens. What's not to like?

The first bison cow and bull to enjoy the urban paradise of Golden Gate Park were named Sarah Bernhardt and Ben Harrison.

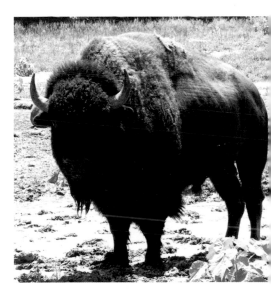

Begin: Sunset Boulevard and Martin Luther King Jr Drive
          (Golden Gate Park)
End: Martin Luther King Jr Drive at Stow Lake Drive
Distance: ROUTE: 2.5 miles — 4,800 steps — 50 minutes
          LOOP BACK: 1.5 miles — 3,400 steps — 30 minutes

Hill Rating:

2

Sites you will pass on today's walk include:

MILE 28

1. **Chain of Lakes**
   Chain of Lakes Dr E

2. **Bercut Equitation Field** Chain of Lakes Dr E

3. **Buffalo Paddock** JFK Dr

   `DETOUR`

a. **Golden Gate Angling and Casting Club– Angler's Lodge and Fly-Casting Pools**

b. **Fred C. Egan Memorial Police Stables**

c. **Athletic Fields– Polo Fields**

MILE 29

4. **San Francisco Model Yacht Club** 36th Ave and JFK Dr

5. **Spreckels Lake**

6. **Marx Meadow** 898 JFK Dr

7. **Speedway Meadow, Hellman Hollow** 50 Overlook Dr

8. **Lloyd Lake and Portals of the Past**

MILE 30

9. **Mothers Meadow** 501–599 MLK Dr

d. **The San Francisco Botanical Garden** entrance on JFK Dr (1199 9th Ave)

Cartoon Trivia
- In the 1949 cartoon *Bushy Hare,* Bugs Bunny pops up in Golden Gate Park in front of Portals of the Past at Lloyd Lake.
- Mel Blanc, the famous voice-over actor who provided voices for Bugs Bunny and over 400 other cartoon characters, was born in San Francisco in 1908.

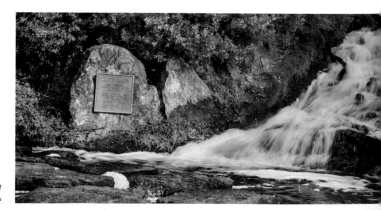

Water flowing into Lloyd Lake

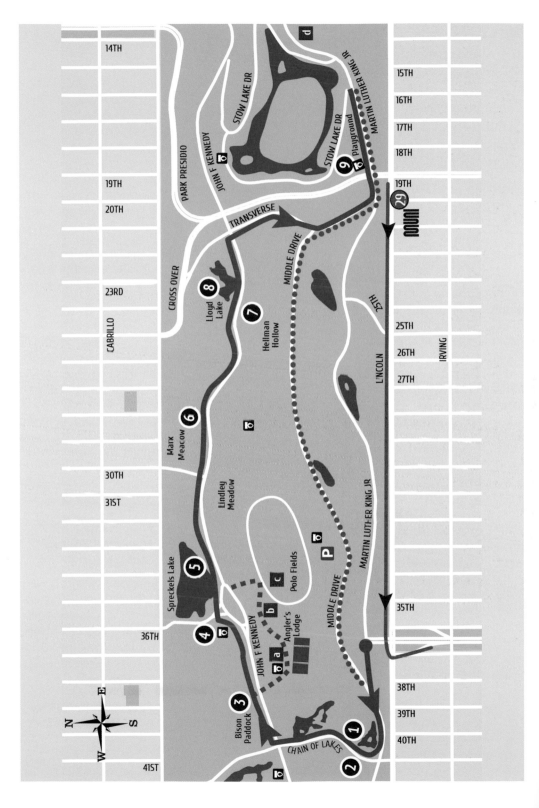

MILE 28

Begins on MARTIN LUTHER KING JR DR at SUNSET BLVD

Continuing from SUNSET BLVD on Walk 9, turn left (west) on MLK DR

Right on CHAIN OF LAKES

1. Chain of Lakes
Chain of Lakes Dr E

Of the original 14 marshy lakes nestled in the dunes destined to become Golden Gate Park, only the North, Middle, and South Chain of Lakes survive today (though they've been reshaped). The rest of the park's 10 lakes are artificial. You'll pass two on your right and the third is to your left as you cross JFK Drive.

2. Bercut Equitation Field
Chain of Lakes Dr E

Horse jumping and training corral. In case you have a horse in the garage that needs exercising, no permit is required to bring horses into the park or ride on designated bridle paths. NOTE: There is a water bottle refill station located right outside Bercut Equitation Field.

In 1915 Charlie Chaplin filmed scenes for two movies in Golden Gate Park and attended the Pan-Pacific Expo.

Cross the street and turn right on JOHN F. KENNEDY (JFK) DR

3. Buffalo Paddocks
JFK Dr

Okay, so technically they're really bison. People called them buffalo back in the 1890s when they transported the first cow and bull here from the Great Plains in an attempt to save them from extinction. Births and imports grew the herd to 30 by 1913, but eventually they all died off from disease. U.S. senator Dianne Feinstein's husband bought a new herd of bison to celebrate her birthday in 1984. Seven more joined in 2011. San Francisco Zoo staff takes care of them today. (HINT: Some days the bison wander out in the meadow; other days finding them is like playing a game of Where's Waldo. They like to hide up in the pen area.)

The Klingon starship in *Star Trek IV: The Voyage Home* (1986) lands in Golden Gate Park. *NOT!* It was actually filmed at Will Rogers State Historic Park near Los Angeles.

Take detour or continue east on JFK DR, veering left with the road around the median toward Spreckels Lake

DETOUR

To see three park gems hidden from view, watch for a small road on the right-hand side of JFK Drive across from the bison. Cross JFK Dr to the entrance of Anglers Lodge. Continue on trails heading east toward the horse stables and Polo Fields, which lead you back out to JFK Dr.

a. Angler's Lodge and Fly Casting Ponds

Founded in 1896, the lodge moved to this location from Stow Lake in 1938. These folks love fly casting so much they offer free lessons, free use of the pools, and even loan rods to anyone who wants to learn fly casting. The shallow concrete pools are not stocked with fish—only targets for fly-casting practice. Note the bench honoring Ernest C. Voight that states, "He treated every fish as if it were big."

b. Fred C. Egan Memorial Police Stables

The horse stables were constructed in the 1930s and named for a longtime police department horse trainer. Today the mounted unit's strength is one sergeant, four officers, and nine Horses.

c. Former Polo Fields, now The Athletic Field

In between the polo and buggy-racing events of yore and the

soccer and music festivals of today, the Polo Fields became a cultural icon when she hosted 30,000 hippies at the mind expanding, drug experimenting, and authority questioning **"Human Be-In"** that launched the **1967 Summer of Love**.

MILE 29

Begins on JOHN F. KENNEDY DR at SPRECKLES LAKE (36th AV entrance to Park)

Cross street to Spreckels Lake

4. San Francisco Model Yacht Club (SFMYC)
36th Av and JFK Dr

Established in 1898, SFMYC is the oldest club in the Americas devoted to model yachts. SFMYC welcomes visitors into her WPA-era clubhouse during monthly meetings to view the beautiful and extensive collection of model boats. Find the clubhouse on your left, before you reach Spreckels Lake.

5. Spreckels Lake

The nautical battle between model boat lovers and full-size boat sailors competing for space on nearby Stow Lake was averted when Adolph Spreckels donated this reservoir for model boat racing in 1904. The Dutch Windmill you passed on Walk 7 pumped water from the underground aquifers near Ocean Beach to fill the lake. Model boat racing continues here today. Electric and steam powered models: Mon., Wed., Fri., 10 a.m.–1 p.m. Gasoline-fueled models: Tues., Thurs., Sat., 10 a.m.—1 p.m. Sailboats: 1 p.m.—4 p.m. every day.

> Adolph Spreckels: sugar magnate, captain of transportation industry, builder of the Legion of Honor, shooter of *Chronicle* co-owner Michael de Young (over alleged slander), donator of Golden Gate Park lands west of 25th Avenue, husband of hot young model Alma de Bretteville, and SF parks commissioner. Busy guy!

Continue on JFK DR to TRANSVERSE DR (the street just before the PARK PRESIDIO BLVD overpass bridge)

6. Marx Meadow
898 JFK Dr

In case you've always wondered, it was not named for Karl or Groucho but rather a park donor from Napa: Johanne Augusta Emily Marx. Jimi Hendrix played here. You are invited to play here also—play disc golf, that is. The 18-hole course, played with Frisbee-like discs, is open to the public and free. To learn about volunteering or playing in San Francisco Disc Golf tournaments visit: SFDiscGolf.org

7. Speedway Meadow, renamed Hellman Hollow on JFK Dr
(50 Overlook Dr)

Once a spot for horse-racing events, today this grassy plain—along with Lindley Meadow (you just passed) and Marx Meadow (across the street)—overflows with picnics, Frisbee golf, and awesome music festivals such as the:

- Eco-friendly **Outside Lands Music & Arts Festival** (think: **Red Hot Chili Peppers, Kanye West, Tom Petty, Macklemore**), and

Dry Branch Fire Squad performing at the Hardly Strictly Bluegrass festival in Golden Gate Park, which is held annually the first weekend in October. PHOTO: GREY3K (OWN WORK)

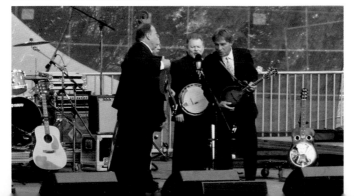

- **Hardly Strictly Bluegrass** festival (think: **Emmylou Harris, The Blind Boys of Alabama**), a free, non-commercial music festival, held every year in October since 2001, founded and subsidized by the late, wonderful Warren Hellman (so we renamed the meadow for him!). Let's do what it takes to keep this festival going!

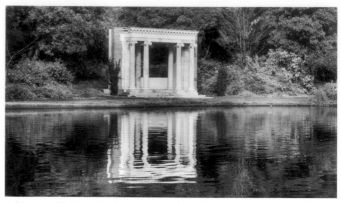

White-marble Portals of the Past earthquake ruins at Lloyd Lake

8. Lloyd Lake and Portals of the Past

Look for the Greek columns across Lloyd Lake to your left. After the 1906 quake and fire these entryway columns were all that remained of Alban Nelson Towne's mansion on Nob Hill. The ruins of City Hall could be seen through the portals. Arnold Genthe snapped a picture of the view, which quickly became an iconic earthquake photo. In 1909 the doorway was dubbed Portals of the Past and moved to the park. (NOTE: Towne's mansion was on California Street where the Masonic Auditorium stands today—you pass it on Walk #2.)

MILE 30

Begins on TRANSVERSE DR at JOHN F. KENNEDY DR

. . . .

Go right on TRANSVERSE DR (no street sign but there is a 49 Mile marker)

Next stop sign, at the intersection with MIDDLE DR, cross street, turn left to continue on TRANSVERSE DR

Next stop sign, left on MLK

Continue on MLK across CROSSOVER DR (19th AVE)

. . . .

9. Mothers Meadow
501–599 MLK Dr

Offering a grassy field, trees, a playground, and picnic area, Mothers Meadow was originally created as a safe haven for parents and their children when Golden Gate Park formally accommodated more hazardous pastimes in the park, such as racing horses.

. . . .

End at 49 MILE MARKER

. . . .

The walk ends at the 49 Mile marker at the intersection of MLK Drive and Stow Lake Drive, just below Stow Lake, but feel free to finish your afternoon off with a stroll through the Botanical Garden or grab a snack at the Tea Garden before heading back (they both can be found by walking a bit farther on MLK Drive past the 49 Mile marker). Walk 11 covers the Japanese Tea Garden and the museums around the Music Concourse.

d. The San Francisco Botanical Garden
entrance on JFK Dr (1199 9th Ave)

Formerly Strybing Arboretum, the Botanical Garden was named for Helene Strybing who willed funds for its creation in 1926. San Francisco's unique microclimate allows the garden to re-create conditions of the high-elevation tropical cloud forests, thus allowing them to grow and conserve plants from all over the world. 55 acres. 8,000 plants. (Free for SF residents with ID)

WALK BACK LOOP SCOOP

A quick Muni ride or walk along Lincoln Blvd will have you back to the beginning quickly, or, to spend more time in the park, take the designated walk-back loop.

NEED TO KNOW

TO GET THERE
Muni N, 29

PARKING
Parking in Golden Gate Park can be very crowded on weekends, in which case you may have to look all along the beginning of the route: Middle Drive West, Martin Luther King Jr. Drive, or Chain of Lakes Drive. During less crowded times, there will be plenty of street parking right by the beginning of the walk.

PUBLIC RESTROOMS
- JFK Dr., 1 block west of Chain of Lakes Dr
- Angler's Lodge (off JFK)
- JFK Dr. outside SF Model Yacht Club
- Lindley Meadow (off JFK)
- Mother's Playground, MLK (past 19th)
- South Polo Field (Middle Dr West)

TURN–BY–TURN INSTRUCTIONS
Begin: MARTIN LUTHER KING JR DR (MLK) at SUNSET BLVD
- Continuing from SUNSET BLVD on Walk 9, turn Left (west) on MLK DR

- Right on CHAIN OF LAKES
- Cross the street and turn right on JOHN F. KENNEDY DR
- Take detour east on JFK DR, veering left with the road around the median toward Spreckels Lake
- Continue on JFK DR to TRANSVERSE DR (the street just before the PARK PRESIDIO BLVD overpass bridge)
- Go right on TRANSVERSE DR (no street sign but there is a 49 Mile marker)
- Next stop sign, at the intersection with MIDDLE DR, cross street, turn left to continue on TRANSVERSE DR
- Next stop sign, left on MLK
- Continue on MLK across CROSSOVER DR (19th AVE)
  - Pass the playground on your left
  - At the intersection with STOW LAKE DR you'll see the 49 Mile marker pointing to the Stow Lake entrance (the sign comes before the entrance of the arboretum farther up on your right and the Japanese Tea Garden to your left.

End: 49 MILE MARKER on MARTIN LUTHER KING JR DR at STOW LAKE DR

HOW TO GET BACK
Muni
- Walk to NW corner 19th Ave & LINCOLN WAY
- Board bus 29 (toward FITZGERALD AVE)
- Get off at SUNSET BLVD and IRVING ST

Other Muni routes: 5, 21, 44, 71

OPTIONAL WALK–BACK LOOP DIRECTIONS
Distance: 1.5 miles, 3,400 steps, 30 minutes

Rating:

Begin: MLK DR below Stow Lake (U-turn back the way you came)
- Head toward CROSSOVER DR (19th AVE)
- Cross over 19th AVE
- Right on TRANSVERSE DR
- Veer left on MIDDLE DR
- You'll pass above the Polo Fields on your right
- Left on MLK JR DR

End: MLK DR and SUNSET BLVD

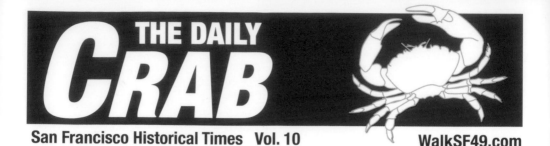

ROBBING THE PARK FROM THE PEOPLE!

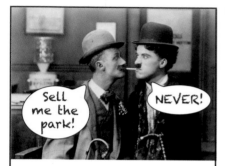

Charlie **Chaplin**, seen here in *His New Job*, filmed part of *A Jitney Elopement* in the western end of **Golden Gate Park**, which includes scenes of the **Murphy Windmill** blades turning and a high-speed chase along an unpaved **Great Highway**.
—Sparkletack.com

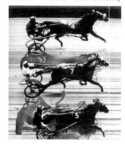

"**C**urmudgeon with a heart of gold," is how **Herb Caen** described Golden Gate Park historian, enthusiast, and protector, **William H. Clary**. Clary's books document the many, many ways greedy folks have tried to use GG park—which people like us paid for, built, and desperately need in the crowded City—for their personal profit, or political agendas, or ego fulfillment. Clary points to examples, such as:

1. The **"Big Four Robber Barons"**—Stanford, Hopkins, Huntington, and Crocker—trying to build their own racetrack in the Park
2. An SF Supervisor trying to sell off two blocks of the park to housing developers
3. A dishonest contractor trying to convince the City that the Park's hills should be leveled to create a flat landscape… of course, he would get the contract to do the work and the resulting sand and rubble would be the free landfill he needed for another project
4. Wealthy people "donating" statues, monuments, and buildings to the park—usually named after themselves and for which they get tax write-offs—which the City then has to pay to maintain forever
5. Our **Board of Supervisors** giving away pieces of the Park each time a new museum or recreational or Expo site is needed—instead of procuring land elsewhere in the city for it!

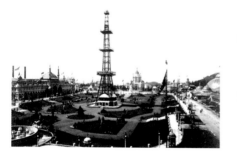

Park superintendent John McLaren did not approve of tearing up 20 acres of parkland to build the **1894 California Midwinter International Expo** (pictured above). To his horror, the expo quickly ballooned to 160 acres with hundreds of temporary structures built to represent cultures from around the world.

But to the delight of 2 million visitors, a 50¢ admission let you enter an exotic fantasyland including colorful minarets, castles, pyramids, igloos, a Hawaiian volcano, Cairo street scenes

with camels, African villages with topless natives, and a gold mine with stagecoach rides (robbed daily by bandits). Additional 10¢–25¢ tickets bought amusement rides (Dante's Inferno, the Haunted Swing), dances, picnics, concerts, acrobat and animal shows (oops, Parnell the Man-Eating Lion killed one of his trainers).

Afterward McLaren tore up and replanted every inch he could. The Music Concourse area is all that remains today.

DISNEYLAND SF?

The early creators of the park envisioned wide-open spaces, a retreat from city crowds and noise. But by the turn of the century, **Golden Gate Park** brimmed with attractions ranging

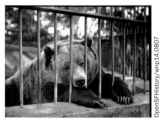

Monarch the Bear was the model for the bear on the California state flag. The bear pit was situated near the west end of what is now AIDS Memorial Grove. By H.S. Hoyt.

from wild animals (elk, moose, caribou, bear, zebra, camel, elephant), birds (chickens, ostriches, pheasants, peacocks), and lush plantings to museums and numerous recreational and athletic activities. Despite its location far from where the populace lived, everyone came.

One weekend in 1886, streetcars delivered **47,000 people to Golden Gate Park in a single afternoon** (out of a population of 250,000 in the city).

Today, Golden Gate Park hosts **13 million visitors each year** and ranks the third most visited park in America—beaten only by **New York's Central Park** and **Chicago's Lincoln Park.**

—SFHistoryEncyclopedia.com

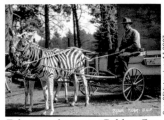

Zebras and cart in Golden Gate Park (circa 1925)

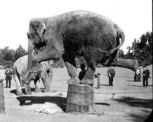

Elephants performing at Children's Playground, by T. H. McAllister

FROM DUST TO LUSH. *How on earth did they do it?*

In 1870, engineer **W. H. Hall** created the blueprint for Golden Gate Park. In 1887, Hall hired **John McLaren**, a horticulturalist trained in Scotland's world-class gardens. Together these tenacious visionaries:

- started by planting grasses, such as barley and yellow lupine, which can grow in sand
- scoured the world for trees and shrubs that could tolerate the conditions

- planted 155,000 trees (by 1889), mostly eucalyptus
- designed winding roads to slow down the ocean winds
- built an engineering wonder of an irrigation system, powered by windmills (for a time)
- constantly fought off politicians and entrepreneurial schemes to sell or repurpose the land

With the help of 400 gardeners and the vocal support of San

Franciscans, they succeeded in creating this 1,017-acre park of gardens, playgrounds, lakes, picnic groves, trails, monuments, and athletic fields for all of us to enjoy. Today their work continues under the jurisdiction of the **SF Recreation and Park Department**, which hires hundreds of gardeners to maintain over 220 parks, playgrounds, and open spaces throughout San Francisco and two outside the city limits.

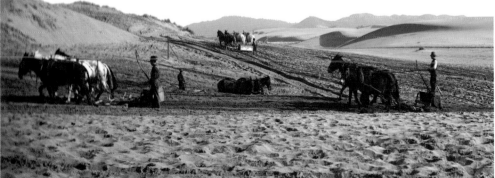

Crews grading the Outsidelands sand dunes (future Richmond District) to create Golden Gate Park

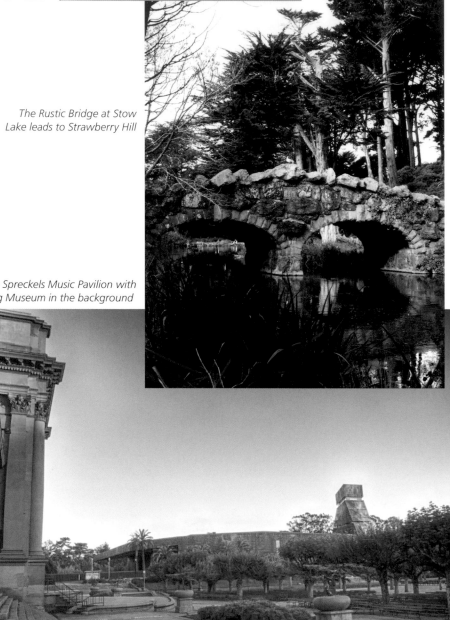

The Rustic Bridge at Stow Lake leads to Strawberry Hill

Profile of the Spreckels Music Pavilion with the de Young Museum in the background

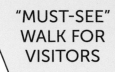
Wow, a jam-packed 2.8 miles of scenic, historic, cultural, and recreational San Francisco awaits you on the second Golden Gate Park walk, the entertainment and attraction eastern half of the park. Today, you'll complete a loop around Stow Lake, skirt passed the museums, Japanese Tea Garden, and band shell that sit on the site of the 1894 California Midwinter International Exposition, peek in at the country's oldest lawn bowling club, and pay homage to the Oakland Raider's and San Francisco 49er's first stadium. Except for the walk up to Stow Lake and the stairs back down, this walk is a flat, easy, eye-catching meander through the heart of the park. Nice!

For visitors who want to see more of SF's famous sites, there are a number of mini-loop options such as crossing to Strawberry Hill on Stow Lake; the Midwinter Expo loop with close-ups of the de Young Museum and Academy of Sciences; the Memorial AIDS Grove detour; and a quick peek at the 1912 wooden-horse carousel.

The end of the walk gives you a number of options also. You can simply cross the street to begin your own exploration of the Haight–Ashbury District. Or take our scenic loop back with a quick trip down Haight and the Panhandle, back through the park past the Conservatory of Flowers and Dahlia Garden on JFK Drive, and through the Midwinter Expo mini-loop on Music Concourse Drive and end your walk with tea at the Japanese Tea Garden (admission required). HINT: You can also stop by the de Young Museum for a free elevator ride to the observation deck, which has great views, including of the living roof on the Academy of Sciences building across the plaza. Or hop on Maya Angelou's old Muni line back to the beginning.

Bottom line: Superintendent John McLaren fought till he was 96 years old to transform this sand dune, waste land into an outdoor space of lakes, trees, flowers, and green, open park space for the likes of you and me—the least we can do is get out and enjoy it.

Begin: Martin Luther King Jr Drive at
Stow Lake Drive

End: Stanyan Street at Frederick Street

Distance: ROUTE: 2.8 miles — 5,500 steps — 1:00 hour
LOOP BACK: 2.4 miles — 4,800 steps — 50 minutes

Hill Rating:

Sites you will pass on today's walk include:

MILE 31
1. **Stow Lake**
   50 Stow Lake Dr

a. **Strawberry Hill**

MILE 32

DETOUR

(Option: View these at the beginning of the walk or on the walk-back loop.)

2. **Japanese Tea Garden** 75 Hagiwara Tea Garden Dr

3. **De Young Museum** 50 Hagiwara Tea Garden Dr

4. **Spreckels Temple of Music and Music Concourse**

5. **California Academy of Sciences** 55 Music Concourse Dr

DETOUR
6. **National AIDS Memorial Grove** Nancy Pelosi Dr

7. **San Francisco Lawn Bowling Club** Bowling Green Dr

DETOUR
8. **Koret Children's Quarter Playground** MLK Dr

MILE 33
9. **Kezar Stadium** 670 Kezar Dr

10. **McLaren Lodge** in the park, near Stanyan St and Fell St

11. **Haight Street**

WALK-BACK LOOP
b. **Amoeba Music** 1855 Haight St

c. **The Panhandle** between Oak St and Fell St

Hidden Stairways
The 49 mile route crosses over a few of the city stairways that are so wonderfully detailed in **Adah Bakalinsky's** *Stairway Walks in San Francisco*— such as at Stow Lake and on the Twin Peaks Walk 13.

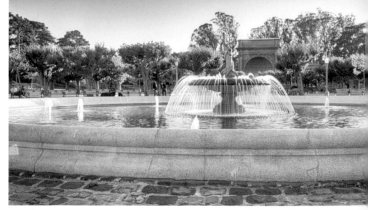

The Music Concourse's central fountain, Rideout Fountain, was built in 1924.

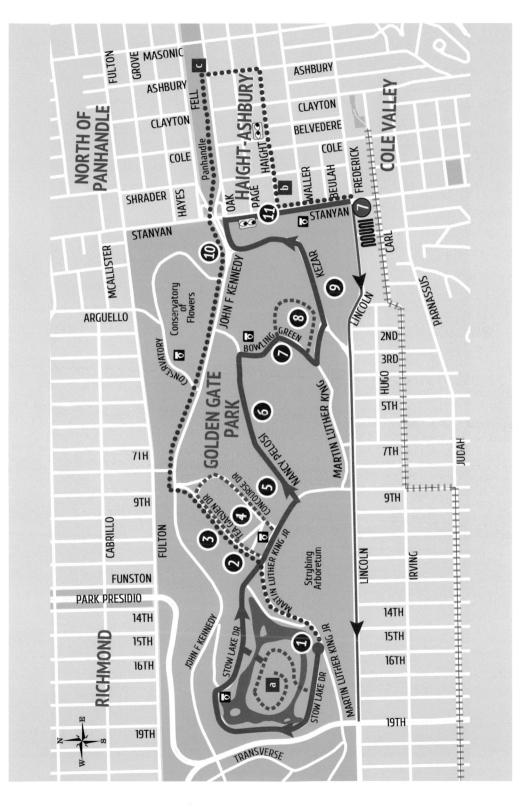

MILE 31

Begins at entry sign to STOW LAKE on MLK DR

· · · · · · · · · · · · · · · · · ·

Turn left

Follow the 49 MILE MARKER up STOW LAKE DR

(NOTE: The sidewalk begins about 50 ft. up on your right.)

Circle the lake clockwise

· · · · · · · · · · · · · · · · · ·

1.   Stow Lake
    50 Stow Lake Dr

The largest man-made lake in the park provides an oasis for picnickers, plus paddleboat, rowboat, bike, and surrey rentals, and a refreshment stand for visitors. Ducks, geese, and turtles call the lake home. In April, May, and June, blue herons build their nests in the trees near the boathouse. Strawberry Hill in its center hosts a concrete pagoda (a gift from San Francisco's sister city, Taipei, in 1981 to commemorate early Chinese settlers), an electrically pumped waterfall, the ruins of a pre-quake observatory, and, at top, views of the Golden Gate Bridge and a reservoir that supplies water hydrants in the city.

MINI-LOOP OPTION
a.   Strawberry Hill

Situated in the middle of Stow Lake and measuring 430 feet

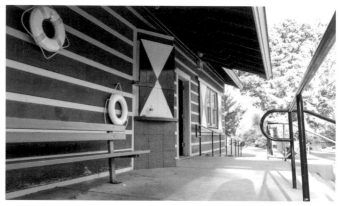

Stow Lake Boathouse

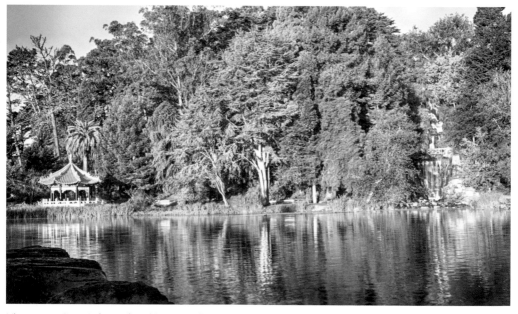

View across Stow Lake to the Chinese Pavilion on Strawberry Hill

high, the island rises as the highest point in the park.

- Cross the Rustic Bridge or the Roman Bridge on either side of the lake.

- Hike the stairs or trail to the top to see views of the Golden Gate Bridge and Mount Tamalpais to the north or the Transamerica Pyramid downtown.

- Or follow the path around the bottom of the island past the waterfall and Chinese Pavilion, where you are welcome to stop for a moment of meditation if you like.

- Cross the same bridge you began with and continue on the route.

Continue circling the lake clockwise

Pass the BOATHOUSE, pass the BRIDGE

As the road makes a sharp right to follow the lake, head to your Left

On your left you'll find a pedestrian stairway leading down to the JAPANESE TEA GARDEN

Follow the stair and path to MLK DR, turn Left on MLK DR

Fit & Fabulous

If you see a group of toned and fit men and women running in little black dresses, you've stumbled upon Frontrunners, the nations first LGBT running club. Most weeks they wear regular jogging clothes as 25–100 runners meet across from the Stow Lake Boathouse on Saturday mornings to walk or run one- to five-mile routes. Founded in 1973, Frontrunners inspired a worldwide network of clubs. Its annual Pride Run raises funds for a different community nonprofit each year.

MILE 32

Begins on MLK DR at HAGIWARA TEA GARDEN DR

Head east on MLK DR, or take detour

DETOUR:

MIDWINTER EXPO LOOP

- Turn left on HAGIWARA TEA GARDEN DR.

- Walk past the de Young Museum.

- Follow TEA GARDEN DR clockwise to CONCOURSE DR.

- Pass the Academy of Sciences.

- Left on MLK DR to rejoin the route

You can walk the Midwinter Expor Loop at the beginning of this walk and return to the main route, or view it as part of the larger return loop through the park at the end of the walk.

2. Japanese Tea Garden (on Midwinter Expo loop) 75 Hagiwara Tea Garden Dr

The oldest public Japanese garden in the United States was created in Golden Gate Park as a Japanese village for the 1894 expo. The exhibit proved so popular that the city hired Makoto Hagiwara to turn it into a permanent tea garden. Makoto invented the fortune cookie here. Today the garden's five acres of Japanese landscaping include a teahouse, Zen garden, pagoda, drum bridge, and moments of pure tranquility. The cherry trees blossom in March and April. Free admission before 10:00 a.m. on Mon., Wed., Fri.

The California Midwinter International Exposition of 1894 was the brainchild of *San Francisco Chronicle* newspaper founder M.H. de Young. He hoped it would stimulate the economy and show off San Francisco's mild climate. Remnants of that event include the eponymous de Young Museum, Music Concourse, and Japanese Tea Garden. The Academy of Sciences moved here in 1916.

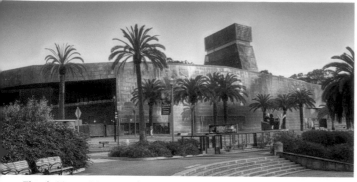

The de Young Museum showcases American art from the 17th through the 21st centuries.

3. De Young Museum (on Midwinter Expo loop) 50 Hagiwara Tea Garden Dr

Another remnant of the 1894 Midwinter Expo, this fine art museum was originally guided by *SF Chronicle* co-owner, M. H. de Young, and was renamed for him in 1921. The original Egyptian motif building gave way to a modern structure in 2005, including an entirely copper exterior and an earthquake-withstanding ball-bearing system that will allow the building to safely slide three feet. (Muni riders get a discount on admission price. Yay, Muni!)

> **FREE CONCERTS ON SUNDAYS: APRIL–OCT., 1 P.M.**

4. Spreckels Temple of Music, the Bandshell (on Midwinter Expo loop)

The Spreckels Temple of Music and the open-air plaza have served as a stage for numerous performers over the years from Luciano Pavarotti and the Grateful Dead to impromptu gatherings like the **Ukulele**

Fortune Cookie Court

As all San Franciscans know, Makoto Hagiwara invented the modern-day fortune cookie when he adapted and begin serving a version of Japanese "fortune tea cakes" in the Japanese Tea Garden at the 1894 Midwinter Expo. However, two jealous rivals, Seiichi Kito, the founder of Fugetsu-Do of Little Tokyo in Los Angeles, and David Jung, founder of the Hong Kong Noodle Company in Los Angeles, both claimed that they had invented the cookie. Ha!

Let the court decide! San Francisco's mock Court of Historical Review, presided over by a real-life federal judge from San Francisco, attempted to settle the dispute in 1983. A summary of the brilliant case made by SF follows:

SF Attorney: "First, your honor, we can show that Japanese bakeries in LA and SF sold the confections to Chinese restaurants until WWII, when 11,000 Japanese were interred, and Chinese bakeries took over making the cookie."

"Second, we would like to submit this fortune cookie into evidence. Would you please open it and read the fortune to the court."

Judge (opens cookie, reads fortune): "'S.F. Judge who rules for L.A. Not Very Smart Cookie.'" After reviewing the evidence I rule that the fortune cookie originated with Makoto Hagiwara of San Francisco."

Sound effects: Gavel bangs. Court erupts in applause.

To save face, the city of Los Angeles subsequently condemned the decision—but San Franciscans know the truth—and we love our activist judges!

—*The History of the Fortune Cookie*, by Borgna Brunner

Rebellion Meet Up Group. The Golden Gate Park Band, currently under the direction of Michael L. Wirgler, has been giving free band concerts here since 1882.

5. California Academy of Sciences (on Midwinter Expo loop)
55 Music Concourse Dr

The museum of natural history, Steinhart Aquarium, and Morrison Planetarium were completely rebuilt in 2008. In addition to the totally cool albino alligator, rain forest dome, and new planetarium show, the academy boasts an environmentally friendly building. With features such as wall insulation made from scraps of denim, the use of recycled water, and a 2.5-acre rooftop garden, it became the world's greenest museum and the largest public building in the world to receive a Platinum environmental rating.

Orson Welles shot a scene from *The Lady from Shanghai* (1947) in Steinhart Aquarium, the old Academy of Sciences building.

. . . .

Continue east on MLK DR

Left on NANCY PELOSI DR (formerly Middle Dr, backside of the academy)

Right on BOWLING GREEN DR, or take detour

. . . .

DETOUR

As you approach Bowling Green Dr, veer right and follow the paved path down to the AIDS Grove, then come back out the other side onto Bowling Green, turning right to continue on route.

San Francisco Lawn Bowling Clubhouse

6. National AIDS Memorial Grove
Nancy Pelosi Dr

The grove is a dedicated space and place in the national landscape where the millions of Americans touched directly or indirectly by AIDS can gather to heal, hope, and remember. Thousands of community volunteers and many generous donors have helped create, maintain, and improve its gardens since 1988.

7. San Francisco Lawn Bowling Club & Field
Bowling Green Dr

Established in 1901, the San Francisco Lawn Bowling Club holds the title as America's oldest municipal lawn bowling club. (HINT: Grab a free lesson on Wednesdays at noon.)

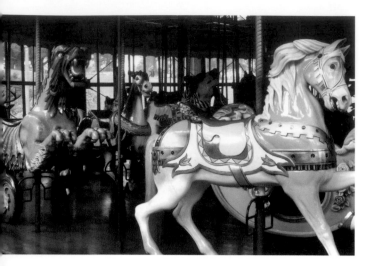

MILE 33

Begins on KEZAR DR at MLK DR

· · · · · · · · · · · · · · · · · ·

Left on MLK DR

Cross the street at KEZAR DR

Left on KEZAR DR, using the official bike/walking path on the right-hand side

Continue on KEZAR DR out of the park

· · · · · · · · · · · · · · · · · ·

DETOUR

8. Koret Children's Quarter, formerly the Children's Playground MLK Dr

Built in 1888 this playground may be the first public playground in the nation and is certainly the oldest and biggest in the city. It features a revamped 1912 Herschell-Spillman carousel. To see the hand-carved carousel animals up close:

> From BOWLING GREEN AVE, as you pass the lawn bowling area, cross the crosswalk on BOWLING GREEN.
> Walk through the parking lot, veering right toward the stone Sharon Art Building.
> Go around the Sharon Art Building; the carousel is behind it.
> Return the way you came to BOWLING GREEN AVE.
> Turn left on BOWLING GREEN AVE to rejoin route.

9. Kezar Stadium
670 Kezar Dr

Named for Kezar family pioneers, this stadium opened in 1925 and has remained "sports central" for nearly 90 years. It has hosted track-and-field competitions, motorcycle racing, auto racing, rugby, lacrosse, soccer, baseball, boxing, cricket, Gaelic football, women's football, high school and college football, and the NFL—plus community events, like music concerts, and movie shoots! A smaller, upgraded 10,000-seat stadium replaced the original 60,000-seat stadium in 1989.

The denouement of *Dirty Harry* (1971) with Clint Eastwood takes place in Kezar Stadium. (Clint was born in SF in 1930.)

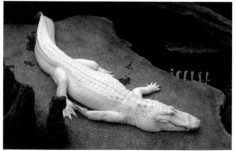

Claude, the albino alligator, lives at the Academy of Sciences. Born in 1995 weighing 2 ounces, today he is 9 feet 5 inches long and has 76 teeth.

10. McLaren Lodge
in the park, near
Stanyan St and Fell St

Park superintendent John McLaren lived in this lodge from 1896 until his death in 1943. The Moorish-Gothic design includes exterior walls of 18-inch-thick ashlar basalt masonry and sandstone quoins (corner blocks). At McLaren's request the ginormous cypress tree in front sparkles with Christmas lights each December. Today it holds the Recreation and Parks Department office.

Right on STANYAN ST

11. Haight Street (as in Haight-Ashbury)

It's time to "turn on, tune in, and drop out" or go shopping. The Haight-Ashbury District grabbed the nation's attention as the center of the 1960s free love, free thought, free drugs, and psychedelic hippie revolution. The 1967 Summer of Love drew youth here from

Maya Angelou: A Muni First

In 1944, 16-year-old Maya Angelou (who later became a renown poet and author) sat in the Market Street Railway Co. office every day for two weeks, seeking her dream job. Finally a man came out of the office and asked her why she wanted the job. Her response, "Because I like the attractive fitted uniforms and I like people," earned her a job as the first female African American streetcar conductor in San Francisco.

Before World War II, nearly all city employees were white. But owing to the shortage of civilian workers during the war, Muni, along with its private competitor, the Market Street Railway Co., began hiring African Americans. Through Maya doesn't specify, she likely worked the 7-Haight line—which is the Muni bus we suggest you would take back to the beginning of Walk 11.

—StreetCar.org

McLaren Lodge

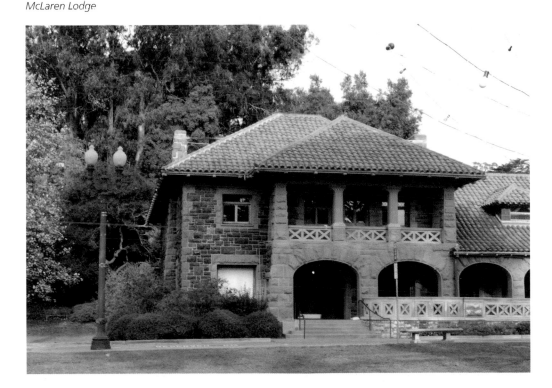

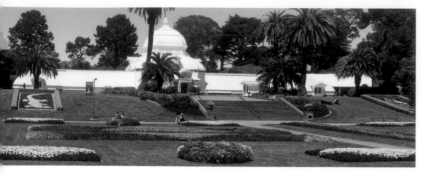

On your walk back take a gander at the Conservatory of Flowers—a greenhouse and botanical garden that houses a collection of rare and exotic plants and is the oldest existing public conservatory in the Western Hemisphere.

all over the country. Janis Joplin and members of Jefferson Airplane and the Grateful Dead all lived here. Today it still has a bohemian ambience with a thriving center of independent local businesses—though lots of chain stores are popping up.

Lovin' the Haight

The Haight, as locals call it (pronounced "hate"), began as a resort area where the wealthy built their summer homes. It was untouched by the 1906 earthquake. The neighborhood declined during the Depression, became the inexpensive housing option for African Americans moving in for wartime jobs, then cheap housing for the growing youth culture of beats, followed by hippies, on to punk and rave, and then circled back to more mainstream shops.

WALK–BACK LOOP SCOOP

The historic 49 Mile Scenic Drive continues on a five-mile uphill climb to the top of Twin Peaks from here (Walks 12 and 13). But if you'd rather take a break, and get a full San Francisco experience of this neighborhood, take this walk-back loop through the historic hippie Haight-Ashbury District for some good eats and one-of-a-kind shopping opportunities, and then meander back through a different section of Golden Gate Park past the SF Conservatory of Flowers and Dahlia Garden.

b. Amoeba Music 1855 Haight St

Located in a converted bowling alley since 1990, Amoeba Music sells hundreds of thousands of music titles, some on actual records. Records: 12-inch-round vinyl discs on which music can be recorded and played.

c. The Panhandle between Oak St and Fell St

This ¾-mile-long-by-one block wide sliver of grassy park at the far, east end of Golden Gate Park was the experimental strip of land used to test suitable plants for the park sand dunes. It is on the northern border of the Haight-Ashbury District. (Note the basketball court named for former Golden Gate Warrior Nate Thurman, the first player in NBA history to record an official quadruple-double.)

The Conservatory of Flowers appears in the movie *Harold and Maude* (1971).

END at STANYAN ST at FREDERICK ST (edge of park)

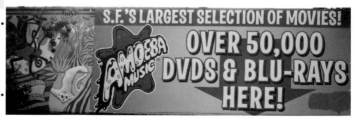

WALK 11 NEED TO KNOW

TO GET THERE
Muni N, 5, 21,44, 71

PARKING
Street Parking is available on MLK BLVD and can be very easy at the Stow Lake Boathouse. Parking can be difficult on weekends during the high tourist season.

There is also paid parking at the underground Golden Gate Parking Garage (1 Music Concourse Dr). South entrance: From Martin Luther King Dr turn onto Music Concourse Drive.

PUBLIC RESTROOMS
- Stow Lake, behind the boathouse
- Bands Shell (78 Music Concourse)
- Tennis courts (at Pelosi and Bowling Green)
- Stanyan (Waller)
- Conservatory of Flowers (Conservatory Dr)

TURN–BY–TURN INSTRUCTIONS
Begin: MARTIN LUTHER KING JR (MLK) DR at STOW LAKE ENTRANCE

- Turn left to follow the 49 MILE MARKER up STOW LAKE DR
  - (NOTE: The sidewalk begins about 50 ft. up on your right.)
- Circle the lake clockwise

- Pass the BOATHOUSE, pass the HISTORIC BRIDGE
- As the road makes a sharp right to follow the lake, head to your left
- On your left you'll find a pedestrian stairway leading down to the Japanese Tea Garden
- Follow the stair and path to MLK DR, turn left on MLK DR
- Left on NANCY PELOSI (formerly Middle Dr, backside of the academy)
- Right on BOWLING GREEN DR
- Left on MLK DR
- Cross the street at KEZAR DR
- Left on KEZAR DR, using the official bike/walking path on the right hand side
- Continue on KEZAR DR out of the park
- Right on STANYAN ST

End: STANYAN ST at FREDERICK ST (edge of park)

HOW TO GET BACK
Muni

- Walk to the north corner of HAIGHT ST and STANYAN ST
- Board Muni 71 (toward Ortega St)
- Get off at LINCOLN ST and 9th AVE walk into park to TEA GARDEN DR

See also free Weekend/ Holiday park shuttle

Other Muni routes: 5,21,33,71

OPTIONAL WALK-BACK LOOP
Distance: 2.4 miles, 4,800 steps, 50 minutes

Rating:

Begin: FREDERICK ST and STANYON ST

- Turn around. Backtrack to HAIGHT ST
- Right on HAIGHT ST
- Left on ASHBURY ST
- Cross OAK ST into PARK PANHANDLE
- Turn left on the first PATH in the PANHANDLE
  - The south side of park is for pedestrians, the north side for bicycles
- Take path to end of PANHANDLE
- Cross over to STANYON ST at the traffic light into GOLDEN GATE PARK
  - FELL turns into JOHN F KENNEDY in the park
- Follow JFK DR
- Left on HAGIWARA TEA GARDEN DR
- Right on MLK DR back to

End: MLK DR at STOW LAKE DR

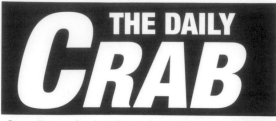

THE DAILY CRAB

San Francisco Historical Times Vol. 11

Cyclists Rule Golden Gate Park!

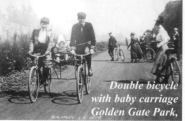

Double bicycle with baby carriage Golden Gate Park,

NEWFANGLED AND DANGEROUS!

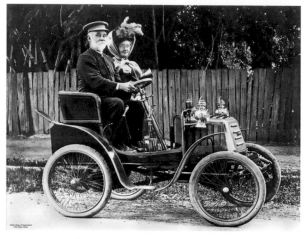

Initially the city banned those "fast and noisy machines that frighten horses and bicyclists" from Golden Gate Park. Finally, in 1904, automobiles were admitted into the park through the Page Street Gate —and they've been scaring horses and bicyclists ever since.

This couple looks well dressed for a spin in a 1902 Linon voiturette with a single cylinder, 3½-horsepower De Dion-Bouton engine, made in Belgium. (photo location unknown)

WAR & PEACE

The **Hagiwara family** lived in and maintained the **Japanese Tea Garden** until 1942, when Executive Order 9066 forced them to relocate to an internment camp with thousands of other Japanese American families. The garden was renamed the "Oriental Tea Garden" and fell into disarray.

In 1949, the **S & G Gump Company** gave the garden a large bronze Buddha (originally cast in Tajima, Japan, in 1790). The city officially reinstated the name Japanese Tea Garden in 1952. In 1953, the Zen Garden, designed by **Nagao Sakurai**, and a 9,000-pound Lantern of Peace were added as a goodwill gesture.

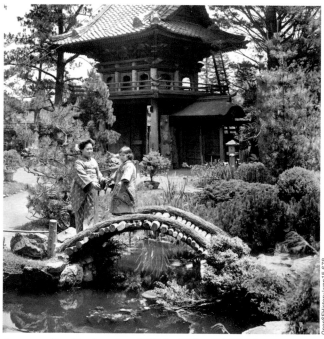

Japanese Tea Garden circa 1912 by Willard E. Worden

DAMN DALLAS COWBOYS!

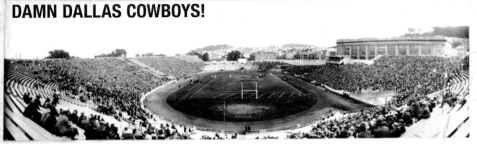

Courtesy of San Francisco History Center, San Francisco Public Library

Football game at Kezar Stadium, 1948

Both the **San Francisco 49ers** and the **Oakland Raiders** held their opening seasons at Kezar Stadium. After SF lost the 1970 NFC Championship to the **Dallas Cowboys**, 17–10, we moved to Candlestick on January 3, 1971. The Cowboys took us down again in '71 and '72, but in 1981 we came back with "The Catch"— 49er **Joe Montana**'s game-winning pass to **Dwight Clark** in the final minute of the NFC Championship Game—one of the most famous games in NFL history. By the time the Niners left for Santa Clara's Levi's Stadium in 2014, we were tied with Dallas at **five Super Bowl rings each.** The rivalry continues.

COVER UP

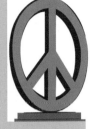

Golden Gate Park founding superintendents **William Hammond Hall** and **John McLaren** firmly believed that statuary does not belong in a pastoral park. Each time a statue was installed in the park, McLaren planted bushes all around it, letting nature envelop the statue as quickly as possible.

In honor of McLaren's 65th birthday, the city gifted him with a life statue of himself! Horrified, he hid it in a box, and it was not seen again until after he died.

After McLaren's death, the statues hidden under his reign were rediscovered, trees and hedges were trimmed to reveal the artworks, and the press was invited to make them known to a generation who hadn't seen them before. Today, the park discourages installation of monuments, suggesting in-

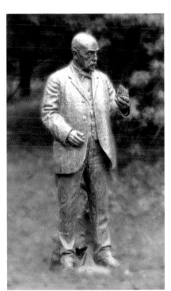

John McLaren, by Melvin Earl Cummings

stead that donations be directed toward enhancement of the existing park.

Of note, unlike every other statue in the park, McLaren's likeness stands directly on the ground instead of on a pedestal.

REJECTED

Proposed statues that didn't make it into the park include:

- **Peace Sign:** 24-foot-high stainless steel, in the Panhandle—rejected because it would draw a "bad element"
- **Vasco Núñez de Balboa:** a monument to the explorer, looking out over the Pacific—rejected because the Spanish-American War kicked up anti-Spanish sentiment
- **Leif Eriksson:** a heroic-size statue of the Scandinavian explorer—rejected because the Depression wiped out the funds

"Who Are You Calling Old, Sonny?"

When park superintendent **John McLaren** refused to retire from his city job at the customary age of 60, he received a public outpouring of support. When he reached age 70, the city gave up and passed a charter amendment exempting him from forced retirement. He lived in and managed the park until his death in 1943 at age 96.

49
MILE

SCENIC
DRIVE

Cole Valley

UCSF

Laguna Honda

Garden for the Environment

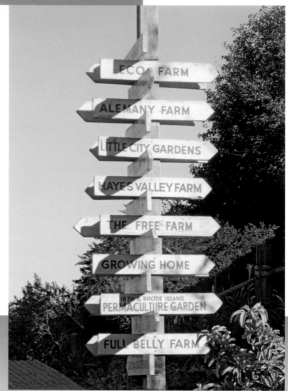

View of Kezar Stadium, St. Ignatius Church, and downtown from UCSF

Are you up for a vigorous three-mile climb to the base of Twin Peaks today? This segment of the Historic 49 mile route connects Golden Gate Park with Twin Peaks via a few neighborhoods tourists rarely visit. You'll start at the edge of Haight-Ashbury and Cole Valley, pass the campus of the second-largest employer in the city, and see life in the fashionable, foggy, family-friendly Inner Sunset.

On the trek up Mount Sutro, via traffic-heavy Laguna Honda Boulevard, you'll get a glimpse of Sutro Tower and the Laguna Honda Forest and Reservoir (and find out if it's real or man-made), plus learn the history of the giant green retaining wall on 7th Avenue, and pass the oldest subway station west of Chicago.

If you can handle this uphill trek with ease, you are welcome to continue on for another mile of steep off-road hiking all the way to the top of Twin Peaks to one of the best viewing spots in the entire city (see Walk 13 for details). Or save the full Twin Peaks walk for another day and trek back to Golden Gate Park over hilly, sleepy Clarendon Heights to quaint, quiet Cole Valley for lunch or a well-deserved treat.

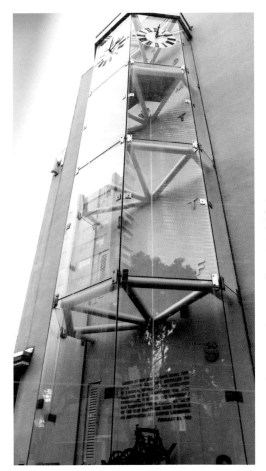

Peek inside the UCSF Clock Tower

Begin: Stanyan Street at Frederick Street (edge of GG Park)
End: Portola Drive at Twin Peaks Boulevard
(bottom of Twin Peaks)
Distance: ROUTE: 2.4 miles — 4,800 steps — 50 minutes
LOOP BACK: 2.7 miles — 5,000 steps — 1 hour

Hill Rating: **5**

Sites you will pass on today's walk include:

MILE 34

1. **UC San Francisco** 505 Parnassus Ave

2. **Hippocrates Statue** 400 Parnassus Ave

3. **Historic Clock in Toland Tower** 500 Parnassus Ave

4. *Bear and Cubs Statue* 530 Parnassus Ave

THE INNER SUNSET

MILE 35

FOREST KNOLL

5. **Garden for the Environment** 1590 7th Ave

6. **Seasonal Pumpkin Patch and Christmas Tree Lot** 7th Ave and Warren Dr

7. **Giant Green Retaining Wall** 7th Ave

FOREST HILL and FOREST HILL EXTENSION

8. **Laguna Honda Reservoir** Laguna Honda Blvd and Clarendon Ave

MIDTOWN TERRACE

MILE 36

9. **Forest Hill Muni Station** Laguna Honda Blvd

10. **Laguna Honda Hospital** 375 Laguna Honda Blvd

11. **Juvenile Justice Center** 375 Woodside Ave

12. **Ruth Asawa San Francisco School of the Arts** 555 Portola Dr

a. **Glen Park Canyon**

NOTE: Seventh Ave turns into a major, loud, multilane thoroughfare after Lawton St. Fortunately, if you cross to the right-hand (western) side of the street, there is a bike lane between you and the cars, which also gives you space to stop and view Laguna Honda Reservoir.

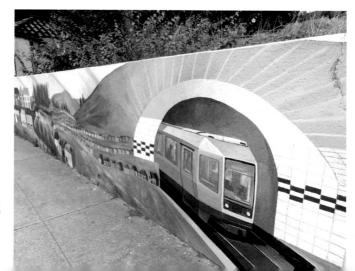

New Precita Eyes mural outside Laguna Honda Hospital

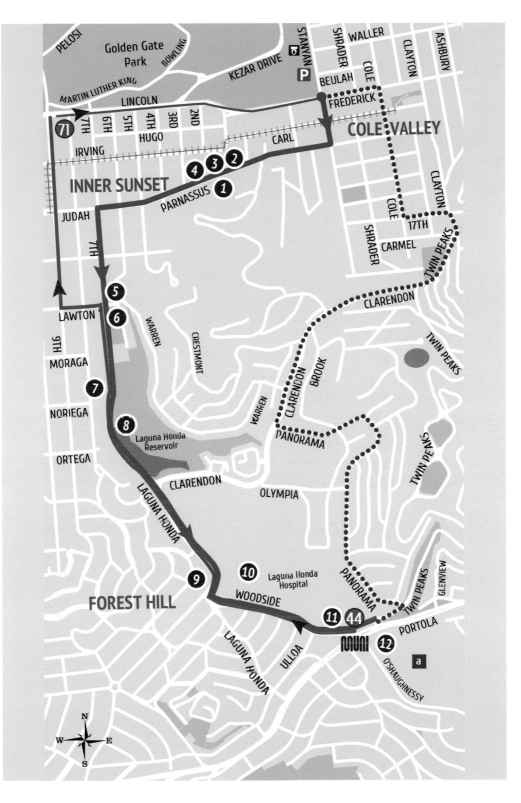

MILE 34

Begins on STANYAN ST at FREDERICK ST (edge of park)

. . . .

Continue from GOLDEN GATE PARK walking south on STANYAN ST

Right on PARNASSUS AVE, staying on the even-numbered north side of the street

. . . .

1. **UC San Francisco**
    most of the buildings you see on Parnassus

One of the 10 University of California campuses, UCSF focuses exclusively on health, specifically research, patient care, and graduate-level education. *U.S. News & World Report* consistently ranks it among the top 10 hospitals in the nation. (NOTE: You will pass two of UCSF's three campuses on the 49 mile walk: Parnassus Heights here on Parnassus and Mission Bay on Walk 16.)

2. **Hippocrates Statue**
    400 Parnassus Ave

Born around 460 B.C., Hippocrates is credited with being the first person to believe that diseases were caused naturally and not as a result of superstition and gods. He believed and argued that disease was not a punishment inflicted by the gods but rather the product of environmental factors, diet, and living habits.

While little is known about who originally wrote it, the Hippocratic Oath has been historically taken by doctors swearing to practice medicine ethically.

In 1987 John Pappas, who immigrated from Greece in 1905, and his wife, Jennie Pappas, donated this statue in appreciation of San Francisco.

3. **Historic Clock in Toland Tower**
    500 Parnassus Ave

The Seth Thomas Clock atop of the 1897 College of Medicine traveled via ship around Cape Horn, South America to get here—and survived the 1906 quake. Today the inner workings of the original clock run three clock faces enclosed in a three-sided glass wall, four stories high, sitting outside the Millberry Union.

4. **Bear and Cubs Statue**
    530 Parnassus Ave

Though UCSF has no sports teams, it does have a mascot, the bear. SF character and artist Benny Bufano sculpted this *Bear and Cubs* in his signature rounded style. Bufano's statues can be found all over the city (you pass his *Penguin's Prayer* on Walk 8).

THE INNER SUNSET

The Inner Sunset—all the homes you see on your right-hand side—has a village-esque

Quick Facts About UCSF
- As the second-largest employer in San Francisco, UCSF generates more than 32,000 jobs.
- On September 15, 1874, the school opened its doors to female students.
- Five UCSF faculty are recipients of the Nobel Prize (for Physiology and Medicine).
- UCSF is training 2,940 students, 1,620 residents, and 1,030 postdoctoral scholars representing 94 countries.
- Mayor Adolph Sutro donated 13 acres for the original hospital in 1898. Today the campus has grown to 107 acres.

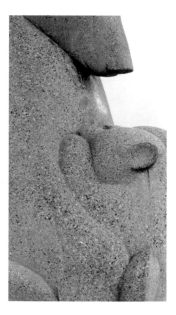

feel created by its walkability and dense commercial corridor centered at 9th Avenue and Irving Street—all shrouded in fog. Yes, it has gentrified, but the *Chronicle Neighborhood Report* agrees it has kept its funky edge, ethnic diversity, and great restaurants. Statistically, the population is about 55% families, 45% homeowners, 23% between ages 25 and 34, 26% foreign born, 53% white, 34% Asian, and 95% high school graduates. Golden Gate Park is their playground. Official borders: Lincoln Way to the north, Arguello Boulevard to the east, Quintara Street to the south, and 19th Avenue to the west.

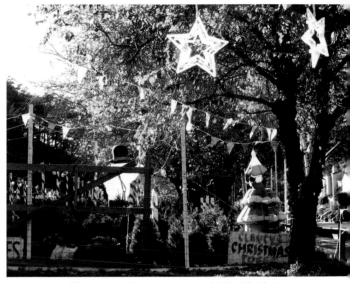

Santa's elves fill the empty lot at Lawton and 7th with Christmas trees every year.

MILE 35

Begins on 7th AVE at PARNASSUS AVE

. . . .

Turn left (south) on 7th AVE

7th AVE turns into LAGUNA HONDA BLVD at LAWTON ST

. . . .

❗ LOOK

SUTRO TOWER VIEW

As you turn onto 7th Avenue look up for a glimpse of the three-pronged, "aviation red"-and-white-colored steel Sutro Tower on the top of Twin Peaks. On Walk 13 you'll climb to a spot pretty close to Sutro Tower—which first opened on July 4, 1973, to enhance the Bay Area's TV viewing and radio listening pleasure. *Thank you!* (Note: If you take the walk-back loop you will be standing almost directly under Sutro Tower in less than an hour from now.)

FOREST KNOLL

To your left (east)—along 7th Avenue between Kirkham and Clarendon—lies Forest Knoll, a truly quiet, tranquil neighborhood snuggled at the foot of steep, forested Mount Sutro next to the UCSF campus.

5. Garden for the Environment
1590 7th Ave

This half-acre urban organic garden offers hands-on composting and sustainable-landscaping classes.

6. Seasonal Pumpkin Patch and Christmas Tree Lot
7th Ave and Warren Dr

Officially named the White Crane Springs Community Garden, this empty lot on 7th Avenue and Warren Drive transforms into a holiday wonderland from October through December.

. . . .

At LAWTON ST, cross 7th AVE—from the garden side of the street to the odd-numbered side

This is the beginning of 1.4 miles of steady uphill climbing

. . . .

TREE-HUGGER HEROES

From the 18th-century explorers to Soviet Union premier Nikita Khrushchev (who visited SF in 1959), people have described the San Franciscan landscape as "treeless." Take a look at the Marin Headlands, Potrero Hill, Twin Peaks, or San Bruno Mountain to get an idea of the grassy, windswept hills the early pioneers first saw. Mike Sullivan describes it well in his book *The Trees of San Francisco*. Even after the tree-planting successes, such as Golden Gate Park, San Francisco streets remained tree-bare until the environmental movement of the 1960s and 1970s. Later Friends of the Urban Forest volunteers began organized, intentional city-street tree planting, and have planted 50,000 trees so far! *Thank you, tree-hugging friends!*

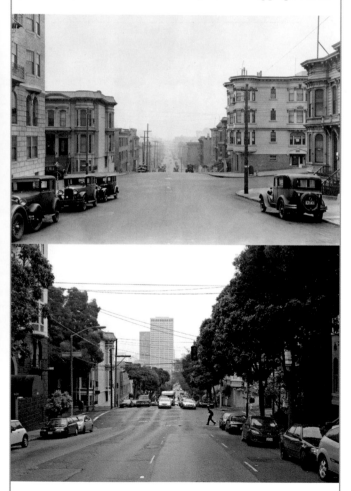

1929 vs. 2010: Street trees have transformed the intersection of Fell and Buchanan Streets (facing east). Images: (top) San Francisco History Center, San Francisco Public Library, (bottom) Hoodline.com

7. Giant Green Retaining Wall
7th Ave

In 1989, the Loma Prieta earthquake caused the sandy soil here to compact and shift, thus severely damaging homes on 8th Avenue. To protect the remaining homes and allow reconstruction of the homes that had to be demolished, the Department of Public Works used Federal Emergency Funds (FEMA) to build this slope stabilization retaining wall.

FOREST HILL AND FOREST HILL EXTENSION

Running from the giant retaining wall to the top of the hill (Portola), the neighborhood you see on the right-hand (western) side of the street is Forest Hill. After the 1906 earthquake, a private firm purchased this area from the heirs of Adolph Sutro and developed Forest Hill. Renowned architects such as Bernard Maybeck, Julia Morgan, Frank Lloyd Wright, and Henry Hill designed many of the homes. All have a view—of either the ocean or downtown.

The unusually wide, curved, and often extravagantly landscaped streets were designed for horse and carriage—not to city street-grading codes—so the city did not begin maintaining them until 1978. One of the least densely populated neighborhoods in San Francisco, Forest Hill has no condominium

or multi-tenancy developments yet has a 100-year-old, active homeowners' association. Forest Hill Extension, located to the south, above it, has more moderately priced and smaller homes.
—Wikipedia.com

8. Laguna Honda Reservoir
Laguna Honda Blvd and Clarendon Ave

You can jog its trails and walk your dog here, but, nope, you can't swim in this lake—because we drink this water (and have been since 1865)! Laguna Honda, which is Spanish for "deep lake," has been modernized with a concrete bottom and a retaining wall, but for the most part, the 19 acres of reservoir land at the base of Mount Sutro, along with the neighboring Laguna Honda Forest (stretched along the west side of Laguna Honda Blvd), have remained a bucolic natural setting for most of the last century. The SF Public Utilities Commission, which manages it, recently cleared a small section for equipment storage. Neighbors weren't too happy about that.

MIDTOWN TERRACE ON YOUR LEFT FROM CLARENDON TO THE END OF THIS WALK

Twin Peaks was once covered in a sea of wildflowers—not a tree to be found—until the

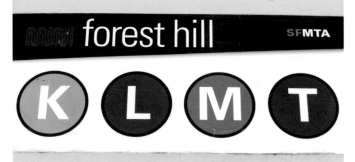

non-native eucalyptus trees planted by Adolph Sutro created Sutro Forest. Carl and Fred Gellert of the Standard Building Company saw that barren landscape on the western side of Twin Peaks and imagined it covered with a new neighborhood. They graded seven levels of streets to give every home a view and built 650 modest single-family homes between 1953 and 1960. No stores, little traffic, almost no Muni service, plenty of trails, great views, starting at $13,000—Midtown Terrace sold out.

MILE 36
Begins at FOREST HILL MUNI STATION

• • • • • • • • • • • • • • • • • •
At the Forest Hill Muni Station crosswalk, cross the street to the Laguna Honda Hospital side of street
• • • • • • • • • • • • • • • • • •

9. Forest Hill Muni Station
Laguna Honda Blvd

This is the oldest subway station west of Chicago. It serves these lines:

Streetcars
• K Ingleside
• L Taraval
• M Ocean View
• S Castro Shuttle
• T Third

Buses
• 36 Teresita
• 43 Masonic
• 44 O'Shaughnessy
• 52 Excelsior
• L Owl

10. Laguna Honda Hospital
375 Laguna Honda Blvd

Opened in 1867 to care for indigent Gold Rush pioneers, today Laguna Honda Hospital and Rehabilitation Center is California's first green-certified hospital. It has 780 beds and provides acute care, skilled nursing care, and rehabilitation care. Managed by the City and County of San Francisco.

Cigarettes Construct Healthy Hospital
The finance package to remodel Laguna Honda Hospital included $141 million in revenue from consumer protection lawsuits filed against the tobacco industry by (former) city attorney Louise Renne in the late 1990s.

. . . .

Follow sidewalk to turn left with LAGUNA HONDA BLVD

which turns into WOODSIDE AVE

Continue on WOODSIDE AVE to the top of the hill

Left on PORTOLA DR
. . . .

NOTE: At the intersection of Portola and Woodside, two taxpayer-supported institutes for youth sit catty-corner to each other: the San Francisco Juvenile Probation Department's Juvenile Justice Center and the Ruth Asawa San Francisco School of the Arts public high school.

11. Juvenile Justice Center
375 Woodside Ave

Juvenile Hall is a short-term, 24/7, youth detention facility for up to 132 youth awaiting investigative action, further court hearings, and court ordered placement. Youth in custody receive educational, medical, and mental health services. They also receive training in socialization skills and general counseling from staff.

12. Ruth Asawa San Francisco School of the Arts (SOTA)
555 Portola Dr

Formerly McAteer High School, SOTA delivers college prep courses in the morning and a preprofessional arts training program in the afternoon. It has no athletic program. Admission is by rigorous audition. SOTA alumni have gone on to attend the Juilliard School and other esteemed art schools and conservatories. (Built on the slope of Glen Park Canyon, the school marquee is about all you can see of it from across the street.)

a. Glen Park Canyon
O'Shaughnessy Blvd and Elk St

The site shows no sign of its years as the former location of San Francisco's zoo (circa 1898). Today, this 70-acre, 500-foot-deep, steep slope canyon below Portola Drive gives you a glimpse of SF before development in the 19th and 20th centuries. The park incorporates free-flowing Islais Creek and extensive grassland with adjoining trees that support breeding pairs of red-tailed hawks and great horned owls. The attached neighborhood at the base of the canyon, **Glen Park**, is an adorable little hidden village of homes with shops on Diamond Street—and its own BART station!

Glen Park Zoo and Scheme to Sell Homes
The 1898 Grand Opening of the 145-acre Mission Park and Zoo in Glen Park garnered 15,000 visitors. The zoo continued as a wildly popular Sunday excursion. The location of the city zoo (and funds to build it) had been hotly contested, but the owners of vast land tracts in Glen Park Terrace fought hardest for it and won. They knew their hilly, far-from-the-city-center subdivision would be useless without access to public transportation. They figured having the city's zoo on their land (plus amusement park, castle, shooting range, high-wire acts, hot-air balloons, lion tamers, vaudeville acts, and more) would bring in people and trains and a chance to sell houses. Woohoo—but it didn't work. By 1905, they gave up, sold off the lots, and let the zoo go. Then a year later the 1906 quake hit and people rushed to buy homes in Glen Park. (*Bummer, dudes!*) —*Tramps of San Francisco*, by Evelyn Rose

END: PORTOLA DRIVE and TWIN PEAKS BOULEVARD

WALK-BACK LOOP SCOOP

Unless you start dating someone from this neighborhood you may never have reason to walk or even drive through this area again – so why not go for it now? See details in Walk-Back turn-by-turn section.

WALK 12 NEED TO KNOW

TO GET THERE
Muni N, 33, 37, 43, 71

PARKING
Street parking or pay lot at Stanyan and Beulah

PUBLIC RESTROOM
Stanyan and Waller

TURN-BY-TURN INSTRUCTIONS
Begin: Continue from GOLDEN GATE PARK walking south on STANYAN ST

- Right on PARNASSUS AVE, staying on the even-numbered north side of the street
- Turn left (south) on 7th AVE
  - 7th AVE turns into LAGUNA HONDA BLVD at LAWTON ST
  - At LAWTON ST, cross 7th AVE— from the garden side of the street to the odd-numbered side
  - This is the beginning of 1.4 miles of steady uphill climbing
- At the Forest Hill Muni Station crosswalk, cross the street to the Laguna Honda Hospital side of street

- Follow sidewalk to turn left with LAGUNA HONDA BLVD, which turns into WOODSIDE AVE
- Continue on WOODSIDE AVE to the top of the hill
- Left on PORTOLA DR

End: PORTOLA DR and TWIN PEAKS BLVD

TO GET BACK
- Board bus 44 (toward California) at the north corner of WOODSIDE AVE and PORTOLA DR
- Get off at 9th AVE and LINCOLN WAY on southeast corner
- Transfer to bus 71 (toward Beale St)
- Get off at HAIGHT and STANYAN

Other Muni routes:
- 36 to Forest Hill Station, then K, T, M, L
- 48, 52

OPTIONAL WALK-BACK LOOP DIRECTIONS
Distance: 2.7 miles, 5,000 steps, 1 hour

Rating: 5

Yes, it's a little hilly, but quiet and tree-lined, and the

directly-underneath-Sutro-Tower-neck-craning view is pretty cool. Clarendon Heights, just north of Midtown Terrace, boasts the highest house in San Francisco—but we won't make you walk to the top. Cole Valley's three-block commercial strip at the bottom of the hill is waiting to reward you with more than a dozen restaurants and cafés, some of which draw visitors from around the Bay Area.

Begin: PORTOLA DR at TWIN PEAKS BLVD (bottom of Twin Peaks)

- Left onto TWIN PEAKS BLVD
- Left at PANORAMA DR
- Right on CLARENDON AVE, which become TWIN PEAKS BLVD
- Left at TWIN PEAKS BLVD and CLAYTON ST to 17th ST
- Left 17th ST to COLE ST
- Right to COLE ST
- Left on FREDERICK ST

End: STANYAN ST at FREDERICK ST (edge of GG Park)

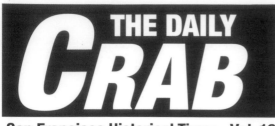

THE DAILY CRAB

San Francisco Historical Times   Vol. 12

In the 1950s Beatniks were "hip." Black people were "hip." But by Beat standards, the new generation of young white kids moving into the Haight in the mid-'60s were cheap imitators of the Beat movement. Not really cool enough to be called "hip," these new kids were junior hip, or "hippies." **SF Examiner's Michael Fallon** is credited with the first contemporary use of the term in 1965.

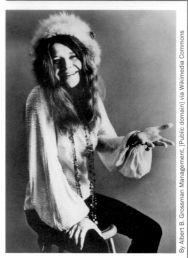

Super hip, Janis Joplin lived in The Haight (photo: 1970)

By Albert B. Grossman Management, [Public domain] via Wikimedia Commons

ALL-AMERICAN GIRL

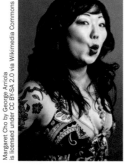

Margaret Cho by George Arriola is licensed under CC BY-SA 2.0 via Wikimedia Commons

Korean American comic **Margaret Cho** says of her upbringing in the Sunset and on Haight Street during the 1970s, "There were old hippies, ex-druggies, burnouts from the '60s, drag queens and Chinese people." That makes it seem perfectly normal that she performed a Samba to **Barry Manilow's** "Copacabana" while wearing a gay-pride-themed dress on **ABC's** *Dancing with the Stars.*

BOOTLEGGING BUILDER

The "Henry Ford of Housing" in the Sunset District, Henry Doelger, was born behind his father's bakery in San Francisco and grew up in the Inner Sunset at the corner of 7th Avenue and Hugo Street. After his father's death, 12-year-old Doelger left school to help support his family—with jobs including running a hot dog stand and a bit of bootlegging. He began speculating on empty property lots in his teens and then moved on to building homes with his brother.

He used assembly-line techniques to build tract homes, and by the time he was done had built 24,000 homes. His crowning achievement: the Westlake neighborhood of Daly City. According to Daly City expert Bunny Gillespie, Doelger claimed Mae West as a relative and named Westlake after her. He died in 1978 at the age of 82.

Sláinte!

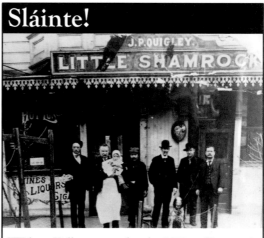

The Kelly-green-colored **Little Shamrock** bar across from GG Park (Lincoln/9th) was established in 1893 to serve the patrons of the **Midwinter Expo**—making it the Sunset District's oldest business and the city's oldest surviving bar.

MENSCHES* MARCH IN
Yiddish for "a good person"

Jews escaping persecution in 19th century Europe, found a welcoming, diverse society in San Francisco that offered equal opportunity for wealth or woe to all (white) newcomers.

The trades Jews were restricted to in Europe, peddler and merchant, were the skills most sought after in the burgeoning new city. Jewish pioneers (**de Young, Fleishhacker, Haas, Hellman, Lilienthal, Stern, Sutro**) got to work creating iconic SF businesses, such as **MJB Coffee, Wells Fargo Bank, City of Paris, Crown Zellerbach, Fireman's Fund, Gump's, I. Magnin, San Francisco Chronicle, S & W Foods**, and the **Levi Strauss Company**.

Jews loved the new American Jerusalem—San Francisco—and gave back generously.

Through three centuries, Jewish philanthropy has had a major impact on San Francisco, from the early days of building the German Hospital in 1858 (later renamed the **Ralph K. Davies Medical Center**) to donating the San Francisco Zoo and creating the **American Conservatory Theater**, and the **Jewish Family and Children's Services** in the 20th century, to the $75 million **Zuckerberg** donation in 2015 to **SF General Hospital**—and so much more. ***Thank you!***

From the Gold Rush era to today, San Francisco has enjoyed a vast diversity of Jewish citizens.

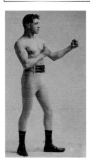

Jewish heavyweight boxer in the 1880s
Joe Choynski, *"The California Terror"*

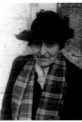

Alice B. Toklas *met her lesbian partner Gertrude Stein shortly after the 1906 earthquake. Later, together, they hosted an avant-garde Parisian salon.*

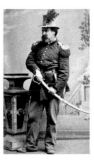

In 1859 San Francisco's favorite eccentric, **Joshua Abraham Norton**, *proclaimed himself Emperor of the United States.*

Explore the City. Get the Gear. Share the Fun.
@walkSF49 *#walkSF49*

SHACKING-UP IN THE SUNSET

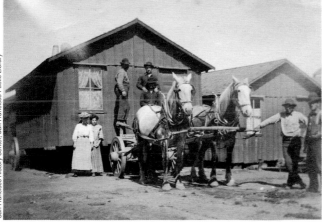

San Francisco History Center, San Francisco Public Library

Moving day. Family hauls earthquake shack to a new neighborhood.

The earthquake and fire of 1906 left approximately two-thirds of the population of San Francisco homeless. A relief fund built 5,610 tiny cottages, now called "earthquake shacks," in parks around the city to house the homeless. Rent ranged from $1 to $2 per month.

By the end of 1906, the city began offering rent rebates to encourage refugees to find vacant lots and move their shacks from public land. Some people moved their shacks to the Sunset, where plenty of lots were available. Many people cobbled together three or four of the 14-by-18-foot shacks to make a home.

49 MILE
SCENIC DRIVE

Twin Peaks Meander to Market Street

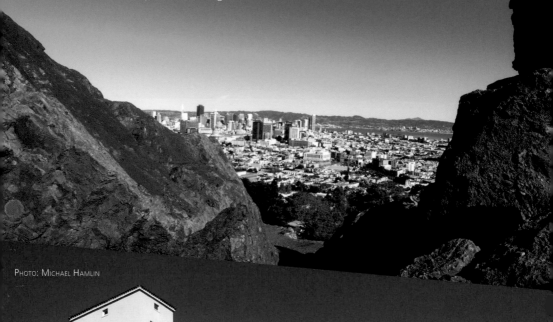

Downtown view from the top of Corona Heights Park

PHOTO: MICHAEL HAMLIN

Alfred Hitchcock shot seven scenes for the movie Vertigo along the 49 Mile Scenic Drive. St. Joseph's Hospital—used as the sanatorium where Jimmy Stewart's character, Scottie, recovered—can be seen from Roosevelt Street.

Stunning. Gorgeous. Repeat this walk with all of your out-of-town guests (or send them on their own). Walking to the top of Twin Peaks is so much more #cool #rad than just driving up to the parking lot. Your hike to the summit will be rewarded with a 360° view of the Bay Area that can't be fully seen from the tourist parking area. The Pacific Ocean, Golden Gate Bridge, Alcatraz, SF skyline, East Bay, Hunters Point shipyards, Mount Diablo, SFO planes flying over San Bruno Mountain, and Mount Davidson can all be seen with the turn of your head. You may find yourself imagining what the Spanish explorers saw and felt from here. You may begin spotting and excitedly pointing out city landmarks that are important to you. You may take too many selfies—but who can blame you?

And then there's more! The short trek down the northern side of Twin Peaks escorts you directly to a thoroughly lovely and romantic stroll past the modern cliff-side homes, old-time city streets, and surprise peekaboo views of Corona Heights, and then winds down to Market Street.

NOTES

1. Wind Warning. When the ocean wind whips over the peaks this hike becomes chilly enough to make you break out your Alaskan parka. Check the weather and go when the forecast calls for clear skies—and no wind!

2. It's a relatively short walk to the top of the peaks, but there are a number of steep ascents and descents to navigate, adding up to a brief but decent workout.

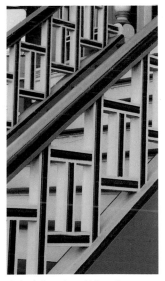

Colorfully painted Victorian stairway. PHOTO: MICHAEL HAMLIN

Begin: Portola Drive at Twin Peaks Boulevard
           (Bottom of Twin Peaks)
End: Market Street at 14th Street
Distance: ROUTE: 3.0 miles — 6,000 steps — 1 hour
           LOOP BACK: 2.5 miles — 5,000 steps — 50 minutes

Hill Rating:

NOTE: The trail up to Twin Peaks traverses the scrub, climbs dirt stairs, and crosses TWIN PEAKS BLVD five times on the way to the top. Please be cautious crossing the street; cars will not be expecting you.

Sites you will pass on today's walk include:

MILE 37
1. **Twin Peaks Summit**
   501 Twin Peaks Blvd

2. **Sutro Tower**
   1 La Avanzada St

MILE 38
Corona Heights

MILE 39
3. **Corona Heights Park** Roosevelt Way
   and Museum Way

DETOUR
a. **Randall Museum**
   199 Museum Way

4. **CPMC Campus**
   Castro St and 14th St

5. **Market Street**

WALK-BACK LOOP: THE CASTRO
b. **GLBT History Museum**
   4127 18th St and Castro St

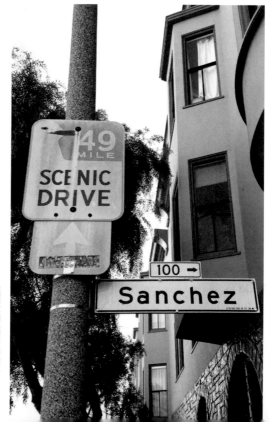

PHOTO: MICHAEL HAMLIN

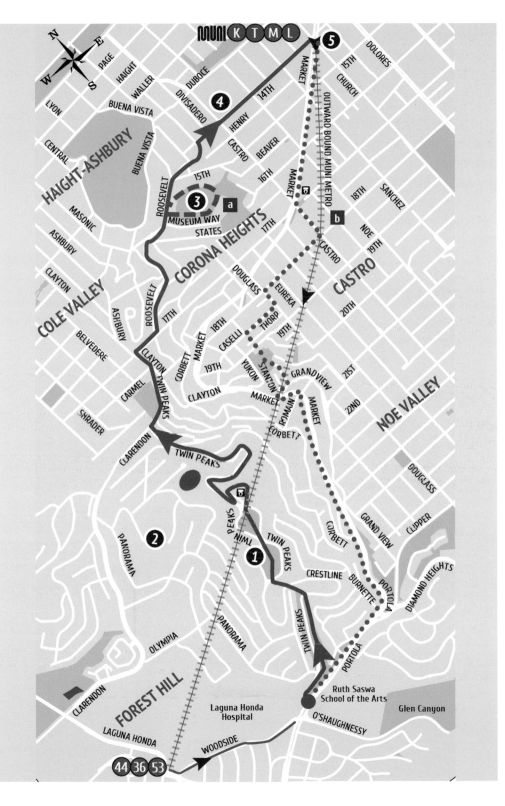

MUNI K T M L

N W E S

PAGE
HAIGHT
WALLER
DUBOCE
DIVISADERO
14TH
MARKET
15TH
DOLORES
CHURCH
OUTWARD BOUND MUNI METRO
LYON
BUENA VISTA
HENRY
4
CENTRAL
BUENA VISTA
CASTRO
BEAVER
15TH
16TH
ROOSEVELT
18TH
SANCHEZ
MASONIC
3
MUSEUM WAY
STATES
a
17TH
CORONA HEIGHTS
NOE
19TH
ASHBURY
CLAYTON
b
CASTRO
CASTRO
HAIGHT-ASHBURY
DOUGLASS
EUREKA
20TH
COLE VALLEY
ASHBURY
ROOSEVELT
18TH
THORP
19TH
21ST
BELVEDERE
MARKET
CASELLI
YUKON
STANTON
GRANDVIEW
CARMEL
CLAYTON TWIN PEAKS
19TH
MARKET
ROMAIN
22ND
NOE VALLEY
SHRADER
CLAYTON
CORBETT
CLARENDON
TWIN PEAKS
GRANDVIEW
MARKET
DOUGLASS
6
CORBETT
CLIPPER
PANORAMA
2
TWIN PEAKS
TWIN PEAKS
CORBETT
GRAND VIEW
PORTOLA
DIAMOND HEIGHTS
1
CRESTLINE
BURNETTE
OLYMPIA
PANORAMA
TWIN PEAKS
PORTOLA
FOREST HILL
CLARENDON
Laguna Honda
Hospital
Ruth Saswa
School of the Arts
Glen Canyon
LAGUNA HONDA
O'SHAUGHNESSY
WOODSIDE
44 36 53

MILE 37

Begins on PORTOLA DR at TWIN PEAKS BLVD

On the right-hand side of TWIN PEAKS BLVD is a dirt path along the guardrail

Walk up the dirt path (trail maps call this CREEKS TO PEAK TRAIL)

Bay Area Bay Ridge Trail
In 1987 a coalition of hiking-outdoor enthusiasts got together to discuss a potential trail covering a 550-mile route for hikers, mountain bikers, and equestrians along the mountain ridgelines surrounding the entire SF Bay. Since then volunteers, municipalities, city departments (such as the SF Recreation and Parks and SF Planning Departments), corporate leaders, trail experts, and private land holders have worked, cooperated, negotiated, raised money, and miraculously completed 360 miles of the trail. *Thank you!* The 49 mile route crosses the Ridge Trail three times— including today's hike on the Creeks to Peak Trail to the top of Twin Peaks. Join the fun at RidgeTrail.org.

OPENING no. 1: Watch for a trail sign, a rubber mat with yellow dots on the road, and an opening in the guardrail

Carefully cross the road to the opening on the other side of the street

Head uphill on trail

When you reach the guardrail at the top of the hill, turn left and follow narrow path along guardrail to:

OPENING no. 2: Watch for a trail sign, a rubber mat with yellow dots on the road, and an opening in the guardrail

Carefully cross the road to the opening on the other side of the street

Head up the hillside stairs

OPENING no. 3: Watch for a green hiking sign and an opening in the guardrail

Carefully cross the road to the green hiking sign, "summit" arrow, and opening on

the other side of the street

Climb to Peak no. 1 and enjoy

Follow dirt stairs down the other side of the peak

Carefully cross the road to the hillside stairs on the other side of the street

Climb to Peak no. 2 and enjoy

Follow dirt stairs down the other side of the peak

Carefully cross the road onto CHRISTMAS TREE POINT

Walk past the radio towers to Twin Peaks Lookout and enjoy

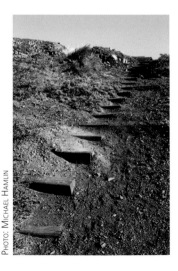

PHOTO: MICHAEL HAMLIN

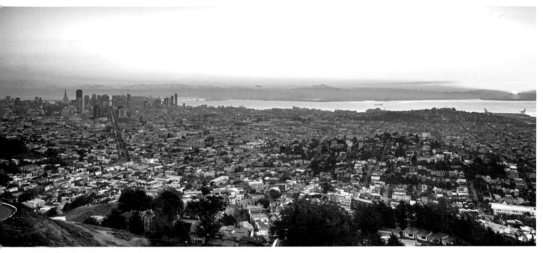

Twin Peaks view at sunrise

1. Twin Peaks Summit
501 Twin Peaks Blvd

With an elevation of 922 feet, these peaks are the second-highest points in the city, but they provide the number one view. (Mount Davidson, to the south, just beats them out for elevation.) The north and south peaks (named Eureka and Noe) stand about 660 ft. apart. That reservoir you see to the north is part of the independent water hydrant supply system created for the San Francisco Fire Department after the 1906 earthquake and fire.

Hike down to the parking lot main viewing area. At the telescope platform you can find a great view through the downtown skyscrapers of Market Street running all the way to the Ferry Building. Another great site: From sunset to sunrise the streetlights of Market Street parallel the car lights of the Bay Bridge.

2. Sutro Tower
1 La Avanzada St

The Bay Area's most visible icon, the antennas on Sutro Tower's 977-foot-high, three-pronged tower deliver clear television and radio station signals throughout the San Francisco Bay Area. A two-person cage elevator transports workers to the top—but, alas, the tower's elevator and views are not open to the likes of you and me. Bummer!

Breasts of the Indian Maiden?
Yes, the 18th-century Spanish conquistadors took one look at these two identical hills and named them Los Pechos de la Chola ("breasts of the maiden"). When the Americans took control of the city in the 19th century, they renamed the girls Twin Peaks.

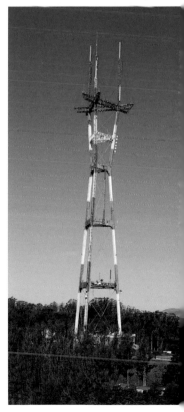

Sutro Tower. Photo: Michael Hamlin

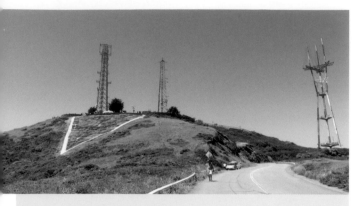

Friends of the Pink Triangle

Every June volunteers climb to the top of Twin Peaks at dawn and hammer 5,000 spikes into 175 pink tarps covering nearly an acre of ground to create a giant pink triangle that can be seen seven miles away.

It serves as a reminder both to never forget the past *and* to celebrate how far we have come.

The pink triangle symbol—now reclaimed as a symbol of pride—was once used by Nazis in concentration camps to identify and shame homosexuals. Other groups were given similar identifying triangles by the Nazis: brown for Gypsies, green for criminals, purple for Jehovah's Witnesses, and a double yellow for Jews.

The Twin Peaks triangle, which stays up for an entire week, has been a part of San Francisco's annual LGBT Pride celebration since 1995—and you are welcome to come help put it up or take it down. —ThePinkTriangle.com

CORONA HEIGHTS

Once called Rock Hill, this neighborhood above Eureka Valley was first developed as a quarry. Wide streets had been carved out of the rock to accommodate large transport vehicles, so, when the quarry closed, the streets made an ideal location for building houses. The cross-town views and proximity to transportation and amenities also made the location prime real estate. Many upscale view homes have been added through the years.

For example:

- In late 2013 a one-bed, one-bath, 960-square-foot abode in Corona Heights sold for $1,010 per square foot.

- A flipper home purchased for $1.1 million in 2012 hit the market in 2015 asking $4.995 million—nearly a fivefold increase in three years.

MILE 38

Begins at TOP of TWIN PEAKS BLVD

• • • • • • • • • • • • • • • • • •

Follow the viewing platform walkway around the towers, out of the parking lot

Right on TWIN PEAKS BLVD

Walk on the road (TWIN PEAKS BLVD), winding downhill, watching both for traffic and great views

Right on CLARENDON AVE (the T at the bottom of TWIN PEAKS BLVD)

Merge left onto CLAYTON ST

Right on 17th ST, 1 block

• • • • • • • • • • • • • • • • • •

MILE 39

Begins on 17th ST at ROOSEVELT WAY

• • • • • • • • • • • • • • • • • •

Left on ROOSEVELT WAY, cross to right-hand side of street as you continue winding downhill

(NOTE: Be sure to veer right with ROOSEVELT WAY and not go straight onto Loma Vista Terrace)

• • • • • • • • • • • • • • • • • •

3. Corona Heights Park
Roosevelt Way and Museum Way

Off-leash dog park, recreation areas, amazing city views, Randall Museum—and a rocky red mountaintop that looks like the surface of Mars. NOTE: SF has 220 city parks and open spaces!

Rock Blasting, Double-Dealing, and Death in Corona Heights
George and Harry Gray established their quarry and brick factory on Rock Hill (Corona Heights) in 1899. They also ran quarries on Telegraph Hill and Billy Goat Hill. The wealthy Gray brothers were notorious for their shoddy workmanship, not paying their workers, dangerous conditions—and squirming out of lawsuits. Rock-blasting debris regularly flew through the air, injuring adults and children and damaging homes. The substandard bricks they sold to the city for building cable car beds crumbled and had to be ripped out and replaced.

In 1914, a 26-year-old former employee, Joseph Lococo, confronted George Gray demanding $17.50 in back wages. When Gray refused, Lococo murdered him. A sympathetic jury acquitted the defendant, and the quarry finally closed.

Follow ROOSEVELT WAY to the left around Corona Heights Park, or take Randall Museum detour

Right on 14th ST, head to bottom of hill

---

4. CPMC Davies Campus Castro St and 14th St

California Pacific Medical Center (CPMC) ranks as one of the largest private, not-for-profit, academic medical centers in California and for many years has been recognized as a

"Leader in LGBT Healthcare Equality" in the Healthcare Equality Index, an annual survey conducted by the Human Rights Campaign (HRC) Foundation. The 49 mile route passes CPMC's newest campus (on the site of the former Jack Tar Hotel) on Walk 1, and the CPMC St. Luke's Campus on Walk 15.

5. Market Street

Designed as San Francisco's first major transit artery in 1847, three-mile-long Market Street begins at the Ferry Building and ends at the intersection with Corbett Avenue up on Twin Peaks.

DETOUR

Enter Corona Heights Park, follow the path to the right to pass the museum, then head left up to the top of the bluffs, then return to the entrance.

a. Randall Museum, located in Corona Heights Park
199 Museum Way

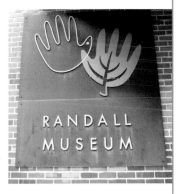

Here you'll find a newly renovated, kid-friendly museum focusing on the arts, sciences, and natural history; a theater; a replica earthquake shack; and classes for all. Its highly capable namesake, Josephine Dows Randall, graduated with a master's degree in zoology from Stanford University in 1913, organized the first Girl Scout and Camp Fire Girl troops in the United States, and became the first superintendent of recreation for San Francisco's Recreation Department. As superintendent she secured hundreds of acres of open space for playgrounds, sports, and artistic programming for the children and families of San Francisco.

Market Street has always reflected SF, following the booms and bust of financial and natural disasters, falling in and out of favor with shoppers, torn up and prettied up, both the healthiest and most clogged transit artery.

Yet when it comes time to come together, Market Street is where San Franciscans gather to mark global, local, and world-shaking events—from opening the Panama-Pacific International Exposition and marking the end of world wars to celebrating (many!) baseball, football and basketball championships and the turn of the millennium, to hosting over a million guests at the annual Gay Pride Parade.

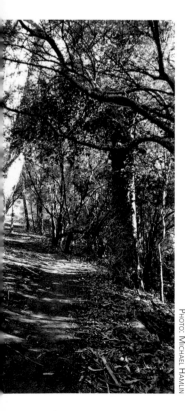

PHOTO: MICHAEL HAMLIN

Over the years Market Street has transported San Franciscans in every conveyance Muni has ever offered: omnibuses, horse-drawn carriages, cable cars, electric streetcars, electric trolleybuses, diesel buses, hybrid bio-diesel buses—and then for fun added back heritage (antique) street cars from around the world.

• • • • • • • • • • • • • • • •

Cross CHURCH ST, cross MARKET ST veering left to stay on 14th ST

END on 14th ST at MARKET ST (near CHURCH ST)

• • • • • • • • • • • • • • • •

OPTIONAL WALK-BACK LOOP

THE CASTRO

The residents called this neighborhood Little Scandinavia in the 1910s and 1920s, then Eureka Valley during the Irish working-class days from the 1930s to the 1960s, and finally The Castro (after the prominent Castro movie theater) when cheap housing helped it become a gay mecca and center of LGBT activism in the 1970s and 1980s. Though

straight families began moving into the Castro this century, and only the wealthy can afford to buy homes here now, the Castro remains a thriving marketplace for all things gay, lesbian, bisexual, transgender, queer, questioning, intersex and otherwise fabulous!

b. GLBT History Museum
4127 18th St and Castro St

San Francisco's "queer Smithsonian" houses one of the world's largest collections of gay, lesbian, bisexual, and transgender historical material. Open Mon. and Wed.–Sat., 11 a.m.–6 p.m.; Sun., noon–5 p.m.; closed Tuesdays. $5 admission.

America's Gay Church
In 1968 Rev. Troy Perry founded the first and only LGBT Christian denomination in the world—The Metropolitan Community Church (MCC). MCC expanded to San Francisco in 1970, began performing same-sex weddings in 1971, and in 1979 became the first LGBT organization in SF to own its own building (Eureka Street near 18th Street). In 2015, the church moved back to one of SF's first gay neighborhoods, Polk Street, which you will pass on Walk 1.

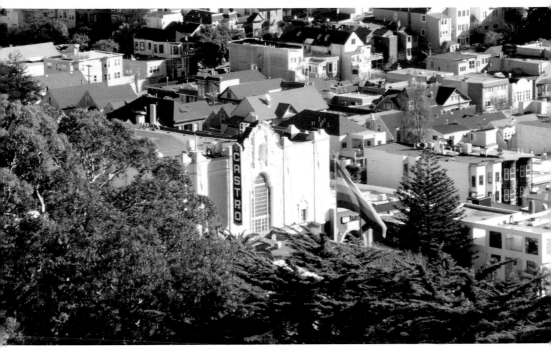

View of Castro Theater and LGBT flag from Corona Heights

WALK 13 NEED TO KNOW

TO GET THERE
Muni K, L, M, or T

- Get off at FOREST HILL STATION
- Transfer to bus 36, 44, or 52 at SW corner outside station
- Get off at the top of the hill, PORTOLA DR

PARKING
Street parking on TWIN PEAKS BLVD

PUBLIC RESTROOMS
- Porta-potty at entry to Twin Peaks parking lot
- On walk back, 2375 Market (just before Castro)

CARS, BIKES, STROLLERS, WHEELCHAIRS:
Follow the road signs to the lookout area (parking lot) at the top (1.3-miles-steep winding road).

There is no sidewalk. It is legal to walk on the road.

TURN–BY–TURN INSTRUCTIONS
Begin: PORTOLA DR at TWIN PEAKS BLVD

- On the right-hand side of TWIN PEAKS BLVD is a dirt path along the guardrail
- Walk up the dirt path (trail maps call this CREEKS TO PEAK TRAIL)

- OPENING no. 1: Watch for a trail sign, a rubber mat with yellow dots on the road, and an opening in the guardrail
  - Carefully cross the road to the opening on the other side of the street
  - Head uphill on trail
  - When you reach the guardrail at the top of the hill, turn left, follow narrow path along guardrail to:
- OPENING no. 2: Watch for a trail sign, a rubber mat with yellow dots on the road, and an opening in the guardrail
  - Carefully cross the road to the opening on the other side of the street
  - Head up the hillside stairs
- OPENING no. 3: Watch for a green hiking sign and an opening in the guardrail
  - Carefully cross the road to the green hiking sign, "summit" arrow, and opening on the other side of the street
- Climb to Peak no. 1 and enjoy
  - Follow dirt stairs down the other side of the peak
  - Carefully cross the road to the hillside stairs on the other side of the street

- Climb to Peak no. 2 and enjoy
  - Follow dirt stairs down the other side of the peak
  - Carefully cross the road onto CHRISTMAS TREE POINT
  - Walk past the radio towards to
- Twin Peaks lookout and enjoy
- Follow the viewing platform walkway around the towers, out of the parking lot
- Right on TWIN PEAKS BLVD
  - Walk on the road (TWIN PEAKS BLVD), winding downhill, watching both for traffic and great views
- Right on CLARENDON AVE (the T at the bottom of TWIN PEAKS BLVD)
- Merge left onto CLAYTON ST
- Right on 17th ST, 1 block
- Left on ROOSEVELT WAY, cross to right-hand side of street as you continue winding downhill
  - (NOTE: Be sure to veer right with ROOSEVELT WAY, and not go straight onto Loma Vista Terrace)
  - Follow ROOSEVELT WAY to the left around Corona Heights Park

- Right on 14th ST, head to bottom of hill
- Cross CHURCH ST, cross MARKET ST veering left to stay on 14th ST

End: 14th ST at MARKET ST (near CHURCH ST)

TO GET BACK
Muni

- At Market St and Church St enter CHURCH STREET STATION
- Take K, T, M, L outbound
- Get off at FOREST HILL STATION
- Immediately outside the station, transfer to any bus going up to Portola: 36, 44, 53
- You can also catch outbound K, L, M, and T at the CASTRO STREET STATION if you take half the walk-back loop

OPTIONAL WALK-BACK LOOP DIRECTIONS:
Distance: 2.5 miles, 5,000 steps, 50 minutes

Rating: 5

WALK-BACK LOOP SCOOP
Walk 13 just skirts the edge of the Castro. If you are up for a long, continual uphill climb back to the beginning, the walk-back loop goes right through the heart of the Castro District (which is totally worth a return trip to explore in full another day) on its way back up Market St to Twin Peaks.

One strategy for an easier walk-back with maximum site seeing: Follow the walk-back directions to the Castro, drop in to the GLBT History Museum, peek in a few stores, then make a U-turn back the way you came to Castro and Market Sts. Catch the Muni K, L, M, or T outbound to Forest Hill Station.

Begin: 14th at MARKET ST (near CHURCH ST)

- Head west (right, uphill, back toward Twin Peaks) on MARKET ST
- Left onto CASTRO ST
- Right on 18th ST
- Left on DOUGLAS ST
- Right on CASELLI AVE, stay on left hand side of street
  - Two-thirds of the way up the block, watch for a stairway on your left, CLOVER LANE
  - Go up CLOVER LANE STAIRWAY, cross THORP ST and continue up stairway
  - The street you come out on is 19th ST
  - Cross 19th ST, turn right, in about 10 steps, to your left, along the side of a brick house, you'll see a narrow alleyway, with crumbling mismatched stairs heading upward
  - Be brave, walk carefully up the alley/stairway to an open field—this is KITE HILL
- Head up toward the green bench, then veer left upward toward another bench at the end of a cul-de-sac road (GRAND VIEW TERRACE)
- Take GRAND VIEW TERRACE to end of block
- Right on GRAND VIEW, cross to left side of road and take stairs up to MARKET ST
- Left on MARKET ST to pedestrian crossover bridge at ROMAIN st
  - Take BRIDGE across MARKET ST
- Continue uphill on MARKET ST (left), which turns into PORTOLA DR at the top of the hill

End: PORTOLA DR and TWIN PEAKS BLVD

THE SECRETS OF SAN FRANCISCO'S VICTORIAN ARCHITECTURE By Katharine Holland

Walking down a San Francisco street is like entering a time machine. Step inside the time machine and dial year 1888 and you see a charming slanted-bay Italianate Victorian Painted Lady that will remain standing to be on today's National Register of Historic Places. Dial year 1906 and you see Dolores Park filled with earthquake shacks, providing temporary housing after the 1906 San Francisco earthquake and fire. Dial year 2016 you see a modern skyscraper with elevators taking you up to the 60th floor.

As you walk past all of this historic and modern architecture, wouldn't you love to take a peek inside these different styles of homes?

With many of its homes 50 to 150 years old, the city's architecture certainly provides a window into its past—and showcases the evolution of city homes and city life. For example:

- A century ago, tearing down the outhouse and installing a bathroom with a claw-foot tub on the back porch was the height of modern living.
- Modernizing your house once meant running gas pipes through your walls to the "high-tech" gas lamps installed to light your home. Today, the rewired electric lights in a 100-year-old home can be controlled from your cell phone.
- In Victorian homes, coal was the source of heat. These fireplaces no longer heat our homes, but many remain as a "decorative" architectural detail in modern living rooms—or have been retrofitted into gas fireplaces that can be turned on by pressing a button.

Duck and Cover

Victorian fireplaces had a "summer cover" (door) that was completely removable and was taken off when there was a fire burning in the cast-iron grate.

During World War II, a massive amount of metal was needed to build tanks, ships, weapons, and planes. The government came through neighborhoods collecting scrap metal to use for the war effort. Fireplace summer covers were often donated to the cause—making them rare to find in San Francisco's homes today.

- As horse-drawn carriages gave way first to tiny Model T Fords, on to huge 1950s Buicks, then electric cars requiring recharging stations in the garage, the houses had to change with each new revolution in transportation. The old horse stable may now be an apartment. Many families had their entire house lifted up so workers could dig a garage space below it to accommodate the family car.

San Francisco homes contain hints of all of these innovations over the years. It all started in 1849 as San Francisco Bay filled up with tall sailing ships bringing in tens of thousands of gold and silver prospectors. Wagon trains arrived daily bringing thousands more. Although these fortune seekers were heading to the Sierra Foothills to prospect, their commerce massively expanded this port city—increasing its size from approximately 1,000 people in 1848 to 15,000 in 1849 and doubling to 30,000 in 1850. By 1856 San Francisco was the largest city in the West with almost 50,000 people.

Giddy with their riches, successful prospectors favored elaborately embellished homes based on the Victorian architecture styles all the rage in London. Features that had previously been used on churches and palaces, along with some new flourishes, were piled onto houses to create a home that said, "I have wealth and status." Queen Victoria was the namesake for this opulent architecture since it was during her reign (1837–1901) that the British Empire's dominance in global maritime trade brought massive wealth to England. With San Francisco's boom in wealth, but limited geographical area, the Victorians were constructed in row-house style, with homes tightly packed together, allowing more houses per block.

In search of building materials, house builders found the world's best timber lining the California coast—the giant redwood tree. Redwoods are naturally resistant to dry rot and decay and stand up to insects, such as termites, and fire. The use of redwood lumber explains why so many historic homes survived the 1906 earthquake and fire and are still standing today.

The Mystery of the Tiny Closets
Why are the closets so small? Is it because there was a tax on closets? Or because people did not own as many clothes? In fact, all of the homes in San Francisco were built with closets. They are just tiny and not in every bedroom. Forget about a coat closet. The homes do have built-in shelving used for general storage purposes in the dining room or living room, not for clothing. Clothes were not hung on hangers; clothes hangers were not used routinely until 1906 or later. Instead, they were folded and kept in a chest of drawers or armoire, or hung on hooks or nails. Even a well-to-do woman would have just a few dresses.

This guide will help you identify the different styles as you walk by them on the 49 Mile Scenic Walk—and will give you a hint of what these homes are like inside.

FLAT–FRONT ITALIANATE VICTORIAN: EARLY 1870s

If you see a home that looks different from all of the rest, it is usually a **flat front Italianate Victorian**. At the time these homes were built, people rode on horseback and many of the homes were either farmhouses or storefronts. You can spot this style as it looks like something out of an old Western movie—with a "false-front" vertical extension beyond the roofline. This feature made hastily built buildings look more impressive.

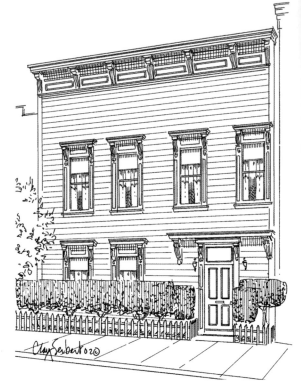

This style often stands alone on a street. You don't see rows of them, like other Victorian-era styles. Exterior decoration is minimal with plain, lapped siding and simple window hoods. No indoor plumbing existed—an outhouse was used. The owner would go to a bathhouse to bathe.

Flat-front Italianate Victorian in Noe Valley on 25th Street

Parlez-vous Parlor?

The English word *parlor* comes from a French word *parler*, "to speak."

In Victorian times, the parlor was the best room of the house, reserved for notable occasions or special visitors, and contained family photographs and other treasured possessions. The furniture, while the nicest that the family could afford, was made for looks rather than comfort.

In the Victorian era, when a young man had an interest in a young lady, he asked if he could call on her. This may be a foreign concept to the younger generation. Maybe I should explain. He didn't text-message her. He didn't ask for her phone number. He asked whether he could call on her at her home. This involved coming to her house, sitting a modest distance away from the young lady and conversing politely, perhaps in the presence of a chaperone. This "speaking" was done in the parlor.

Liquor in the Loo
Old outhouse pits from the 1880s are excellent places for archeological excavations, offering up a treasure trove of common objects from the past. For example, it is especially common to find old liquor bottles, which seemingly were secretly stashed (or trashed), so their contents could be privately imbibed. These time capsule may also contain valuables such as dentures, dolls, eyeglasses—even guns—that fell in the muck.

SLANTED-BAY ITALIANATE VICTORIAN: LATER 1870s TO 1890

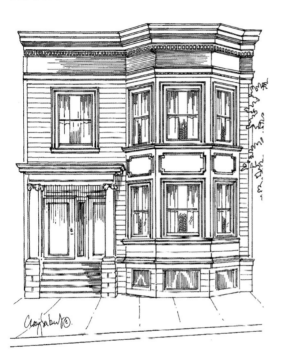

This slanted-bay Italianate stands right across the street from Dolores Park (Walk 14).

The **slanted-bay Italianate Victorian** evolved and pushed out the flat-front style by adding slanted or square bay windows and oversize cornices (molding just below the roof) along the rooftop. Classic columns around the front door, a flat roof, Douglas fir softwood floors, and sometimes a tiny Juliet balcony over the front porch are characteristics of this style.

Bathrooms were added at a later date, and many owners converted the back porch for this purpose—often resulting in the bathroom being located right off the kitchen. Tiny closets were common during this period as it seems people used armoires for their clothes instead of closets. Despite small bathrooms and closets and no garage, these charming homes are hot sellers today. Home buyers gladly fit their modern lives into these historic, cottage-like homes.

As you start looking closely at these two types of Italianate Victorians you will see many remodels and additions visible from the outside. Often, a garage has been added by having a construction crew raise up the house and put a garage underneath. Sometimes an apartment has been added downstairs. Parking is in such short supply in San Francisco, you know the owners must love their home and the city to be living here—with no garage, only two closets, and a bathroom off the kitchen!

How Many Victorians remain?
In 1973, Judith Lynch went on a hunt for Victorian homes in San Francisco. Funded by a grant from the National Endowment for the Arts, Ms. Lynch, who would later help create City Guides, did a painstaking survey of nine San Francisco neighborhoods. By her count, there were 13,487 Victorian era structures still standing.

SAN FRANCISCO STICK: 1860s TO 1880s

The quickest way to spot the **San Francisco stick** style is to look for its squared bay windows, repetitive use of finely detailed surface decoration, and strong vertical trim on sides of windows. False mansard roofs (also called a French roof) and gabled roofs (a simple roof design shaped like an inverted V), a wide band of trim under the cornice (molding just below the roof), and sunbursts in gables all cry out, "I have money."

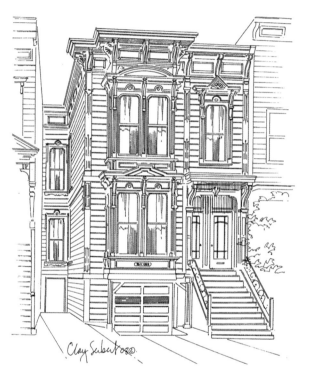

Many homeowners of the past read about the style in national magazines and asked their builder to make one for them.

San Francisco stick on 17th Street in the Mission

Bay Windows
Although not invented in San Francisco, the bay window is so common here that it is synonymous with San Francisco. They increase the light (welcome in the ever-present fog and frequent absence of side windows) and square footage—creating a perfect spot for a cozy window seat and storage underneath it.

Bay windows were identified as a defining characteristic of San Francisco architecture in a 2012 study that had a machine-learning algorithm examine a random sample of 25,000 photos of cities from Google street view.

QUEEN ANNE VICTORIAN: 1880s – LATE 1910s

The most recognizable architectural style is the **Queen Anne Victorian**. Elaborate, ornate, and eccentric, Queen Annes include turrets or round towers, a steep and gabled roof, rounded or arched windows, spindles, stained or leaded glass, elaborate 3-D pressed wood decorations, and rows of shingle siding (icing), all combined to make this style.

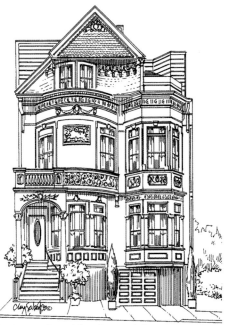

There are two types: **tower** and **row**. Tower homes have a tower or turret and are rare with fewer than 400 remaining today. Row houses are pressed together, one after another in a row.

The floor plan inside a Victorian house can seem cluttered and convoluted. Instead of open spaces, you may find a series of small rooms connected by a maze of hallways and doors.

And then there's the bathroom. Although indoor plumbing was available at the turn of the century, the bathrooms (called water closets in Victorian days) are usually cramped compared to our bathrooms of today. Many of them have a split bathroom—where the toilet is in one room and a sink and claw-foot bathtub in the other room. Many owners today combine these two rooms into one bathroom.

This Queen Anne Victorian, and the ones next to it, that you will pass on Post Street (Walk 2) were picked up and moved here in the 1970s.

Many Queen Annes have a double parlor, fireplaces with tile surround and threshold, coved ceilings, elaborate ceiling cornices around light fixtures, sliding pocket doors, wainscoting, and crystal chandeliers.

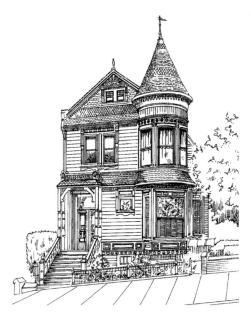

You will pass one of the 400 remaining Queen Anne Victorian tower homes on Walk 14.

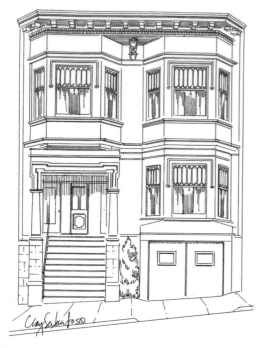

Edwardian on Stanyan Street

EDWARDIAN—1900 TO 1915

Victorian buildings were the biggest losers in the 1906 earthquake and fire. The newer style of home, the simpler, stripped-down **Edwardian**, was just coming into vogue and so Edwardians were built to replace the destroyed Victorians. Recognizable by the canted bay window (flat front and angled sides), Edwardians have window seats inside those bay windows, larger closets, hardwood oak floors, and garages. Formal dining rooms have built-in shelves for dishes, wood paneling, and box beam ceilings.

Take the Quiz
On page 199, test your knowledge of Victorian architecture on Walk 14 down Dolores Street.
Correct answers: 1-b, 2-b, 3-b, 4-a, 5-a, 6-b, 7-b, 8-a, 9-b, 10-a, 11-a, 12-b, 13-a, 14-a, 15-a

Architectural Styles: Approximate Number Still Standing

Victorian = 13,487
Queen Anne row house = 5,500
Stick = 3,600
Flat-Front Italianates = 1,900
Italianate bays = 1,200
Queen Anne tower = 400
Earthquake shacks = 100

Katharine Holland has been selling homes in San Francisco since 2003 and loves her work. KatharineHolland.com

Illustrations courtesy of Clay Seibert Rendering and Fine Arts. Clay specializes in drawing, painting, and photographing San Francisco homes. ClaySeibert.com

Painted Ladies

Early San Franciscans loved painting their Victorian and Edwardian homes in three or more colors to embellish or enhance their architectural details.

As one newspaper critic noted in 1885, ". . . red, yellow, chocolate, orange, everything that is loud is in fashion . . . if the upper stories are not of red or blue . . . they are painted up into uncouth panels of yellow and brown."

During World War I and World War II, many of these houses were painted battleship gray with war-surplus navy paint.

According to Wikipedia, in 1963, San Francisco artist Butch Kardum began combining intense blues and greens on the exterior of his Italianate-style Victorian house. Some neighbors criticized his house, but other neighbors began to copy the bright colors on their own houses. Kardum became a color designer, and he and other artists/colorists such as Tony Cataletich, Bob Buckner, and Jason Wonders began to transform dozens of gray houses into Painted Ladies (the new term for the colorful look). By the 1970s, the colorist movement, as it was called, had changed entire streets and neighborhoods. This process continues to this day.

One of the best-known groups of Painted Ladies is the row of Victorian homes at 710–720 Steiner Street, across from Alamo Square Park. It is sometimes known as Postcard Row.

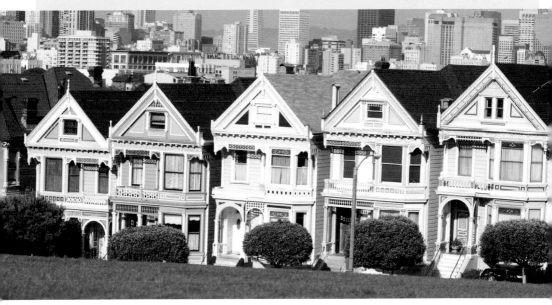

The Painted Ladies, San Francisco. PHOTO: ALEX PROIMOS

49 MILE
SCENIC DRIVE

The Mission:
Dolores Street to
Cesar Chavez Street

Dolores Park was not named after Mission Dolores! Details to follow . . .

Latin, sunny, artsy, and vibrant, The Mission is the oldest settled area of the city. This bustling "city within the city" has historically been working class—with each generation of workers moving on as the next group of workers moved in.

The historic 49 mile route runs through the neighborhood's calm elegant edge along Dolores Street. Today you'll follow the route along this undulating, grand boulevard of towering palms past stately old churches, historic buildings, a cemetery, and classic Victorian and Edwardian homes—including Dolores Park and Mission Dolores.

Look up and down streets you pass for surprise views, explore all the eateries around Dolores Park, stop to catch your breath at the top of the hills, especially the steep section between 22nd and 25th, and absorb the beauty.

Then, if you're up for a real San Francisco Mission experience after your calm stroll—have we got a fantastic walk-back loop for you. Just a few blocks away, the Latino, hipster side of one of the city's most colorful neighborhoods awaits you. The total loop is just over three miles, and the return streets are flat, so don't miss it—take the Mission walk-back loop!

The loop back spends a few blocks walking past Mission Street's corner bodegas and outdoor produce bins and then turns up to Valencia Street, allowing you to see the exploding boutique, artisan, multicultural foodie corridor of the new urban, affluent tech workers—all with a bit of Latin flavor. Enjoy.

Explore inside Mission Dolores.

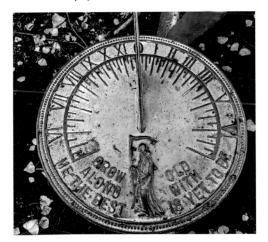

Begin: Market Street at 14th Street
End: Cesar Chavez Street at Mission Street
Distance: ROUTE: 1.9 miles — 3,800 steps — 40 minutes
LOOP BACK: 1.9 miles — 3,800 steps — 40 minutes

Hill Rating: 3

Sites you will pass on today's walk include:

MILE 40

1. **Dolores Street**

2. **Tanforan Cottages** 214 and 220 Dolores St

3. **Sha'ar Zahav and First Mennonite Church of San Francisco** 290 Dolores St

MUST-SEE

4. **Mission Dolores** 3321 16th St

5. **Mission High School** 3750 18th St

6. **Mission Dolores Park** 19th St and Dolores St

a. **Hidalgo's statue stands high over Dolores Park today**

b. **Golden Fire Hydrant** Church St and 20th St

MILE 41

7. **Integral Yoga Institute** 770 Dolores St

8. **Views** at Jersey St and 25th St

9. **Salvation Army Rehab Center** 1500 Valencia St

10. **St. Luke's Hospital** 3555 Cesar Chavez St

11. **3435 Army Sign** Cesar Chavez St and Mission St

MUST-SEE

ON WALK-BACK LOOP

MISSION STREET

c. **Yummy Food** Mission St at 25th St

VALENCIA CORRIDOR

d. **Dandelion Chocolate Factory** 740 Valencia St at 18th St

e. **Good Vibrations,** 603 Valencia St at 17th St

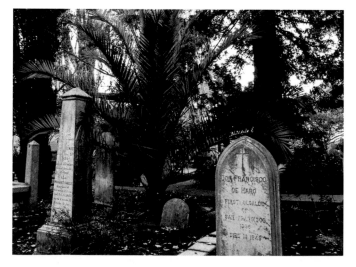

Alcalde Francisco de Haro's tombstone at Mission Dolores

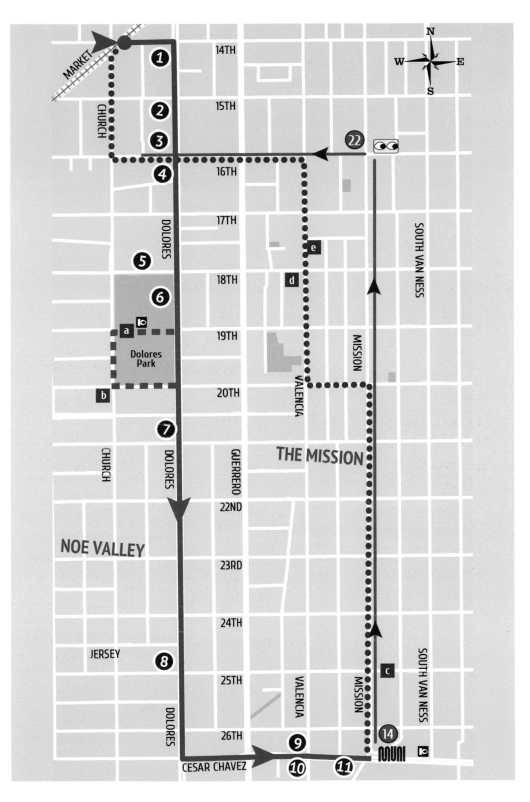

MILE 40

Begins on 14th ST at
MARKET ST

· · · · · · · · · · · · · · · · ·

At the intersection of
MARKET ST, CHURCH
ST, and 14th ST, start
at the opposite side
of the street from
Safeway.

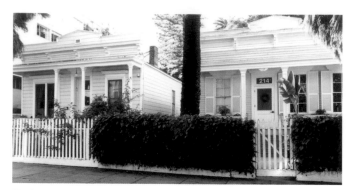

Tanforan Cottages

Head east (downhill)
on 14th ST (away from
Twin Peaks)

Right on Dolores

· · · · · · · · · · · · · · · · ·

1. Dolores Street

This boulevard of rolling hills
adds more than just beauty
to the city. The wide expanse
of Dolores Street created a
life-saving firebreak during
the 1906 earthquake and
fire. Thus surviving Victorians
can be seen on the west side,
while the east side has the
newer Edwardians.

Some historians say Golden
Gate Park superintendent
John McLaren began lining
the median with palm trees
in preparation for the 1915
Pan Pacific Expo. Other
sources claim that the Phoenix
palms that lined Panama
Pacific Avenue of Palms were
transplanted to Dolores Street
when the fair was torn down.
Either way, the towering palms
turned Dolores Street into the
grand lady of the Mission.

Palm Funday

Los Angeles may be
the palm tree capital of
California today, but in 1900
San Francisco had the most
landscaped palms in the
state. We planted a Palm
City for the 1894 Midwinter
Expo, adorned Union Square
with them, and enjoyed the
Palm Garden at the Palace
Hotel. Alas, most fell in the
1906 quake. Some were
replaced. The city chose
Phoenix palms for the 1915
expo (Phoenix being the
symbol of SF), but the love
affair started growing cold.
The last civic palm planting
projects celebrated the
completion of the Golden
Gate and Bay Bridges, as
well as an obligatory Palm
Avenue at the 1939–40
Golden Gate International
Expo. Los Angeles picked
up the slack. However, for
reasons unknown, the 1989
Loma Prieta quake inspired
a new wave of palm tree
enthusiasm, so someone
needs to go count LA's palms
and see where we stand.

2. Tanforan Cottages
214 and 220 Dolores St

Built in the 1850s, this pair
of redwood cottages built
by the Tanforan ranching
family on land that lay within
the 1836 Mexican grant to
Francisco Guerrero are likely
the oldest residences in the
city. Today, nonprofits use
them for residential treatment
programs.

3. Sha'ar Zahav and the First Mennonite Church of SF
290 Dolores St

"Congregation Sha'ar Zahav is a
progressive Reform synagogue,
established in 1977. We
are lesbian, gay, bisexual,
transgender and heterosexual
Jews, together with family
and friends, both Jewish and
non-Jewish. We worship God
with egalitarian, feminist and
gay-positive Jewish liturgy."
—Shaarzahav.org

"First Mennonite Church of
San Francisco is an Anabaptist
community committed to
joyfully walking in the way of

Jesus in community with each other . . . [we seek] to follow Jesus' example by welcoming [everyone]." —Menno.org

⚠ MUST–SEE STOP, $5

4. Mission Dolores
3321 16th St

Misión San Francisco de Asís, founded in 1776, stands as the oldest surviving structure in San Francisco and the sixth religious settlement established as part of the California chain of missions. The Mission Cemetery remains one of only three burial sites still within the city limits (along with the National Cemetery in the Presidio and the Columbarium). Though many of the original Mission Dolores buildings were secularized after 1835—becoming a hospital, German brewery, saloons, gambling hall, and more—the parish remained active serving the community. If you look into the larger

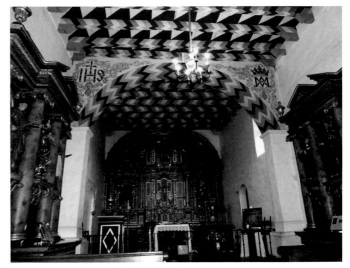

Inside Mission Dolores

basilica parish next door to the mission you may see a *Quinceañera* or wedding taking place as you walk by.

> The padres found the lagoon and site of the original mission on the Friday before Easter—the Day of Sorrows when Jesus was crucified—so they named it Laguna de los Dolores.

5. Mission High School (on 18th St facing Dolores Park)
3750 18th St

Built in 1896, this is San Francisco's oldest high school still sitting on its original site. It was rebuilt in the Spanish baroque style after a fire in the mid 1920s (though seismic retrofitting in the '70s required much of the ornamentation be removed).

Nearly 70% of the students come from low-income families and 50% are learning English. By giving a lot of one-on-one attention to students, including students' leadership skills and community involvement, as well as improving

> *"San Francisco was destined to become a gay mecca. After all, it was named after St. Francis, a sissy."*
> —unknown comic

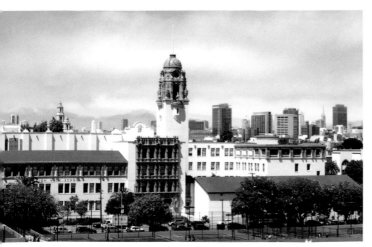

Mission High School

grades, Mission High has become one of SF's big turn-around schools—impressing college admission officers including those at UC Berkeley. *Great job, Mission Bears!*

—*Jill Tucker, SFGATE.com*

"Oye Como Va"
Grammy award–winning musician/guitarist Carlos Santana is an alumnus of Mission High School.

6. Dolores Park
19th St and Dolores St

Formerly the site of a Jewish cemetery (1861–1895) and a camp for 1,600 earthquake refugees in 1906, today this is one of the city's most popular parks—freshly renovated with tennis courts, a new children's playground, plenty of grassy spots for tanning, and an event for everyone including Cinco de Mayo, Dyke March, Film in the Park Night, Dogs Clean Up and

Social, and the over-the-top Sisters of Perpetual Indulgence Easter-time Hunky Jesus Contest. And it is all surrounded by yummy eateries—stop and have a snack.

Dolores Park is NOT named for Mission Dolores!
When Father Miguel Hidalgo rang the church bell in the city of Dolores Hidalgo as a public cry for freedom, his *El Grito de Dolores* ("cry of Dolores") sparked the Mexican Revolution.

18th Street
Heading west for five blocks this corridor will take you to the heart of the Castro; a detour east we'll take you past Bi-Rite's scrumptious ice cream and the startling murals of the Women's Building in the first block as it heads on to Mission Street.

Dolores Street

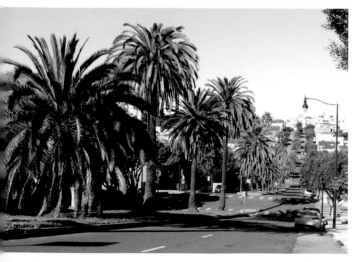

DETOUR

Halfway past Dolores Park, at 19th Street, enter the park, climb the stairs past the Mexican liberty bell and the statue of Father Hidalgo, exit the park, turn left on Church Street, walk up to 20th Street to see the Golden Fire Hydrant, turn left on 20th back to Dolores Street, turn right on Dolores to rejoin the route. (NOTE: There is a restroom halfway up the stairs)

a. Hidalgo's statue stands high over Dolores Park today

❗ SF HIDDEN GEM

b. Golden Fire Hydrant
Church St and 20th St

During the 1906 San Francisco earthquake and its subsequent citywide fires, this "little giant" (one of the few functioning hydrants in the city) saved the historic Mission District from complete destruction. Each year, on the April 18 anniversary of the Great Quake, the fire hydrant receives a new coat of gold paint at 5:12 a.m., the exact time the massive earthquake destroyed 80% of San Francisco.

Victorian Architecture Quiz

Read the architecture chapter and then see if you can correctly identify the style of these Victorian homes on Dolores Street when you go on Walk 14. *(Correct answers are listed on page 190.)*

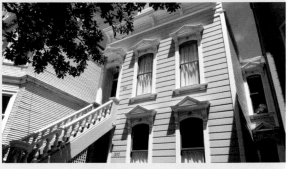

1. 816 Dolores Street
   a. flat-front Italianate Victorian
   b. slanted-bay Italianate Victorian

2. 833–837 Dolores Street
   a. San Francisco stick
   b. Edwardian

3. 839 Dolores Street
   a. San Francisco stick
   b. flat-front Italianate Victorian

4. 890 Dolores Street
   a. Slanted Bay Italianate Victorian
   b. Queen Anne Victorian

5. 945–947 Dolores Street
   a. San Francisco stick
   b. flat-front Italianate Victorian

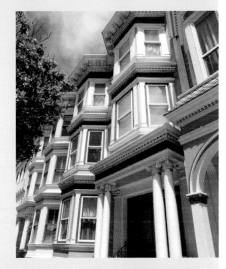

6. 987-991 Dolores Street
   a. Queen Anne Victorian
   b. Edwardian

7. 1074–1076 Dolores Street
   a. Edwardian
   b. San Francisco stick

8. 1083 Dolores Street
   a. Queen Anne Victorian with turret
   b. San Francisco stick

9. 1157-1161 Dolores Street
   a. flat-front Italianate Victorian
   b. Edwardian

10. 1191–1193 Dolores Street
    a. Queen Anne Victorian
    b. slanted-bay Italianate Victorian

11. 1200 Dolores Street
    a. Queen Anne Victorian with turret
    b. Edwardian

12. 1249 Dolores Street
    a. Queen Anne Victorian
    b. San Francisco stick

13. 1257–1261 Dolores Street
    a. Edwardian with curved windows
    b. San Francisco stick

14. 1273–1275 Dolores Street
    a. Queen Anne Victorian
    b. Edwardian

15. 1285–1287 Dolores Street
    a. flat-front Italianate Victorian
    b. San Francisco stick

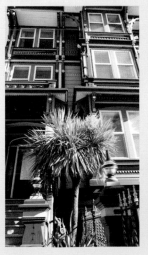

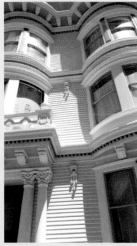

Noe Valley—24th Street Corridor

José de Jesús Noé, the last Mexican *alcalde* ("mayor") of Yerba Buena, sold his rancho to John Horner, a Mormon immigrant, in 1854. Horner laid out the area for development. The city assessor's office still calls it Horner's addition today. At first home to Scandinavian dairy farmers, German and Irish workers soon joined them—moving into the row houses built specifically for working-class families who couldn't afford the upscale areas of the city.

Today it is an upscale, gentrified neighborhood but retains its low-crime, family-oriented village charm. Heading west (right) up **24th Street** for a few blocks takes you to Noe Valley's main shopping corridor.

MILE 41

Begins on DOLORES ST at 22nd ST

7. Integral Yoga Institute
770 Dolores St

A spiritual community (ashram) offering classical Hatha Yoga instruction to the public daily—in a converted Victorian mansion. What's not to like? Open to all. Bliss.

▌ LOOK

8. Views
  • at Jersey St look right for Twin Peaks view on Dolores St
  • at 25th Street look left . . .

See how the next few streets run toward the bay? The next street over, 26th Street, skirts Potrero Hill and, before the freeway went in, ran all the way to the Navy Pier so it was originally named Navy Street.

Army Street (later renamed Cesar Chavez Street) ran to the Army Pier.

. . . .
Left CESAR CHAVEZ
. . . .

▌ LOOK

Three old-time San Francisco institutions sit across from each other on Cesar Chavez.

9. Salvation Army Adult Rehabilitation Center
1500 Valencia St

Motivated by its spiritual convictions, the Salvation Army has been offering food, shelter, and a helping hand to the underserved in San Francisco since 1883. In fact, the famous red Christmas kettle tradition began here in 1891 when Captain Joseph McFee set out a giant iron pot at the Ferry Building to collect funds to deliver Christmas dinner to destitute San Franciscans. The "Army" serves about 70,000 people a year in SF. One of 16 in the city, this center on Valencia Street, provides clinical treatment and rehabilitation for men and women battling substance abuse and chemical dependency.

10. St. Luke's Hospital
3555 Cesar Chavez St

St. Luke's Hospital, serving the medical needs of the community since 1873, merged with California Pacific Medical Center in 2007. The original St. Luke's building crumbled in the 1906 earthquake, so the hospital moved for a while to a tent under the grandstand of the New California Jockey Club Race Track.

Name Game

Many Noe Valley streets were laid out and named by landowner John Horner. Elizabeth Street, after his wife, and Jersey Street, after his home state, retain their original names. However, when the city decided to simplify and organize city street names after the 1906 quake city by turning them into numbered streets and avenues, his Park Street, Temple Street, and Navy Street became 24th, 25th, and 26th Streets, respectively. Army Street retained its name for nearly a century, but became Cesar Chavez Street in 1995.

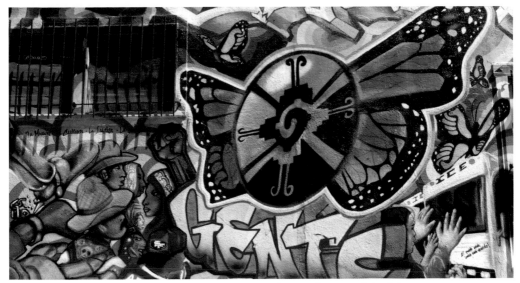

Mission and 25th Street mural. You'll see even more murals on Walk 15's walk-back loop.

11. 3435 Army Sign, former Sears Building

Cesar Chavez St and Mission St

Look up toward the top of the big squat building to your right, just past Valencia Street. The "3435 Army Street" address sign identifies the former Sears Roebuck department store, which sold goods to San Franciscans from 1926 to 1975. Now the building houses the EDD Human Services Agency and other groups.

· · · · · · · · · · · · · · · · · · · ·

END CESAR CHAVEZ STREET at MISSION STREET

· · · · · · · · · · · · · · · · · · · ·

WALK-BACK LOOP SCOOP

For authentic cultural and SF experiences, good food, and one-of-a-kind stores in one of the city's most vibrant neighborhoods, this is a must-

see walk-back loop. See details on page 203.

MISSION STREET

Rougher and far more Latino than neighboring Valencia Street, this section of Mission Street has been a commercial corridor for Latino families since the 1940s—and many of the clothing and jewelry shops, bakeries, and grocery stores look as though they haven't been remodeled since. Shopping here makes for a

Waves of Workers

The oldest-known occupants of San Francisco were the Yelamu (Ohlone) Indians who had lived here for 2,000 years before the Spanish missionaries came. The peaceful natives were pressed into building the Mission in the 18th century and within 30 years were essentially wiped out from abuse and disease. Irish and German immigrants came with the Gold Rush in the 19th century, followed by Polish immigrants in the 1920s. Mexican immigration flourished in the 1940s–1960s, followed by an influx of Central and South Americans in the 1960s–1980s. Tech boom workers and young urban professionals have been the most recent wave in the 1990s–2010s.

The Mission's Latin flavor took permanent hold with the "white flight" beginning in the 1940s. Now, with the recent dramatic rise in rents and home prices in this historically blue-collar neighborhood, the Latin population has dropped by about 20% in recent years.

real adventure, and the food selection takes you around the globe—Senegalese, Italian, Mediterranean, Japanese, Indian, French, Thai, Mexican. You'll even find vegan restaurants.

c. Yummy Food
Mission St at 25th St

Between the banana cream pies at the 21st-century Mission Pie (2007) and the rum cakes of the historic Italian bakery, Dianda's (1962) sits highly rated La Taqueria, one of the first taquerias to open in the area (1973). (All three contribute to Kristine's waistline—Carolyn's weakness is Cosmopolitans.)

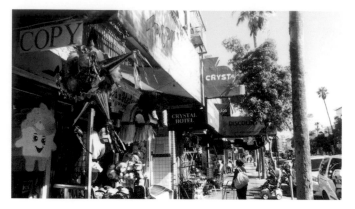

VALENCIA CORRIDOR

Not so long ago, Valencia Street was a funky mix of car-repair shops, seedy dives, nonprofit media centers, and women-owned businesses catering to the urban poor and Latino communities. Today, its vibrant mix of pupuserias, art galleries, restaurants, and nightlife and the spirit of independent design have been greatly influenced by an explosion of new "hipster" restaurants, bars, and furniture, fashion, and artisan shops which have cropped up to cater to the newest Mission tech-sector residents.

For example:

d. Dandelion Chocolate Factory 740 Valencia St at 18th St

A bean-to-bar craft chocolate factory. Dandelion has been roasting the beans and hand-wrapping each bar of chocolate right there since 2010.

e. Good Vibrations
603 Valencia St at 17th St

This sex-positive erotica store has been run by and for women since 1977.

Both offer tours and classes!

16th and Valencia: the epicenter of Tech-Worker and Mission Vibe Hipdom

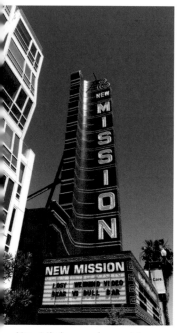

New Mission condos next to restored historic Mission Theater marquee

24th Street Corridor (on return loop)
This commercial corridor starts in the lower Mission at Potrero Street with businesses by and for Latino families, then passes the 24th Street BART Station on Mission Street continuing north over the hill through the upscale family community and shops of Noe Valley (which you just passed). Walk 15 return-loop takes you up the eastern, Latino portion of 24th Street.

WALK 14 NEED TO KNOW

TO GET THERE
Muni, K, L, M, T, F-Line, 22, 37 to CHURCH STREET STATION

PARKING
It can be challenging at times to find street parking here, and when you do it will be limited to 2 hours.

PUBLIC RESTROOMS
- Dolores Park at 19th St stairway (on detour)
- Cesar Chavez (South Van Ness)

TURN–BY–TURN INSTRUCTIONS
Begin: at MARKET

- At the intersection of MARKET ST, CHURCH ST, and 14th ST, start at the opposite side of the street from Safeway.
- Head east (downhill) on 14th ST (away from Twin Peaks)
- Right on DOLORES ST
- Left on CESAR CHAVEZ ST

End: CESAR CHAVEZ ST at MISSION ST

TO GET BACK
Muni

- Board 14 (towards STEUART ST) at NE corner of 26th ST and MISSION ST
- Get off at 16th ST and MISSION ST
- Transfer to 22
- Get off at NE corner of 16th ST and CHURCH ST

Other Muni transit routes: 12, 27, 36, 49

WALK-BACK LOOP DIRECTIONS
Distance: 1.9 miles, 3,800 steps, 40 minutes

Rating:

This must-see walk-back loop is fascinating for all the reasons mentioned in the points-of-interest section, plus it's an easy, flat 1.9 miles. BUT NOTE: The farther you get down MISSION ST, the rougher it gets, so this walk turns off MISSION ST early, at 20th ST. If you choose to walk all the way to 14th ST or take the Muni

transfer at 16th ST, you will be passing homeless people and drug addicts. Stay aware.

Begin: CESAR CHAVEZ ST and MISSION ST

- Left (north) onto MISSION ST, going in the direction you came from
- Left on 20th ST
- Right on VALENCIA ST
- Left on 16th ST
- Right on CHURCH ST
- Right on MARKET ST

End: 14th ST and MARKET ST

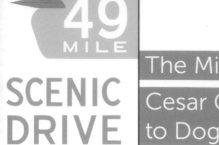

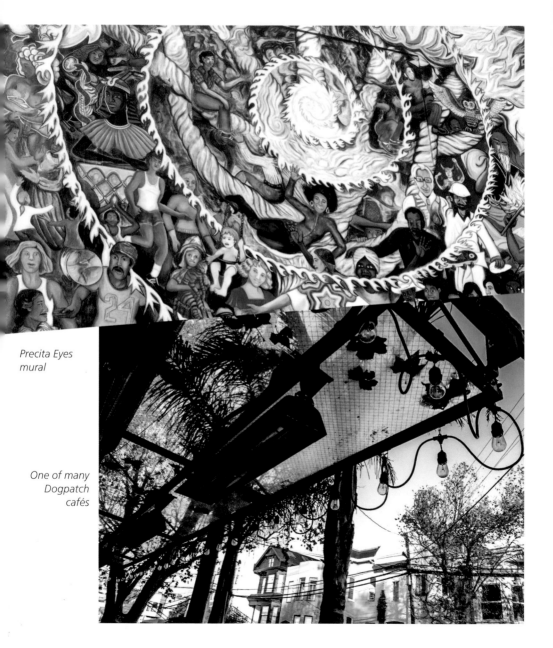

Precita Eyes mural

One of many Dogpatch cafés

Are you ready for a rough and raw, urban adventure? The historic 49 Mile route takes us nearly the entire length of Cesar Chavez Street—the dividing line between four neighborhoods: the Mission and Bernal Heights, then Potrero Hill and Bayview-Hunters Point. Historically, these have been the neighborhoods where the blue-collar workers who built the city live.

This multilane road on the outer edges of town inclines toward run-down and industrial, but the hike begins with a stroll along the newly constructed Cesar Chavez Sewer & Streetscape Improvement Project. This long-sought-after neighborhood upgrade includes a tree-lined median, bike lane, pedestrian bulb-outs, left-turn pockets, new sewer lines to replace century-old pipes, and Sí Se Puede Plaza, named for the motto of Cesar Chavez's United Farm Workers union.

If you aren't an experienced city hiker, the second half of this walk may feel a bit dicey as you follow the cement trail under U.S. 101, walking along the truck thoroughfare through the industrial, warehouse second mile of Cesar Chavez—but you'll be rewarded. First we peek at the hidden playground of the Department of Public Works, and then we ignore the official 49 mile route signs directing traffic onto the freeway and instead veer off for a surprise ending in charming Dogpatch. Plus, this walk has a "must see" walk-back loop through the historic, tree-lined, mural-laden stretch of 24th Street known as El Corazón de la Mission, "the heart of the Mission."

NOTE: At Indiana Street the official 49 mile route markers direct automobiles to the 280 freeway. Walkers: Ignore the official sign on Indiana Street. Follow the directions here to explore Dogpatch.

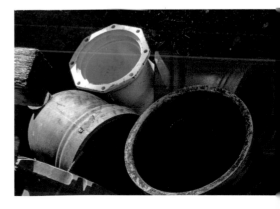

Begin: Cesar Chavez Street at Mission Street
End: 3rd Street at 22nd Street
Distance: ROUTE: 2.3 miles — 4,600 steps —45 minutes
LOOP BACK: 0.9 mile — 1,800 steps — 20 minutes

Hill Rating:

2

Sites you will pass on today's walk include:

MILE 42

1. **Cesar Chavez Street**

2. **Mission Street**

3. **St. Anthony of Padua Church and School** 299 Precita Ave at Folsom St

4. **Mission Murals** 3125 Cesar Chavez

5. **Precita Park** Precita Ave between Folsom St and Alabama St

BERNAL HEIGHTS

MILE 43

6. **U.S. 101/Bayshore Freeway**

7. **Bayshore Boulevard**

8. **Eagle-Warrior Sculpture** Cesar Chavez St and Bayshore Blvd

9. **DPW Maintenance Yard** 2323 Cesar Chavez St

POTRERO HILL

BAYVIEW-HUNTERS POINT

10. **San Francisco Yellow Cab Co-op** 1200 Mississippi St

11. **Interstate 280**

12. **Progress Park** 1325 Indiana St

13. **Muni Biodiesel Maintenance Yard** Indiana St

DOGPATCH

ON WALK-BACK LOOP
a. **24th Street Corridor**

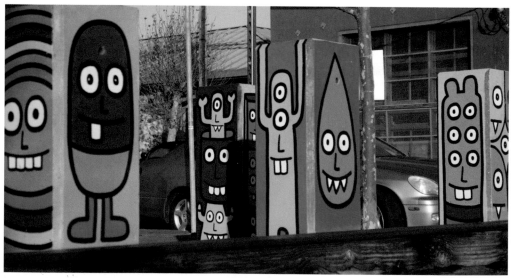

Dogpatch playground art
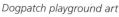

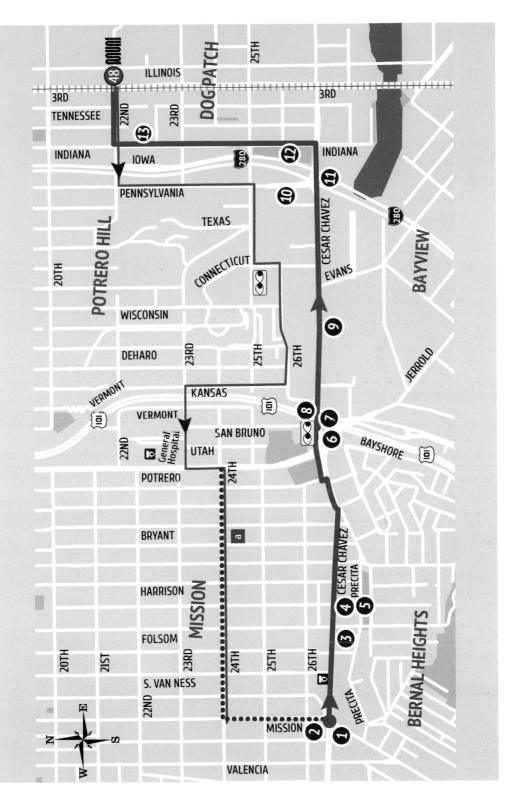

MILE 42

Begins on CESAR CHAVEZ ST at MISSION ST

• • • • • • • • • • • • • • • • • •

Continue walking east on CESAR CHAVEZ ST (on the odd-numbered south side of the street)

• • • • • • • • • • • • • • • • • •

1. Cesar Chavez Street

You've reached the southern border of the Mission District. Once known as Army Street, because it ran to the Army Pier on the bay, this corridor was re-named for farmworker activist Cesar Chavez, amid much pro-and-con uproar in 1995. In the 1930s and 1940s Army Street was widened into an eight-lane thoroughfare to give cross-town traffic a way to access the newly planned 101 Bayshore Freeway—which basically turned a residential street into a noisy, dangerous, freeway-on-the-ground. Recently, the neighborhood campaigned to have the city turn the street into a more safe, livable neigh-borhood thoroughfare, and the neighborhood won.

NOTE: A 22-minute documen-tary about Cesar Chavez Street by Susie Smith, *People Live Here,* debuted in Precita Park in 2013 at the annual Bernal Heights Outdoor Film Festival (you can find it on vimeo.com)

2. Mission Street

This 7.2-mile arterial thorough-fare is the city's longest and nearly oldest street. It runs from San Francisco Bay at the city's northeast corner all the way to her southern border and then on into Daly City. The southern end of Mission Street is part of the old El Camino Real built to connect all the Spanish missions in California (although Mission Street no longer goes directly to Mission Dolores). Some of the best restaurants and clubs in the city are found at this far southern end of Mission Street you are crossing today.

NOTE: You can read more about the Mission in Walk 14, which loops back down Mission and Valencia Streets.

VIEW: To your right is SOCHA, to your left is NOCHA, the new real-estate designations for south and north of Cesar Chavez.

3. St. Anthony of Padua Church and School
299 Precita Ave at Folsom St

In 1876 Dominican Sisters came to San Francisco to teach Ger-man immigrant children in the Mission. In 1950 they expand-ed to teach Italian immigrant children. After more than 100 years of teaching children in the neighborhood, St. Anthony-Im-maculate Conception School brought in its first lay (non-or-dained) principal in 2008.

4. Mission Murals— Flynn Elementary
3125 Cesar Chavez

Here's another great reason to get out walking even more in

Cesar Chavez

Union leader and labor organizer Cesar Chavez dedicated his life to improving treatment, pay, and working conditions for farmworkers. Stressing nonviolent methods, Chavez drew attention for his causes via boycotts, marches, and his own hunger strikes. He encouraged the Hispanic laborers to join the Filipino grape workers strike and then form the United Farmworkers of America. It is believed that Chavez's several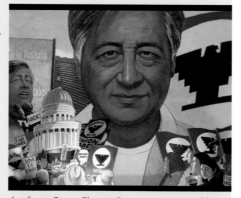

Art from Cesar Chavez Day poster created by the U.S. Department of Labor.

hunger strikes contributed to his death at age 65. His birthday, March 31, is a state holiday in California. —*Biography.com*

the city once you've finished your 49 mile challenge: SF City Guides Free Walking Tours. The Mission Mural Tour (including Balmy Alley) begins up on Harrison Street behind Flynn Elementary School. Don't miss the murals along the side of Flynn Elementary as you walk by.

Precita Eyes Muralists Association

In 1977 Susan and Luis Cervantes started creating community murals to build community, celebrate SF's cultural heritage, prevent graffiti, and teach children about art. You can see their wonderful, colorful gift to San Francisco all through the Mission. *Thank you!*

—PrecitaEyes.org

5. **Precita Park** Precita Ave between Folsom St and Alabama St

A neighborhood park since 1894, this lovely three-blocks long-by-one-block-wide grassy

park offers a playground, butterfly garden, and numerous surrounding cafés. Of note is a memorial bench dedicated to two teenagers who were killed in the park in 1996. The bench was built from cedar and melted guns by John Ricker, whose Peaceful Streets organization invites the public to donate guns, and then melts them to transform them into art.

"Either you were a hoodlum, or you were a puddle on the sidewalk."

—Jerry Garcia, musician, singer/songwriter for the Grateful Dead, born in San Francisco in 1942, lived just beyond Bernal Heights in the Excelsior District until age 11.

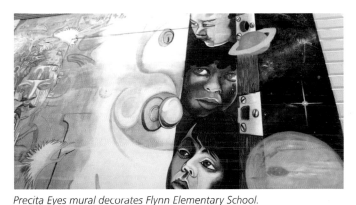

Precita Eyes mural decorates Flynn Elementary School.

BERNAL HEIGHTS

FriendlyNeighborhoodGuide.com lovingly describes Bernal Heights as "where hipsters and lesbians go when they tire of Mission craziness and want to settle down." This formerly affordable area still has a "small-town feel" and an enviable off-leash dog park sitting high on hill with a 360-degree city view—all just minutes from downtown. The

"Who you callin' hipster?"

The moniker "hipster" can refer to any number of bands, people, or situations—yet it's hard to find anyone who self-identifies as a hipster.

- **History:** It began as a term associated with the jazz subculture in the 1940s, "hepsters."
- **Philosophy:** In the 2010s it became the label for a subculture of white, affluent, 20- and 30-year-olds, living in gentrifying big-city neighborhoods, broadly associated with independent thinking, counterculture, progressive politics, and indie-rock, and favoring organic artisanal foods and witty banter, while wearing vintage and thrift store-inspired fashions.
- **Fashion:** As the "effortless, cool, urban bohemian" hipster look became popular—hipster also became a fashion description for any young, bearded guy wearing tight-fitting jeans and thick-rimmed glasses.
- **Attitude:** The perceived "air of superiority and entitlement" of many hipsters has turned the label into a pejorative used to describe someone seen as pretentious or overly trendy.

restaurants, parks, shopping corridor on Cortland, and crime rate have all improved with the slow gentrification over the last few decades.

NOTE: The neighborhood has an active history association: BernalHistoryProject.org.

MILE 43

Begins at CESAR CHAVEZ ST at U.S. 101

To get under the freeway, if you are walking on the south side of the CESAR CHAVEZ ST as you approach 101, take the pedestrian overpass to the north side of the street

▌ LOOK

When you reach the top of the pedestrian overpass, look around. Would you want this freeway in your neighborhood? In the 1950s, 10 such freeways were planned to crisscross and divide the city.

Walk on the narrow sidewalk next to Rolph Playground

Use the crosswalk on POTRERO AVE

Follow the signs to the pedestrian undercrossing (don't use the bicycle path)

Continue on the south side of CESAR CHAVEZ ST

6. U.S. 101/Bayshore Freeway

Built in the 1940s and 1950s, **U.S Route 101** connects San Jose and San Francisco. In the city it is also called the James Lick Freeway.

7. Bayshore Boulevard

Bayshore Boulevard marks the former shoreline of the bay before it was filled in with rubble. In the 1930s Bayshore replaced El Camino Real as U.S. Route 101 into the city but was subsequently replaced by the new, elevated U.S. 101 freeway in the 1950s.

8. Eagle-Warrior Sculpture
intersection of Cesar Chavez St, Bayshore Blvd, and 26th St

For 2,000 years of Mesoamerican civilization, an elite corps of eagle-warriors served as religious and military leaders. This sculpture by Pepe Ozan next to the bicycle path under U.S. 101 honors the Indigenous heritage of this region.

▌ LOOK

9. Department of Public Works Maintenance Yard
2323 Cesar Chavez St

Look through the fence openings and over the railing for the next few blocks. Way cool equipment . . . backhoes, meter maid tri-wheelers, sewage elephants, barricades, grates . . . is that a boat? This is where the essential, unsung equipment that keeps our magnificent city running lives.

POTRERO HILL

"If a giant cat lived in San Francisco, Potrero Hill is where it would pick as its spot to sleep. It's that coveted high cozy corner, peaceful but not too far from the action." — SanFranciscoDays.com

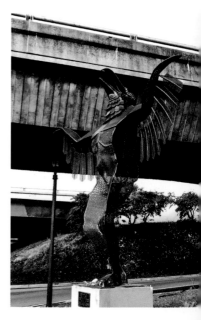

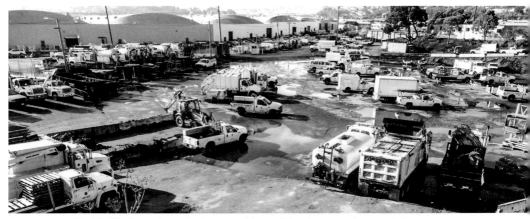

Department of Public Works—where the inner workings of the city go to sleep at night

One of the sunniest neighborhoods in the city, Potrero Hill has two parts. The northern slope: upper-middle-class, family-oriented residential neighborhood with nice restaurants and small businesses. And the southern end: housing projects so badly managed the federal government threatened to step in and take them over. Today, Hope SF is working to update and integrate the housing projects into the community with state-of-the-art mixed-income housing.

Find out about Potrero Hills History Night at PotreroArchives.com.

Athlete, actor, and convicted felon O.J. Simpson lived in the Potrero housing projects as a youth. In the mid-1960s he starred as a football running back at SF City College, including setting a junior college national rushing records and twice winning the title "conference player of the year."

When Artists and Queers Move In
In between its humble working-class past and its gentrified upper-middle-class present, Potrero Hill was an inexpensive, bohemian, creative hub full of artist studios, showrooms, and art schools.

BAYVIEW–HUNTERS POINT

"The door between Bayview and the rest of San Francisco opened slightly with introduction of the Third Street (T) Muni Line, marginally softening its reputation as a toxic and dangerous corner of the city."

—SanFranciscoDays.com

The long-neglected, blighted Bayview neighborhood is also the city's sunniest neighborhood with fantastic city

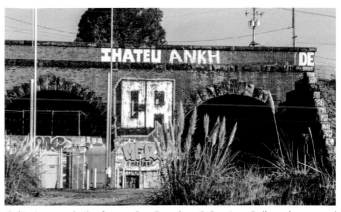

CalTrain tunnel. The former San Francisco & San Jose Railway has served Peninsula commuters since 1864.

views and blocks and blocks of adorable middle-class homes. People are flocking to the very affordable housing (next to the new public transit line), businesses are moving in, the government is actively working to rehab it, the toxic naval shipyard is being cleaned up—and the neighborhood dynamics are shifting.

10. San Francisco Yellow Cab Co-op
1200 Mississippi St

When the former Yellow Cab Company went belly-up in 1976 a group of cab drivers, mechanics, dispatchers, and other local investors purchased it by creating a co-op. Each member put in $5,000 to cover the down payment. Today Yellow Cab Co-op is a completely independent, locally owned operation in San Francisco, boasting that "women, gay and minority

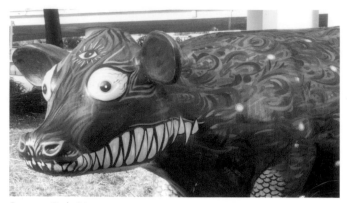

Progress Park. Mooooo.

shareholders comprise about 50% of the membership."

. . . .

At CONNECTICUT ST, cross to the north side of the street

Left on INDIANA ST, stay on the right-hand side of street

. . . .

11. Interstate 280

Conceived in 1955 and completed in 1970, Interstate 280 is the Interstate Highway System route from San Jose to San Francisco. In 2013 urban renewal planners began considering tearing it down and making it San Francisco's third freeway-to-boulevard conversion (as with the Embarcadero and Central Freeways). Stay tuned.

12. Progress Park
1325 Indiana St

There's an odd sliver of land on Indiana Street created

by an I-280 entrance ramp and the elevated freeway. Dogpatch residents have done an amazing job of planting, designing, and turning it into a beautiful neighborhood asset—including an off-leash dog area.

13. Muni Biodiesel Maintenance Yard
1001 22nd St and Indiana St

These new hybrid buses are here to help Muni reach its goal to become 100% emission-free by 2020! Woohoo! Though initially more expensive to acquire ($500,000 vs. $350,000 for old buses), the 30% decrease in fuel cost and savings in maintenance from fewer moving parts will make up the difference. Passengers will appreciate that the hybrid buses are more reliable (fewer broken-down buses!), are lower to the ground for easier boarding, and run more smoothly. Officially called the **John M. Woods**

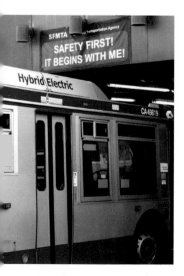

Muni Goal: 100% emission-free by 2020

Motor Coach Center, or "Woods Division," this center is also home of the cable car carpentry shop where skilled Muni tradesmen and women build and repair our historic cable cars.

. . . .
Right on 22nd ST
. . . .

Miss Eastine Cowner, a former waitress, is helping construct the Liberty ship SS George Washington Carver *at the Kaiser Shipyards (1943).*

STRUGGLE AND HOPE

In the 1940s African Americans flocked to San Francisco for wartime work in the shipyards. Many lived in the Fillmore District but were forced out when the city's urban renewal plans bulldozed their "Harlem of the West" neighborhood in the 1960s. Because housing discrimination severely limited African American housing choices, many moved to the Bayview.

As the postwar shipping industry and jobs left Hunters Point, the white population moved to more attractive suburbs. The African American population swelled from 21% in the 1950s to 69% by the 1970s. Meanwhile, freeway construction (both 101 and 280) and poor public transportation cut off the district from the rest of the city. When the last big employer, Hunters Point Naval Shipyard, closed in 1974 the economy of the area collapsed. The polluted, toxic shipyards were unsuitable for any other industry. Isolation, lack of jobs, harsh living conditions, and neglect soon led to poverty, crime, and trouble with drugs and gangs.

From the 1950s through the 1970s Bayview-Hunters Point was a flashpoint of racial conflict and civil rights debates in SF—and then it became the city's forgotten, neglected neighborhood. Yet, in the midst of that, there has always been a large core of home-owning, business-owning middle-class African Americans struggling to keep the culture, neighborhood, and small businesses viable.

Today, the sweeping socio-economic trends of this century have created a spike in density and a major demographic shift in Bayview. This time around, the city's urban renewal plans seem to be better planned including a federal grant to clean up the pollution and develop it into a center for green jobs. The longtime residents hope the Bayview of tomorrow will retain its scrappy charm and commitment to social justice— and its memory of the past.
—BayviewFootprints.org

NOTE: To learn more about Bayview-Hunters Point's complicated, unknown history, search YouTube for the documentary *Point of Pride: The People's View of Bayview/ Hunters Point,* by Dimitri Moore (2014).

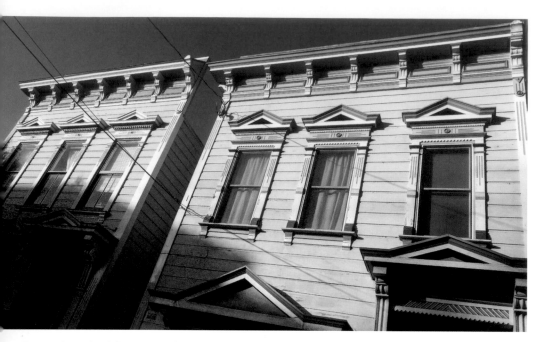

Dogpatch survived the 1906 quake and has some of the city's oldest buildings.

DOGPATCH

Here it is: a neighborhood that *survived* the 1906 earthquake and fire! That's why this formerly thriving industrial waterfront area is still chock-full of historic buildings, including the city's oldest firehouse and public school, and quaint workers cottages built as far back as the 1860s. Its early shipbuilding glory days slipped away after WWII, and by the 1960s it had fallen into urban blight. Bit by bit since the 1970s, warehouses and factories have become artist lofts, upper-middle-class folks have moved down off Potrero Hill into the flatlands, and today gourmet gastronomic pit stops have popped up alongside other entertaining entrepreneurial enterprises, making Dogpatch a #cool #disruptive #maker space.

· · · · · · · · · · · · · · · · · ·

END on 22nd ST and 3rd ST

· · · · · · · · · · · · · · · · · ·

ON WALK-BACK LOOP

a. 24th Street Corridor
beginning at Potrero St

This historic, tree-lined stretch of 24th Street running from Potrero to Mission Street is known as El Corazón de la Mission, or "the heart of the Mission." Many of the oldest shops and bakeries along this street have been here since the 1940s and 1950s, when workers came from Mexico to work in the shipyards and factories and settled. The **St. Francis Fountain and Diner** has been here since 1918. Though "hipster-fication" has seeped through in the form of gourmet ice cream, donut, and coffee shops, the street boasts a vast number of unique stores and restaurants as well as the greatest concentration of murals in the city.

WALK-BACK LOOP SCOOP

Don't. Really. Grab a bus or cab at the end of this walk. But instead of going all the way back to the beginning or just going home, hop over to Potrero and 24th Streets to take the must-see 24th Street Corridow Walk. See details on page 215.

WALK 15 NEED TO KNOW

TO GET THERE
Muni 12, 14, 27, 36, 49

PARKING
Street parking

PUBLIC RESTROOMS
- Cesar Chavez (South Van Ness)
- SF General Hospital (Potrero at 23rd)

TURN-BY-TURN INSTRUCTIONS
Begin: CESAR CHAVEZ ST at MISSION ST

- Walk east on CESAR CHAVEZ ST (on the odd-numbered south side of the street)
- To get under the freeway, if you are walking on the south side of CESAR CHAVEZ ST as you approach 101, take the pedestrian overpass to the north side of the street
  - Walk on the narrow sidewalk next to Rolph Playground
  - Use the crosswalk on POTRERO AVE
  - Follow the signs to the pedestrian undercrossing (don't use the bicycle path)

- Continue on the south side of CESAR CHAVEZ ST
- At CONNECTICUT ST, cross to the north side of the street
- Left on INDIANA ST, stay on the right-hand side of street
- Right on 22nd ST

End: 22nd ST and 3rd ST

TO GET BACK
Muni

- Board bus 48 (toward Great Hwy) on NE corner at 22nd St and 3rd St
- Get off at 24th St and Mission St

Other transit routes:

- Muni K, T
- Caltrain 22nd St Station

OPTIONAL WALK-BACK LOOP DIRECTIONS
Distance: 0.9 miles, 1,800 steps, 20 minutes

Rating:

Hang out and enjoy Dogpatch for a while. Then, don't even think about walking back—most of the alternate streets you could walk back on tend toward unattractive, dangerous, or hilly. But we do have a great partial walk-back for you. Hop on a bus or grab a cab to Potrero Ave and 24th Street for a walk that will steep you in great Mission District ambience as you stroll along the not-to-be-missed 24th St corridor to Mission St. Another option, of course, is to continue on Walk 16—a visitor must see walk along the Embarcadero. But, really, 24th St is great, so do that.

Begin: Take a cab or bus to 24th ST and POTRERO AVE

- Head west on 24th ST (away from General Hospital and the Walgreens on the corner)
- Left on MISSION ST

End: MISSION ST and CESAR CHAVEZ ST

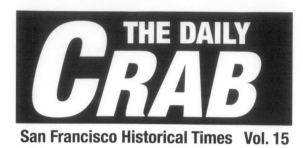

THE DAILY CRAB

FREEWAY REVOLT

San Francisco Historical Times Vol. 15

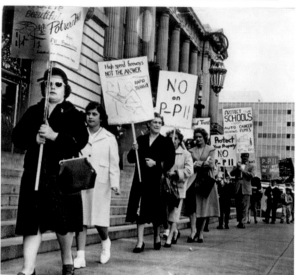

After WWII, the car was king and plans to build highways and freeways to connect us all boomed, especially in California. Neighborhood activists in San Francisco were among the first to realize these freeways would tear up streets and divide neighborhoods—and in 1955 they started a protest movement that spread around the world. By 1959, the SF Board of Supervisors voted to cancel seven of 10 planned freeways (including ones planned to go through the Panhandle, Golden Gate Park, and Glen Park Canyon). *Thank you, fellow citizens!*

1961: Placard-carrying opponents of the Southern Freeway, which would have gobbled up 63 parcels of property, including 26 residences, marched before City Hall to show their united opposition to the freeway.

Murder, Racism, Jingoism: The Founding of Potrero Hill

When Mexico owned California, the government gave the land grant for Potrero Nuevo (*potrero* or "pasture" used for grazing livestock) to **Francisco and Ramon de Haro**, the twin sons of Yerba Buena's first alcalde ("mayor"), **Francisco de Haro**. Two years later, during the Mexican-American War, U.S. Army captain **John Fremont** "caught" three unarmed Mexicans crossing San Francisco Bay. They were the 19-year-old de Haro twins and their uncle, **José de los Reyes Berreyesa**. In what many consider an act of revenge for the deaths of two Americans, Fremont ordered famed frontiersman and adventurer **Kit Carson** to execute them. Carson

protested but, under further orders, shot all three.

Potrero Hill became the property of the twins' father,

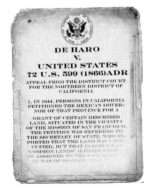

DE HARO
V.
UNITED STATES
72 U.S. 599 (1866)ADR

APPEAL FROM THE DISTRICT COURT
FOR THE NORTHERN DISTRICT OF
CALIFORNIA

1. IN 1844, PERSONS IN CALIFORNIA PETITIONED THE MEXICAN GOVERNOR OF THAT PROVINCE FOR A GRANT OF CERTAIN DESCRIBED LAND, SITUATED IN THE VICINITY OF THE MISSION OF SAN FRANCISCO. THE PETITION WAS REFERRED TO THE SECRETARY OF STATE, WHO REPORTED THAT THE LAND WAS UNOCCUPIED, BUT THAT INASMUCH AS "COMMON LANDS" (EJIDOS) WERE TO BE ASSIGNED TO THE SAID MISSION, HE WAS OF OPINION THAT...

Francisco de Haro. Fearful the U.S. government would strip de Haro of his land rights once California became U.S. property, de Haro's good friend **John**

Townsend convinced de Haro to sell off the land in lots. However, buyers were equally wary of de Haro's legal ownership. Squatters quickly moved in. After de Haro's death, his family fought all the way to the Supreme Court to retain ownership of the land. The court ruled against the de Haros in 1866. Squatters celebrated with a giant bonfire.

As for Fremont, in 1856 he ran as the first candidate of the new Republican Party for president of the United States. However, famed architect **Jasper O'Farrell** and others began publishing their eyewitness accounts of Fremont's unwarranted execution of the popular and unarmed Californios, and Fremont lost the presidential election.

MISSION
TOLL BOOTHS

Originally, Mission Street was the the main path into or out of town. It went partly through a swamp considered to be impassable for vehicles. **Charles L. Wilson** and his associates obtained the rights, leveled, filled, and planked the street—and put in a tollgate. As more roads were built and savvy travelers began detouring down to Folsom Street to skirt the toll, the savvy entrepreneurs built a tollbooth on Folsom, too.

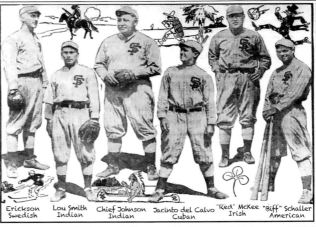

San Francisco Seals baseball team with illustrated nicknames (1917).

Erickson Swedish — Lou Smith Indian — Chief Johnson Indian — Jacinto del Calvo Cuban — "Red" McKee Irish — "Biff" Schaller American

The 280-101
Squeeze!

The majority of the population of the San Francisco Peninsula lives somewhere between Interstate 280 and U.S. Route 101.

"PLAY BALL"

In 1868, the first professional baseball stadium in California was built at Folsom and 25th: **Garfield Square**, capacity 17,000. In the 20th century, two more baseball stadiums went up in the Mission District: **Recreation Park** (14th/Valencia) and **Seals Stadium** (16th/Bryant), where the

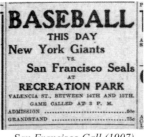

BASEBALL
THIS DAY
New York Giants
vs.
San Francisco Seals
AT
RECREATION PARK
VALENCIA ST., BETWEEN 14TH AND 15TH.
GAME CALLED AT 3 P. M.
ADMISSION 50c
GRANDSTAND 75c

San Francisco Call (1907).

Mission Reds and the **San Francisco Seals** played.

BAYVIEW: BUTCHERS & BATTLESHIPS

If you've ever experienced the sights, smells, sounds, and carnage of a slaughterhouse, you'll understand why San Francisco banned meat-butchering businesses from the city center in 1868. In response, the butchers moved to the farthest southeast reaches of the city and converted 81 acres into "Butchertown"—today known as Bayview-Hunters Point.

The area's isolation, water supply, and open spaces drew a variety of agricultural, fishing, industrial, and shipbuilding activity. It also fostered intermingling of racial and religious groups uncharacteristic of the rest of San Francisco.

In the late 1930s, the U.S. government evicted the Chinese shrimp-fishing community and pushed out many other industries to make way for the WWII military buildup and the **Hunters Point Navy Base.**

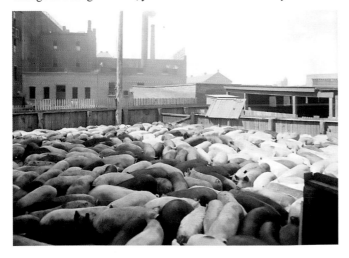

49 MILE
SCENIC DRIVE

Mission Bay

AT&T Park

The Embarcadero

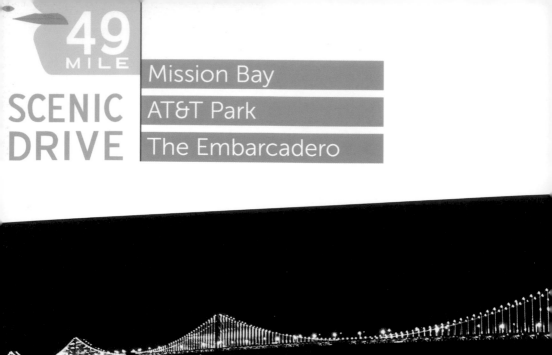

The San Francisco–Oakland Bay Bridge's light show illumines 25,000 LED lights along its 300 cables.

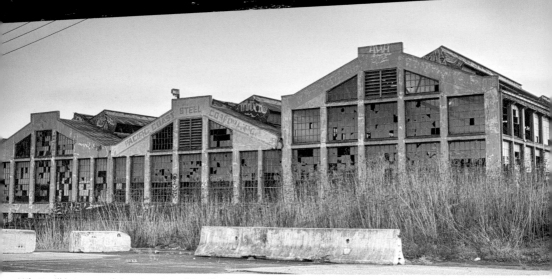

What will become of the abandoned Pacific Coast Steel Company on Pier 70?

Score! This walk begins right along the bay in the rough, rusting, old, shipbuilding, warehouse neighborhood of Dogpatch—see it now before it's gone. Then as you pass the home of the many-time world champion Giants baseball team, the streets transform before your eyes into the burgeoning, slick South Beach neighborhood. But that's nothing compared to the end of the walk along the postcard-perfect Embarcadero, promenading directly under the Bay Bridge, with a final stop at the renovated, historic Ferry Building. The water, breeze, sun, and views alone on this excursion make it worthy of repeat visits.

But you get a bonus urban adventure: Be sure to take the T-line or walk-back loop to the beginning to experience the newest part of San Francisco: Mission Bay. If you haven't been down here in the past 10 years, you won't recognize it. Our eastern waterfront shows how the city rebuilds, revitalizes, and transforms ugly abandoned landfill into commercial success and vibrant neighborhoods.

Mission Bay's blocks and blocks of huge, modern shiny medical buildings, solar-paneled parking structures, and modern condos along 3rd Street look like no other neighborhood in the city, with more green spaces soon to come. In another year it will look different still, and in another 10 years it will be unrecognizable, again.

It's hard to imagine that this area used to be an actual bay, Mission Bay, spanned by a long wooden bridge, called Long Bridge, connecting downtown to Potrero Hill and Hunters Point! Hiking this route will give you an up-close glimpse of both SF history *and* new SF in the making. Enjoy!

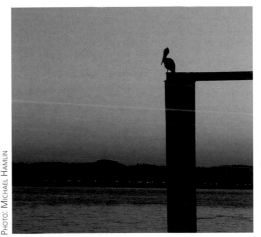

PHOTO: MICHAEL HAMLIN

Begin: 3rd Street at 22nd Street	Hill Rating:
End: The Embarcadero at Market Street (Ferry Building)	
Distance: ROUTE: 3.0 miles — 6,000 steps — 1 hour	
LOOP BACK: 2.9 miles — 5,900 steps — 1 hour	

Sites you will pass on today's walk include:

MILE 44
1. **3rd Street**
2. **Pier 70**
   at the end of 20th St
3. **Mission Rock Bleacher Boards**
   817 Terry A Francois Blvd
4. **Terry A Francois Boulevard**

MILE 45
5. **Former Port of SF building** Pier 50
6. **China Basin Park**
7. **Lefty O'Doul Bridge** 3rd St
a. **Hidden Houseboats**
   Mission Creek at Channel St
8. **AT&T Park**
   24 Willie Mays Plaza
9. **Herb Caen Way**

MILE 46
10. **Java House** Pier 40
11. **The Embarcadero**

12. **Bay Blocking Basketball!?**
   Piers 30 and 32
13. **Red's Java House**
   Pier 30

SOUTH BEACH
14. **San Francisco– Oakland Bay Bridge**
15. **Hills Brothers Old Coffee Factory**
   2 Harrison St
16. **SF Fireboats Station No. 35** Pier 30
17. *Cupid's Span*
   The Embarcadero and Folsom St
18. **Y—M-C-A**
   169 Steuart St

TREASURE ISLAND
19. **The Audiffred Building** 1 Mission St
20. **Ferry Building** 1 Ferry Building, the Embarcadero at Market St

WALK- BACK LOOP
b. **UCSF Mission Bay Campus** 1825 4th St
c. **UCSF Benioff Children's Hospital**
   4th St and 16th St
d. **Carpenters Union Local 22** 2085 3rd St

NOTE: Keep your eyes peeled along the Embarcadero walk by the bay for:

- Viewing platform with history panels
- Black-and-white square columns telling the history of sailing ships
- Tall red poles with quotes from artists about the bay
- Brass rectangles of poems in the sidewalk
- Sea creature sculptures guarding the concrete benches
- Hidden stairs to the bay
- Art installations—temporary ones are added often

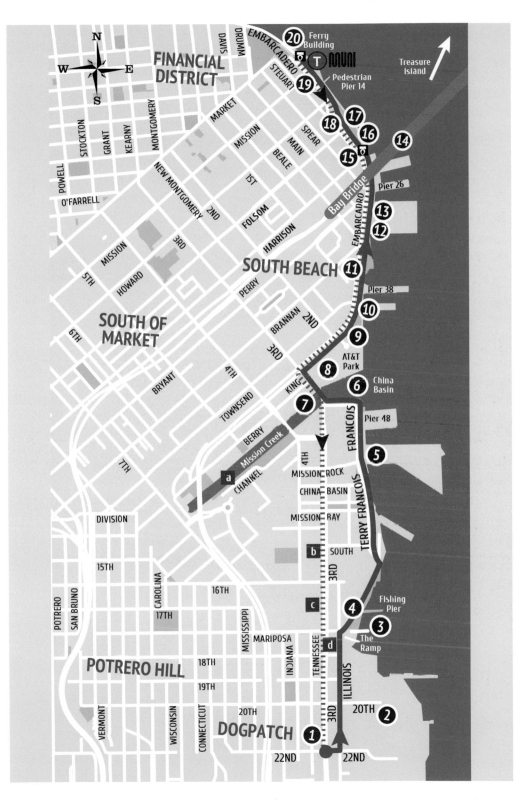

MILE 44

Begins on 3rd St at 22nd St

∙ ∙ ∙ ∙ ∙ ∙ ∙ ∙ ∙ ∙ ∙ ∙ ∙ ∙ ∙ ∙

Continue from Walk 15 walking east on 22nd St

Cross 3rd St

∙ ∙ ∙ ∙ ∙ ∙ ∙ ∙ ∙ ∙ ∙ ∙ ∙ ∙ ∙ ∙

1. 3rd Street

Third Street is *long*—both in length and history. It begins in the Bayview where it was formerly called Railroad Avenue because the railroad route ran along the street (and before that, circa 1878, the stagecoach line ran down the same path). Third Street then crosses Islais Creek Channel into Dogpatch (onto what was once called Kentucky Street) and continues on through Potrero Hill and Mission Bay. Then it crosses over Mission Creek, past AT&T Park to Market Street. But the street itself is actually longer than that. At Market Street, 3rd Street turns into Kearny Street, which runs north, and, after a little hop over Telegraph Hill, runs all the way to the Embarcadero. At the opposite end of town, as 3rd heads south out of the Bayview District, it crosses U.S. 101 and turns into Bayshore Boulevard, which runs all the way to San Jose!

∙ ∙ ∙ ∙ ∙ ∙ ∙ ∙ ∙ ∙ ∙ ∙ ∙ ∙ ∙ ∙

Left on ILLINOIS

∙ ∙ ∙ ∙ ∙ ∙ ∙ ∙ ∙ ∙ ∙ ∙ ∙ ∙ ∙ ∙

2. Pier 70 at the end of 20th St

The oldest working civilian shipyard in U.S., Pier 70 has been a shipyard and industrial site since the Gold Rush. Pier 70 workers built the first steel ships on the Pacific coast. Though it's still one of the largest ship repair yards on the West Coast, many of the buildings are leased to other businesses; many others are crumbling. The Port Authority plans to completely transform these 28 acres of the central waterfront into a new city neighborhood for an estimated $100 million.

∙ ∙ ∙ ∙ ∙ ∙ ∙ ∙ ∙ ∙ ∙ ∙ ∙ ∙ ∙ ∙

Right at TERRY A FRANCOIS BLVD (MARIPOSA ST)

FRANCOIS BLVD eventually curves left and runs back into 3rd ST

∙ ∙ ∙ ∙ ∙ ∙ ∙ ∙ ∙ ∙ ∙ ∙ ∙ ∙ ∙ ∙

3. Mission Rock Bleacher Boards 817 Terry A Francois Blvd

Both The Ramp and Mission Rock Resort serve up great places to take in the sun, sailboats, shipyards, and seafood on a warm afternoon or before a Giants' game, but when you're through looking at the menus, take a look at the numbers carved into the aged siding of Mission Rock. Those colored boards are old bleacher seats from UC Berkeley. *Go Bears!*

Lefty O'Doul Bridge across 3rd Street

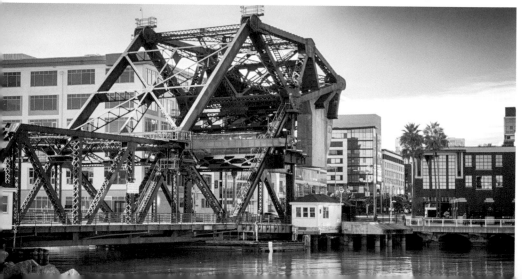

San Francisco Bay Trail
Today's walk along the shore overlaps a section of the SF Bay Trail, a planned 500-mile walking and cycling path around the entire San Francisco Bay shoreline running through all nine Bay Area counties, 47 cities, and across seven toll bridges. Of the 343 miles in place so far, 225 are paved, and 118 miles are natural surface trails. Join the fun: BayTrail.org.

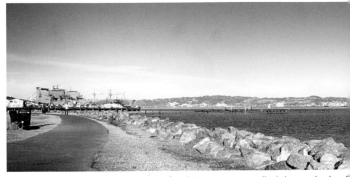

Thank you, San Francisco Bay Trail, for this gorgeous walk right on the bay!

4.   Terry A Francois Boulevard

The rusting industrial repair docks, fishing pier, crumbling old wooden pylons, and views of the huge white shipping cranes across the Bay at the Port of Oakland all take you back to SF's rough and tumble waterfront days. Of course, the manicured jogging path, Bayview Boat Club and Mariposa Hunters Point Yacht Club, yachts, grassy areas, views of the Bay Bridge and poop bag station keep it civilized. And the backside construction views of all the new buildings facing 3rd Street keep it modern. We have the San Francisco Bay Trail Project to thank for this gorgeous nature walk, blessing us with more foghorn blasts than car horn blasts. The tranquil Bay walk is named for the first African American to sit on San Francisco's Board of Supervisors (1974), Terry François.

MILE 45

Begins on FRANCOIS BLVD at MISSION BAY BLVD N

5.   Former Port of SF building (now another business)
Pier 50

The old building is classic, but the current Port of San Francisco headquarters has relocated to Embarcadero 1 (on the other side of the Ferry Building). This public agency manages the 7½ miles of San Francisco Bay shoreline stretching from Hyde Street Pier in the north to India Basin in the south.

6.   China Basin Park

As you sit on the grassy mound with the ballpark looming over your shoulder, staring up at the bronze statue of Giants' legend Willie McCovey backlit by the bay and bridge, you can almost hear the sound of his bat cracking as he hits one of his 521 career home runs. Or maybe that's the sound of the children playing T-ball in

the scaled-down diamond of the Junior Giants Field behind you. Either way, it's a lovely, lovely spot to picnic, enjoy bay views, or watch boaters sitting in McCovey Cove waiting to catch balls knocked out of AT&T Park. This little urban oasis sits in China Basin, whose name comes from the 1860s when clipper ships bound for China tied up here.

Mission Creek
Native Ohlone tribes lived along the area we call Mission Creek and Mission Bay for thousands of years. When the Spanish arrived in the 18th century they discovered ships could navigate up the creek all the way to a lagoon near Mission Dolores. Today nearly all of Mission Creek runs underground.

· · · · · · · · · · · · · ·
Right on 3RD ST

Cross the (cantilever) bridge
· · · · · · · · · · · · · ·

7. Lefty O'Doul Bridge
3rd St

Rechristened in 1969 to honor the famous ball player Francis "Lefty" O'Doul, this drawbridge allows cars and people to cross Mission Creek, aka China Basin Channel, as it runs into McCovey Cove (named for famed Giants first baseman Willie McCovey). Take a peek inside the two old abandoned station houses on either side of the bridge. What year do you guess they were last used?

a. Hidden Houseboats
Mission Creek at Channel St

Just a few blocks from the Giants baseball park, 20 floating homes and 35 small boats sit docked right in the middle of some of the most valuable real estate in the West. Two women, Ruth Huffaker and the perfectly named Betty Boatright, fought

AT&T Park

the city to save the community from eviction in the 1970s and secure a long lease.

Cheap and Easy
The last drawbridge of its kind in the SF area, the Lefty O'Doul Bridge is an inexpensive, easy-to-maintain heel trunnion-type bascule drawbridge designed by Joseph Baermann Strauss, who also designed the slightly better-known Golden Gate Bridge. The design lacked grace, so it was used only where appearance was secondary to cost and efficiency.

· · · · · · · · · · · · · · · · · ·

Right on KING ST (WILLIE MAYS PLAZA)

where it curves to meet the shore, it becomes EMBARCADERO

· · · · · · · · · · · · · · · · · ·

8. AT&T Park
24 Willie Mays Plaza

Welcome to the home of 2010, 2012, and 2014 Baseball Major League World Series Champions. The Giants moved to this $357 million stadium from Candlestick Park in 2000. AT&T Park features glorious bay views, gourmet junk food, a free peekaboo section to watch games from, splash cove, a retro design, and 42,000 seats (which are built slightly wider than in most stadiums). The Giants have a 66-year lease and pay $1.2 million in rent annually to the San Francisco Port Commission.

SF Giants Retired Numbers

#3	Bill Terry
#4	Mel Ott
#11	Carl Hubbell
#20	Monte Irvin
#24	Willie Mays
#27	Juan Marichal
#30	Orlando Cepeda
#36	Gaylord Perry
#42	Jackie Robinson
#44	Willie McCovey

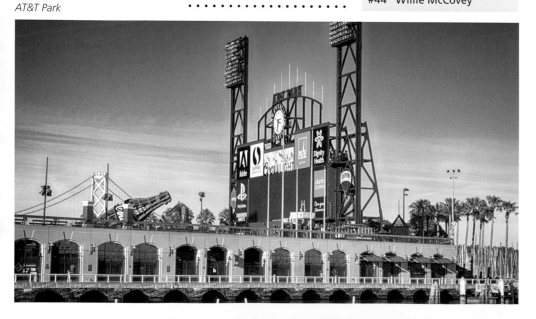

HINT: Free Visit in AT&T Park
You can pretend that you're sneaking into the park and getting away with a slide down the giant Coke bottle, but all you really have to do is show up at the back gate entrance any day from 10 a.m.–4 p.m. during the summer, and M-F the rest of the year—except on game days—and the guard will let you in to wander around the empty stadium. Cool!

• • • • • • • • • • • • • • • • • •

Follow EMBARCADERO
veer right to the inside walkway along the bay (that parallels Embarcadero)
• • • • • • • • • • • • • • • • • •

"Not in history has a modern imperial city been so completely destroyed. San Francisco is gone."
—*eyewitness quote after the 1906 earthquake from author Jack London, who was born in SF near 3rd and Brannan Streets in 1876*

9.   Herb Caen Way...

For 60 years, 1937–1997, Herb Caen's daily column in the *SF Chronicle* provided gossip, satire, and anecdotes of the city he adored. He wrote over a dozen doting books about San Francisco, coined the term "Beatnik" and popularized the word "hippie." To honor this beloved citizen, the city

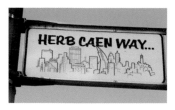

renamed 3.2 miles of the Embarcadero for him—even included three ellipses on the street sign as a nod to Herb's habit of ending his sentences with them. (As you pass the ballpark, look up at the blue streetlights to see the Herb Caen Way... signs.)

MILE 46

Begins on THE EMBARCADERO at PIER 40

10. Java House at Pier 40

Java House has been feeding longshoremen and tourists since 1912. Rumor has it that Red and his brother took over the Java House in the 1950s, but after a fight Red moved down to Pier 30 to open Red's Java House.

11.   The Embarcadero

After the city filled in Yerba Buena cove (from 1867–1869) workers constructed this engineered seawall and roadway atop the landfill to create a new waterfront edge and christened it the Embarcadero, Spanish for "the place to embark."

12. Bay Blocking Basketball!?
Piers 30 and 32

In 2012, the Golden State Warriors of the National Basketball Association announced plans to construct a new 19,000-seat arena to be built on Piers 30–32 near the foot of the Bay Bridge. SF loves the Warriors, but the voters declined to rewrite city waterfront laws to accommodate the proposed enormous, view-blocking "Wall on the Waterfront" stadium and condo complex. Had the vote taken place after the Warriors won the 2015 NBA Championship, who knows what would have happened?! Still determined to move to SF, in 2015 the Warriors purchased a 12-acre plot in Mission Bay—along Terry A Francois Boulevard you just walked down.

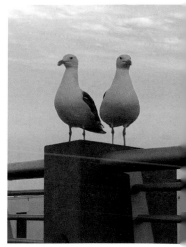

PHOTO: MICHAEL HAMLIN

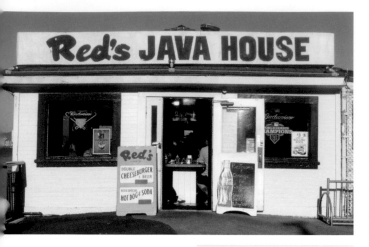

13. Red's Java House
Pier 30

Red's served as the wharf's most famous burger and beer dive for the 20th century. The newest owners fancied up the menu—adding French fries. Rumor has it Red and his brother, from the neighboring Java House, eventually made peace and went back to working with each other.

"Coffee—the favorite drink of the civilized world."
—*Thomas Jefferson*

SOUTH BEACH

This formerly dilapidated waterfront warehouse area's transformation into a high-gloss neighborhood includes shining modern apartment towers packed with luxury suites, surrounded by trendy clubs, chic cafés, and fabulous bay views.

14. San Francisco–Oakland Bay Bridge
(aka: Willie Brown Bridge, or "The Crooked Willie")

When it first opened in 1936, our new "risky" hybrid suspension and truss-cantilever bridge was the longest, most expensive bridge in the world—$77 million.

At a cost of $6.4 billion, our new 2013 "earthquake-proof" eastern span has brought the title of most expensive bridge in the world back to the bay. Yay, us! We deserve it.

In addition to the palm trees down the center, a new bike lane, and a light show every night, our bridge has set two Guinness World Records! The new eastern span has been crowned both the widest (258.33 feet) and the longest self-anchored suspension span bridge in the world (2,047 feet).

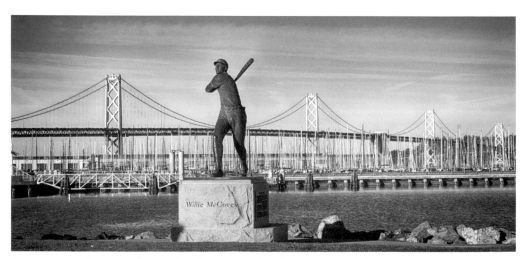

Commuters on the Bay Bridge watch Willie McCovey hit a home run out of China Basin Park.

15. Hills Brothers Old Coffee Factory
2 Harrison St

The Hills Brothers, actual brothers, came to San Francisco in 1873 and quickly joined the city's booming coffee industry. The discovery of vacuum packaging for freshness in 1900 let them become one of the first to ship coffee all over the West. After the 1906 quake, they rebuilt their factory on the Embarcadero. The smell of coffee wafting from the factory is cited by old-time San Franciscans as the quintessential "smell" of the city. A nine-foot bronze statue of their original logo, an Arab drinking coffee, stands outside the building, which closed in 1990. (NOTE: This industry's connection to Central American coffee fields provided the first link between San Francisco and the many Central America laborers who followed the coffee work.)

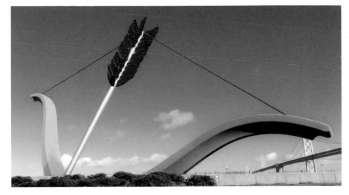

16. SF Fireboats Station No. 35: The *Guardian* and the *Phoenix* Pier 30

In a city once prone to fires, San Francisco fireboat *Phoenix* (hero of the Loma Prieta earthquake) and fireboat *Guardian* are part of maritime lore.

Pier 22½ couldn't be more romantic and picturesque, but the pier is crumbling and the small 1915 fire station built from a leftover building from the Pan-Pacific Expo is so antiquated it doesn't even have a women's bathroom.

17. *Cupid's Span*
The Embarcadero and Folsom St

What's up with that 64-foot-high, painted, fiberglass, and stainless-steel bow and arrow planted in the ground at Rincon Park? Could it be a tribute to the Ohlone natives, or Xena Warrior Princess? No. According to the married artist team Claes Oldenburg and Coosje van Bruggen, the 2002 Cupid's bow was inspired by San Francisco's reputation as the home port of Eros.

18. Army and Navy YMCA 169 Steuart St

In case you were wondering: The 1920's-era YMCA building across the street (at Howard) is not the YMCA branch that inspired the eponymous song by the Village People. That honor goes to the McBurney YMCA Branch that used to be on W. 23rd Street in the Chelsea neighborhood of Manhattan.

Little-Known Bay Bridge Facts
- Prior to its opening in 1936, the Bay Bridge was blessed by the cardinal who later became Pope Pius XII.
- Caltrans operates a bicycle shuttle during peak commute hours for $1 each way.
- The Bay Bridge served 9 million vehicles its first year. Today it carries 102,200,000 vehicles per year.
- Trains ran on its lower deck to the Transbay Terminal until 1962.
- There had been discussion of building a bridge between San Francisco and Oakland since the 1870s, but cost and fear delayed action until the Reconstruction Finance Corporation, with support from President Herbert Hoover, agreed to purchase bonds to be repaid later with bridge tolls.

! LOOK:
TREASURE ISLAND

In 1936–37 the U.S. Army Corps of Engineers built a 404-acre island next to Yerba Buena Island. Speculation that millions of dollars of gold dust had been dredged up from the bay to create the island led to the name Treasure Island. Its purpose was first to host the upcoming Golden Gate International Exposition in 1939 and then to be converted into San Francisco International Airport. However, with war looming in Europe, the U.S. Navy wanted this strategic location in the bay so the island was traded for Mills Field located down on the peninsula that became today's San Francisco International Airport (SFO). Treasure Island served as a naval base until 1996. Today it is being developed for residential and retail space.

19. The Audiffred Building 1 Mission St

Why does this red-brick building with white ornamentation across the street look nothing like the buildings around it? Two reasons: (1) A French immigrant, nostalgic for his homeland, modeled it after a Parisian commercial building in 1889 and (2) Every other building around it, except the Ferry Building, was blown up immediately after the 1906 quake to stop the inferno

raging through the city. How did Hippolite D'Audiffret save his building? By promising two quarts of whiskey and a cart of wine to each fireman— if they didn't destroy the building. After another century of adventure, the Audiffred building became SF Landmark no. 7 and the Zagat-rated restaurant Boulevard.
—Alex Bevk, SF.Curbed.com

20. Ferry Building 1 Ferry Building, the Embarcadero at Market St

This is a great resting spot after your walk. Check Walk #17 for details on the history, upmarket shops, and info about free walking tours.

· · · · · · · · · · · · · · · · · · · ·
END at MARKET ST
(Ferry Building)
· · · · · · · · · · · · · · · · · · · ·

WALK-BACK LOOP (VIA 3RD ST)

b. UCSF Mission Bay Campus 1825 4th St

Just a decade ago this area of town was an abandoned railroad yard. Today the University of California San Francisco (UCSF) Mission Bay thrives as a biotechnology hub where the next generation of scientists, researchers, doctors, nurses, pharmacists, and dentists are trained with the most modern tools available. The sprawling 43-acre Mission Bay campus will eventually include three hospitals,

20 structures dedicated to biomedical research and education, and housing for 9,100 employees. UCSF also pledged to devote eight acres and 1% of its $1 to $2 billion in construction costs to cultural enrichment and recreational facilities for the neighborhood.

c. UCSF Benioff Children's Hospital 4th St and 16th St

Marc Benioff has stepped right into a long history of wealthy, successful, and creative San Franciscans who give back to the Bay Area and the world. His charitable giving reaches far beyond the $200 million he and his wife, Lynne Krilich, have given to build state-of-the-art children's hospitals in Oakland and San Francisco. Marc proclaims everywhere he goes that being wildly successful and being wildly philanthropic go hand in hand. He has lived out that philosophy since day one at his company, Salesforce, and also works hard at encouraging other tech companies to give back to the community and be socially responsible corporate citizens. *Thanks, Marc!*

d. Carpenters Union Local 22 2085 3rd St

Representing the interests of working people while simultaneously elevating the carpentry trades and the construction industry in San Francisco since 1882.

WALK 16 NEED TO KNOW

TO GET THERE
- Muni K, T, 22, 48
- Caltrain: 22nd ST STATION

PARKING
Street parking, some 4-hour zones available

NOTE: During ballgames, many streets become no-parking tow-away zones. Very complicated parking signs are posted to detail the rules. Look for these and follow them.

PUBLIC RESTROOMS
- Public kiosk, Embarcadero at Harrison
- Ferry Building

TURN-BY-TURN INSTRUCTIONS
Begin: 3rd ST at 22nd ST
- Continuing from Walk 15, walk east on 22nd ST
- Cross 3rd ST
- Left on ILLINOIS ST
- Right at TERRY A FRANCOIS BLVD (MARIPOSA ST)
  - FRANCOIS BLVD eventually curves left and runs into 3rd ST
- Right on 3rd ST
- Cross the (cantilever) bridge

- Right on KING ST (WILLIE MAYS PLAZA),
  - where it curves to meet the shore, it becomes EMBARCADERO
- Follow EMBARCADERO
  - Veer right to the inside walkway along the bay (that parallels Embarcadero)
End: at MARKET ST (Ferry Building)

TO GET BACK
Muni
- Walk to the EMBARCADERO METRO STATION
- Board the inbound T–Line
- Get off at 3rd ST and 20th ST

Other transit routes:
- Embarcadero Station
  - BART
  - All Muni inbound trains
- California St Cable Car
- F- Line
- Muni 1, 2, 5, 6, 9, 14, 21, 31, 28, 71
- Golden Gate Transit 4, 56

OPTIONAL WALK-BACK LOOP DIRECTIONS
Follow the bus line marked on the map.

Distance: 2.9 miles, 5,900 steps, 1 hour

Rating: △1

This route along the Embarcadero is so beautiful, and so iconically San Francisco, it's worth seeing it again in the opposite direction. And if you stay on 3rd St once you cross over the Lefty O'Doul Bridge, you'll get the bonus of seeing the shiny new part of Mission Bay and the trendy new stores and restaurants in Dogpatch you missed on the way to the Ferry Building. So take the T-Line back, or just walk the T-Line route on your map. Either way, you'll have an awesome time.

Begin: at MARKET ST (Ferry Building)
- Make a U-turn on EMBARCADERO, returning the way you came
- EMBARCADERO turns into KING ST
- Left on 3rd ST
- Cross the (cantilever) bridge
- Continue on 3rd ST
End: 3rd ST at 22nd ST

THE DAILY CRAB

San Francisco Historical Times   Vol. 16

REAL ESTATE FEVER

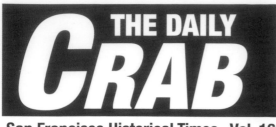

Mission Bay:
Long Bridge to Landfill

In the 19th century, SF's vast tidal coves, such as **Mission Bay** and **Islais Creek,** jutted into the southern portions of the city, which meant **Potrero Hill** and **Dogpatch** down to the **Bayview** and **Hunters Point** had to be reached by boat. In 1865, we built a wooden **Long Bridge** that ran across the waterways to connect San Francisco proper to what was called South San Francisco—all the way to the **Old Clam House on Bayshore.** It was wide enough for horse-carriage tracks and made a great new fishing pier.

But more importantly, Dogpatch's slaughterhouses, glassworks, mills, and dry docks, once deemed too far south, were suddenly a stone's throw away. The Long Bridge, running along what is now **3rd Street**, completely transformed Potrero Hill from a no-man's land to a central hub—complete with waves of real estate speculation.

As part of the wild money-making fever that swept the city throughout the 19th century, speculators, city planners,

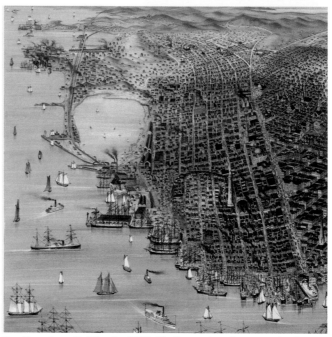

San Francisco, California, 1878. Bird's-eye view facing south, showing the eastern side of the city. SF Bay in the foreground, Market Street to the right, and to the left, Long Bridge crossing Mission Bay, and then connecting Dogpatch to Hunters Point (seen jutting out at the top left). Sketched and drawn by C.R. Parsons. Published by Currier and Ives.

visionaries, and crooks sought to create more land to sell for the booming San Francisco population by filling in the shallow waters and salt marshes of Mission Bay. City hills and sandlots were leveled to create landfill for the bay and as Mission Bay filled

up, Long Bridge was closed. Planked roads, followed by railroads, warehouses, shipping yards, industries, and finally concrete freeways, covered Mission Bay over the next century.

—*A History of San Francisco's Mission Bay,* by Nancy Olmsted

DOG PACK DINER

Before WWII, the **Bayview District,** home to the city's slaughterhouses, was called **Butchertown.** The part of the city in

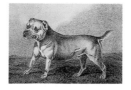

which the butchers dumped all their meat scraps attracted packs of wild dogs, so people called that area "dogpatch"—or so states one theory on the origin of the Dogpatch neighborhood's name.

"DAMBARCADERO FREEWAY"

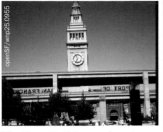

The Ferry Building peeks out over the Embarcadero freeway (1974).

WATERFRONT WAR

During the 1934 **West Coast Waterfront Strike**, the longshoremen's unions organized at Pier 26. The "Bloody Thursday" riots of July 5, 1934, that killed two union workers occurred outside Pier 26. Although the strike was perceived by many to be a failure, it helped secure a critical pay raise for the longshoremen during the darkest days of the Great Depression and cemented the resolve of waterfront unions to protest abuse by their superiors. Each year, the **International Longshore and Warehouse Union** does not work on July 5 in memory of Bloody Thursday.

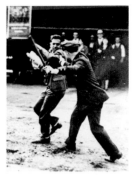

Do you remember the double-decker freeway that ran along the Embarcadero—that also abruptly stopped midair? Called a gray monstrosity by some, an eyesore by others, it blocked our view of the bay and covered up the Ferry Building.

And the traffic jams! Oy! *SF Chronicle* columnist **Herb Caen** summed up the prevailing sentiment best, calling it, "the Dambarcadero Freeway." After the freeway was damaged beyond repair in the 1989 Loma Prieta quake, it was torn down.

Confrontation between a policeman wielding a nightstick and a striker during the San Francisco General Strike (1934).

1939 GOLDEN GATE INTERNATIONAL EXPOSITION

To celebrate and show off the newly completed Golden Gate and SF Bay bridges, the Bay Area threw a giant party: the **Golden Gate International Expo of 1939**. The "Pageant of the Pacific" celebrated the countries, cultures, artists, and engineers around the Pacific Rim. The fair's buildings were brightly and colorfully illuminated at night, which earned her the nickname of "the Magic City."

Ironically, and tragically, the 1939 fair, which opened in celebration of friendship among the Pacific nations of Asia and the Americas, closed in 1940 to the drumbeats of war among nations in the Pacific.

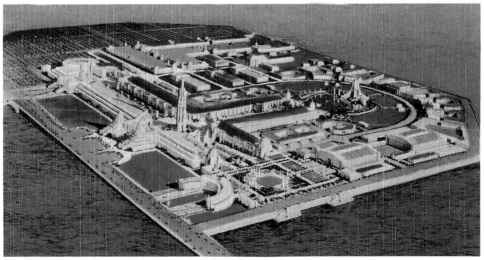

The 1939 Golden Gate International Exposition held at Treasure Island. The theme: The Pageant of the Pacific.

49 MILE
SCENIC DRIVE

Ferry Building
Financial District
South of Market

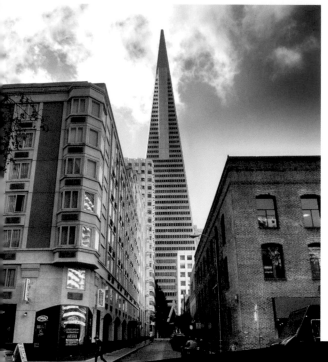

Feel free to detour down to the Transamerica Pyramid building for a closer look.

Winter ice-skating at Justin Herman Plaza. Vaillancourt Fountain on the left.

1915

Skyscraper wealth and homeless grit. Civic triumph and civic failures. Antique buildings and futuristic businesses. The "homestretch" final hike of the historic 49 Mile route draws your gaze upward as you roam through densely packed centers of SF history, finance, and civic life. You can feel the change in neighborhoods block by block as you walk through, including mid-Market area's latest boom industry: tech companies.

You are welcome to begin your adventure with a tour of the Ferry Building—order brunch, explore the Farmers' Market, or just admire the interior. Then, the first mile of your hike is over the bones of buried ships in Yerba Buena Harbor. The city's original shoreline began at Montgomery Street. Watch for the marker at First and Market Streets that shows the original shoreline.

The 1906 quake and fire left very little of downtown San Francisco standing, yet on this adventure you get to stare down Market and see one city icon every survivor of the 1906 quake and fire saw: the Ferry Building. Yep, this walk is the heart of the Phoenix, where the city has burned, rebuilt, flourished, celebrated victories, screamed in protest, made and lost fortunes and continues to re-create herself, over and over.

And if this is your final 49 mile walk—congratulations, you're about to become a little piece of that history! Feel free to run up the City Hall steps and do a little victory dance.

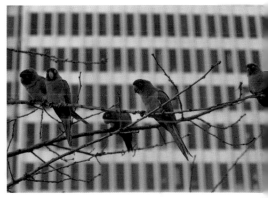

The wild parrots of Telegraph Hill have tripled over the years and can be seen throughout the city.
PHOTO: MICHELLE

Begin: The Embarcadero at Market Street (Ferry Building)   Hill Rating:
End: City Hall Entrance, McAllister Street and
           Dr Carlton B Goodlett Place (Polk Street)
Distance: ROUTE: 2.8 miles — 5,600 steps — 1 hour
           LOOP BACK: 1.8 miles — 3,600 steps — 35 minutes

Sites you will pass on today's walk include:

MILE 47

MUST-SEE
1. **Ferry Building**
   Embarcadero at
   Market St

2. **Justin Herman Plaza** 1 Market St

3. **Vaillancourt Fountain**
   Justin Herman Plaza

4. **Sue Bierman Park**
   Washington St and
   Drumm St

5. **Embarcadero Center**

6. **Transamerica Pyramid Building**
   600 Montgomery St

FINANCIAL DISTRICT
7. **Mechanics Statue**
   Bush St and Market
   St (north side)

a. **Slot Machine Landmark No. 937**
   Battery and Market
   median

b. **Shoreline Historical Landmark No. 83**
   1st St and Market St
   (south side)

MILE 48
8. **Transbay Terminal Construction Site**
   Howard St

9. **Moscone Center**
   between Howard St
   and Folsom St

c. **Keith Haring Figurines**
   3rd St and Howard St

DETOUR
10. **San Francisco Museum of Modern Art**
    151 3rd St

11. **Yerba Buena Gardens**
    between Howard St
    and Mission St

d. **MLK Memorial**

e. **Contemporary Jewish Museum**
   736 Mission St

f. **St. Patrick's Church**
   756 Mission St

g. **Carousel**
   4th St and Howard St

h. **Convention Center**
   747 Howard St

12. **TechShop**
    926 Howard St

13. **6th Street**

MILE 49
14. **Ninth Circuit Court**
    95 7th St

15. **Ninth Street Independent Film Center** 145 9th St

16. **Quaker Meeting House** 65 9th St

17. **Falling Glass Pianos** 55 9th St

18. **Dolby Laboratories**
    1275 Market St

19. **Civic Center Plaza**
    Larkin St and
    Grove St

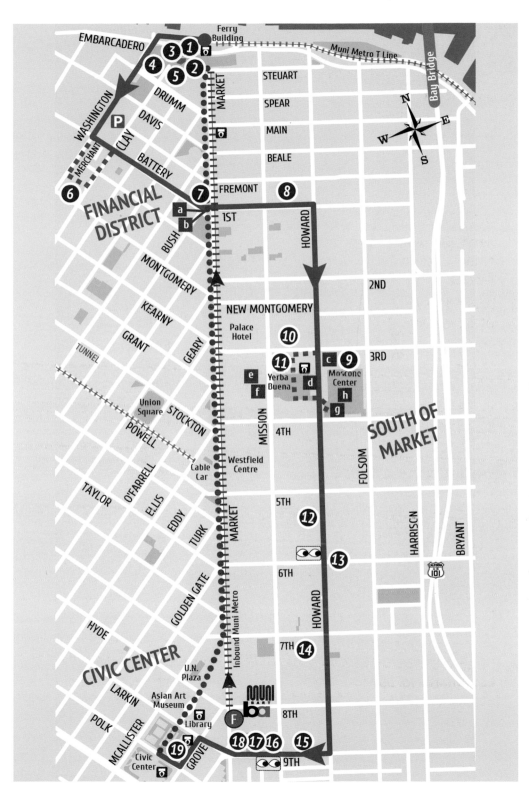

MILE 47

Begins on EMBARCADERO at MARKET ST

1. Ferry Building
Embarcadero at Market St

SF Chronicle columnist Herb Caen once described the Ferry Building as "a famous city's most famous landmark." With her remodel in the 1990s she has again become one of the most visited grande dames in San Francisco. Practically speaking, the Ferry Building serves as a terminal for Sausalito, Oakland, Alameda, Vallejo, and Larkspur ferries. She also marks the even/odd pier division—all odd-numbered piers begin to her west and even-numbered piers to her east.

❗ MUST SEE

If you didn't do it on Walk 16, begin with a walk through the **Ferry Building** to enjoy the bustling crowds, interesting architecture, up-market and un-usual foodie stores (chocolate olive oil, peach-fed pork, Far West Fungi) and tasty aromas wafting out of the many restaurants. Out back you'll find great bay views, a working ferry terminal, statue of Mahatma Gandhi, and outdoor Farmers Market on Tuesdays, Thursdays, and Saturdays. Open nearly every day of the year, usually 10 a.m.–6 p.m. You can even join in on a free tour with the fabulous, amazing SFCityGuides.org.

. . . .

Continue on EMBARCADERO northwest past the Ferry Building
. . . .

2. Justin Herman Plaza
1 Market St

Named for the controversial head of San Francisco's Redevelopment Agency, Justin Herman, this big public plaza across the street from the Ferry Building is the entryway to the Embarcadero Center and flows into Sue Bierman Park just to its west.

3. Vaillancourt Fountain across from the Ferry Building

The grouping of giant square concrete tubes jutting into the air at the edge of Justin Herman Plaza has been called by some "one of the world's most fabulous fountains," and by others a $100-a-day-to-operate eyesore (which is the estimated cost to pump 30,000 gallons of water through the square tubes each day). What do *you* think?

. . . .

Left on WASHINGTON ST
Note the concrete history bunker on the sidewalk as you cross to WASHINGTON
. . . .

4. Sue Bierman Park
Washington St and Drumm St

As you walk past the patch of grass to your left on Washington Street, give a sigh of gratitude for this beloved former supervisor who fought to protect the city's tenants, streetscapes, neighborhoods, and downtown from runaway skyscraper development. Sue began her political career as a quintessential neighborhood activist fighting to stop a freeway through Haight-Ashbury and Golden Gate Park. (Hmmm . . . Justin Herman gets a concrete plaza, Sue gets a patch of grass? Well.)

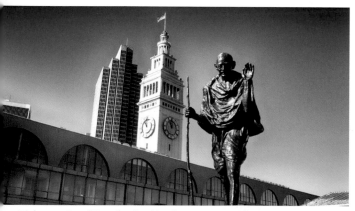

Mahatma Gandhi walks the 49 mile route every day!

Vertical Earthquake

In the 1950s Justin Herman was hired to head San Francisco's Redevelopment Agency. Enacting eminent domain whenever necessary, he set upon an aggressive campaign to tear down hundreds of blocks of aging homes in the city and replace them with modern construction. Critics accused Herman of racism when he tore down 60 blocks of the blighted Western Addition, forcing black residents to move from their homes near the Fillmore jazz district to newly constructed public housing projects, such as near the naval base at Hunters Point. His other plans led to the creation of the Embarcadero Center, the Embarcadero Freeway, Japantown, the Geary Street superblocks, and eventually Yerba Buena Gardens.

The late Herb Caen, longtime *San Francisco Chronicle* newspaper columnist, decried much of the city's "redevelopment" as a "vertical earthquake" of high-rise development threatening to turn a unique city of "breathtaking vistas" and "sacred view corridors" into "any other skyscraper-plagued metropolis."

DETOUR

It's worth a quick jog two blocks farther down Washington Street to the Pyramid building to admire the redwood park—yes, there's a half-acre redwood grove nestled between the skyscrapers in downtown SF. The park, meant as a respite for city workers, has a fountain, benches, and clever brass statues, including one of a group of leaping children holding hands. (Return to Battery St, turn right.)

5. Embarcadero Center

It took 18 years, beginning in 1971, to build this 4.8-million-square-foot commercial complex made up of two hotels and five office towers (30–45 stories tall). This prime 9.8 acres of mixed-use area covers five city blocks from the Embarcadero to Battery Street and accommodates standard retail stores, restaurants, offices, a movie theater, events, parking—and 14,000 workers. It doesn't look like much from the outside, but during the holiday season the towers sparkle with 17,000 lights outlining the towers.

6. Transamerica Pyramid Building
600 Montgomery St

As you head toward the San Francisco Financial District you can get a glimpse of the Pyramid building straight ahead. Though it may soon lose its status as SF's tallest skyscraper (853 feet) to the new Transbay Terminal Tower, its status as a San Francisco icon will remain. NOTE: Visitors *cannot* ascend to the top for a panoramic view.

If you didn't take the detour, turn left (south) on BATTERY ST

VIEW: If you skip the Pyramid Detour, look right at Merchant Alley as you walk down Battery Street for a cool sliver-of-a-view of the Pyramid building.

FINANCIAL DISTRICT

Can you feel the power? Banks, financial institutions, law firms, corporate headquarters, international businesses, skyscrapers, upscale hotels, four-star restaurants, shopping, and tech empires—and 280,000 worker bees keep it all humming.

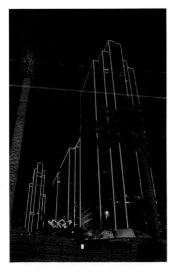

Follow **BATTERY ST** until it veers left into **BUSH ST**

Continue one block to **MARKET ST**

7. Mechanics Statue
Northeast corner of Bush St and Market St

Wow. None of my mechanics ever looked like that. Men were hot in MDCCCXCIX!

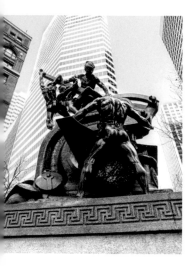

a. Slot Machine Historical Landmark No. 937 median between Bush St and Battery St

Across the street from the Mechanics Statue, on the median between Bush and Battery, is a marker celebrating Charles August Fey, a pioneer and inventor of coin-operated slot machines (still used today), which he built in his 1890s

SF workshop near here (407 Market).

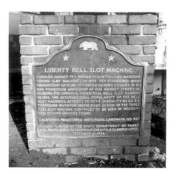

Cross **MARKET ST**, **BUSH ST** becomes **1st ST**

b. Shoreline Historical Landmark No. 83
catty-corner to the Mechanics Statue

If you stand on 1st Street and look down Market Street toward the Ferry Building, everything you see is built on sunken ships and other bay fill. You can also cross to the 49 Mile marker located on Market and 1st Streets and look down

to see a brass plaque located in the sidewalk that details the original San Francisco Bay shoreline as it existed when gold was discovered by James W. Marshall at Coloma, California, January 24, 1848.

MILE 48

Begins on HOWARD ST at 1st ST

8. Transbay Terminal Construction Site
Howard St

Back when commuter trains ran along the lower deck of the Bay Bridge, this area is where they came to drop off commuters. By 1962 all tracks had been replaced with pavement and the Transbay Terminal became a major bus terminal.

The massive new visionary transportation and housing Transbay Transit Center Program, scheduled to open in 2017, wants to be the "'Grand

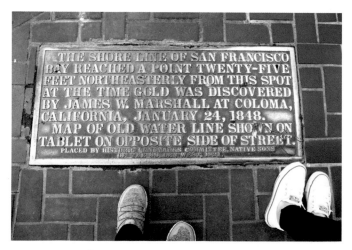

Market Street
- Market Street was laid out by 26-year-old civil engineer Jasper O'Farrell around 1847. He designed it to run parallel to the only road out of town, Mission Street, and, intending to make it the city's main thoroughfare, made it to be the widest street in town, 120 feet between property lines.
- At the time, the right-of-way through Market Street was blocked by a 60-foot sand dune where the Palace Hotel is now, and a hundred yards farther west stood a sand hill nearly 90 feet tall. The city leveled the dunes and used the sand for landfill around Portsmouth Square.
- Market Street cuts a diagonal across the city's north–south, east–west street grid. By design, the city streets south of Market suddenly turn to a diagonal grid to align with Market. Then at Duboce Street, where Mission Street turns left and heads south, the street grid follows it back to a north–south orientation.

DETOUR

At 3rd Street, Howard opens up with Yerba Buena and Moscone Center on each side. You may want to come back another time for a half-day visit fo these sites, but for today it's definitely worth your while to make a quick loop through this two-block area. You'll find public parks, the Children's Creativity Museum, an ice-skating rink, bowling alley, a carousel, cafés, retail space, and the Rev. Dr. Martin Luther King Jr. memorial, the contemporary Jewish Museum, and historic St. Patrick's Church.

Central Station of the West' . . . connecting eight Bay Area counties and the State of California through 11 transit systems . . . allowing more than 100,000 people per day . . . to travel and commute without the need for a car . . . all in the heart of a new transit-friendly neighborhood . . . with new parks . . . a hotel . . . and housing." Wow. And one of its proposed 13 towers will replace the Pyramid building as the tallest tower in the city.

· · · · · · · · · · · · · · · ·

Right on HOWARD ST

Continue to 9th ST or take detour at 3rd St

· · · · · · · · · · · · · · · ·

9. Moscone Center
between Folsom St and Mission St

c. Three Dancing Figures (1989) corner of 3rd St and Howard St

(NOTE: If the statue is not here, it is likely still at the de Young Museum, Walk 11. Famed pop artist Keith Haring completed more than 50 mural and sculpture projects between 1982 and his death from AIDS-related illness in 1990 at the age of 31. He was committed to making accessible public art, and both his easily identifiable style and his political activism earned him international recognition.

Begin on the southeast corner of 3rd St and Howard St

Turn right (northwest) on 3rd St back toward MARKET ST to explore Yerba Buena Gardens, beginning with a peek at:

· · · · · · · · · · · · · · · ·

Scoop on South of Market Area (SOMA)
SOMA refers to the many smaller neighborhoods found south of Market Street. This vast diverse neighborhood was cluttered with warehouses and rundown homes after WWII, where poor elderly people and artists could afford to live. Urban renewal and the tech boom of the 1990s began the gentrification of the area. The area is still a mix of everything from warehouses and tech companies to museums, loft condos, and subculture dance clubs.

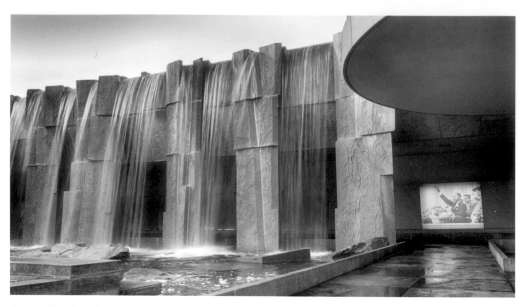

Rev. Dr. Martin Luther King, Jr. Memorial

10. San Francisco Museum of Modern Art 3rd St between Howard St and Mission St

Over 20,000 square feet larger than the Museum of Modern Art in New York, SFMOMA is the largest contemporary art museum in the U.S. (Pop into the gift store for free.)

· · · · · · · · · · · · · · · · · · ·

At the SFMOMA entrance, cross 3rd Street into Yerba Buena Gardens

· · · · · · · · · · · · · · · · · · ·

11. Yerba Buena Gardens between Howard St and Mission St

d. Rev. Dr. Martin Luther King Jr. Memorial

On your left you can walk under the waterfall into the third-largest memorial to **Rev. Dr. Martin Luther King Jr.** in the country.

Also of note, and worth a visit, are the two brick buildings you can see across Yerba Buena's grassy expanse on Mission Street:

e. Contemporary Jewish Museum 736 Mission St

f. St. Patrick's Church 756 Mission St

· · · · · · · · · · · · · · · · · ·

Continue on the path past the MLK monument, turn left up the stairs, and cross the pedestrian bridge over HOWARD ST back to Moscone Center.

· · · · · · · · · · · · · · · · · ·

"Until justice rolls down like water and righteousness like a mighty stream."
Venture behind the 20-foot-by-50-foot Yerba Buena waterfall to experience a "baptism" of water and inspiration at the Martin Luther King Jr. Memorial. The floating walkway leads you past 12 shimmering glass panels set in Sierra granite inscribed with Dr. King's powerful words and images from the civil rights movement.

g. Carousel
4th St and Howard St

Behind the carousel: **Children's Creativity Museum, Ice-Skating Rink, and Bowling Alley.**

h. Convention Center
747 Howard St

The 1984 Democratic National Convention that nominated Geraldine Ferraro for vice president—the first time a woman had ever been nominated by a major party for either office—happened right here at Moscone Center.

RETURN DETOUR

At this point in the walk Howard St will begin looking less like the Financial District and more like the Homeless Shelter District. If your goal is to walk the historic 49 Mile Drive, put your electronic devices in your pocket, walk purposefully, and pay attention to what is going on around you for the rest of the walk. Thousands of people walk these streets daily so you will likely be just fine, but if you are not in the mood for the grittier side of big city life at the moment:

- Turn right on 5th ST
- Turn right on MARKET ST
- Head back to the Ferry Building—by foot, cab, Muni F-Line, or Powell Street underground.

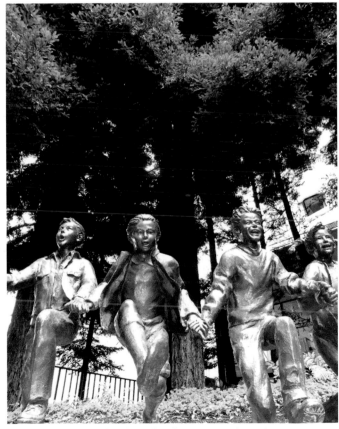

Transamerica Pyramid Redwood Park. Bronze sculpture by Glenna Goodacre.

Today Moscone Center hosts major events from Macworld to the Fancy Food Show. A large solar electricity system installed on the roof of the center by PowerLight Corporation in March 2004 marked San Francisco's first major step toward obtaining all municipal energy from pollution-free sources.

Continue following the route southwest on HOWARD ST

12. TechShop
926 Howard St

This affordable, membership-based do-it-yourself workshop is jam packed with laser cutters, plastics and electronics labs, a machine shop, a wood shop, a metal working shop, a textiles department, welding stations, a waterjet cutter—and classes for every skill level

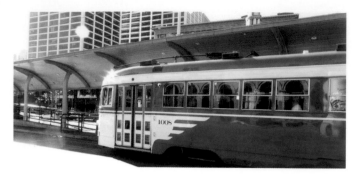

to teach you how to use it all! Woohoo! Whether you are a tinkerer, student, inventor, or entrepreneur, you can make virtually anything at TechShop.

13. 6th Street

While a few blocks away Market Street bustles with tourists and workers, 6th Street is Tenderloin grit: single-room occupancy hotels, urine-soaked entryways, crack addicts, and rescue missions. Hipsters may be willing to brave the dangerous trek to enjoy the uber rad nightlife, but we suggest you follow the sage advice of Virginia Reed, survivor of the ill-fated Donner Party: "Never take no cut-offs and hurry along as fast as you can." And don't park your car here either.

LOOK

As you traverse Howard Street notice the amazing mix of old and new shops and crumbling and restored buildings, and nary a chain store in sight. For example: High-end and trendy shops, such as an organic market, antique store, and brew pub, sit

side by side with warehouses, the inexpensive wares in the household merchandise and underwear store, and AsiaSF (sexy transgender dancers serving Asian cuisine at 9th and Howard).

MILE 49

Begins on HOWARD ST at 7th ST

14. United States Court of Appeals for the Ninth Circuit
95 7th St

With 29 active judgeships given jurisdiction over nine western states, Guam, and the Northern Mariana Islands, the **Ninth Circuit Court** is by far the largest of the 13 courts of appeals. Known for controversial rulings—such as declaring that adding the phrase "under God" to the Pledge of Allegiance violates the U.S. Constitution and upholding Seattle's $15 an hour minimum wage—this is the court that politically conservative U.S. senators and radio commentators love to

decry and ridicule as the most liberal, activist court in the land.

· · · · · · · · · · · · · · · · · ·
Right on 9th St
· · · · · · · · · · · · · · · · · ·

15. Ninth Street Independent Film Center 145 9th St

SF's Indie filmmakers rock! And to ensure that filmmakers have a permanent, secure hub for training, synergy, screening, promoting festivals, affordable office space, and movie-making, the city's leading film organizations bought their own building. Partner organizations include Frameline (lesbian, gay, bisexual, and transgender media arts), Center for Asian American Media (CAAM), SF Jewish Film Festival, National Alliance for Media Arts and Culture (NAMAC), SF Green Film Festival, and The Global Film Initiative.

16. Quaker Meeting House 65 9th St

Home of the American Friends Service Committee (AFSC), which is "a Quaker organization that includes people of various faiths who are committed to social justice, peace and humanitarian service. AFSC's work is based on our belief in the worth of every person, and faith in the power of love to overcome violence and injustice." — SFQuakers.org

17. Glass Pianos Hanging from an Apartment Building
55 9th St

Opera singer Enrico Caruso sang in SF the night before the 1906 quake. Look up. The designers hope that standing under 13 tons of flashing pianos seemingly falling from the sky while listening to recordings of Caruso singing will help you share his earthquake experience. *Caruso's Dream* is the second of two public art installations by Brian Goggin and Dorka Keehn found on SF's 49 Mile Scenic Drive. Lights are choreographed by Gabriel Rey-Goodlatte.

18. Dolby Laboratories
1275 Market St

In 1967, long before tech was cool, Ray Dolby brought his sound lab to San Francisco and began transforming our entertainment experience —especially at the movies. Even if you don't understand words like "oscilloscope" and "biophysical sensory lab," stop outside Dolby's brand-new 16-story lab on the corner of 9th and Market Streets, stare at the 60-foot ever-changing video screen in the lobby and ooh and aah—or better yet, step into the lobby and listen to the Dolby sound.

> The first film with Dolby sound was *A Clockwork Orange* (1971).

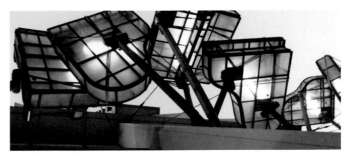

The piano light show starts after dark and responds to the Caruso music on 90.9 FM.

! LOOK

. . . Left down Market Street. The Twitter logo hangs on its headquarters' building, corner of 10th and Market. Tweet out your successful completion of the 49 mile challenge to the world—and tag us **@WalkSF49**— so we can celebrate with you!

. . . .

As 9th St crosses MARKET ST bear right onto LARKIN ST

Left on GROVE ST

Right POLK ST, which turns into GOODLETT PL

. . . .

19. Civic Center Plaza
Larkin St and Grove St

If this is your first visit to Civic Center Plaza, check Walk 1 to read all about the grand buildings here. San Francisco's Civic Center was created to celebrate the city's rise from the ashes of the 1906 quake and fire. Now, over a century later, it would be hard to imagine a type of rally, protest, or festival that *hasn't* taken place in this plaza. Now *you* can use it to celebrate your 49 Mile Scenic Drive walking adventure victory. Go ahead, run down the tree-lined center of the park, do a "Rocky" up the City Hall steps, and give the front door a "high five." You've earned it. *Congratulations!*

. . . .

END on 1 CARLTON B GOODLETT PL, San Francisco City Hall front steps

. . . .

WALK-BACK LOOP SCOOP

Hop on a historic F-Line streetcar on Market Street for a ride past the shopping district, cable car turnaround and Financial District—it should only take about 10 minutes. Or walk down Market and enjoy it all at your own speed. As you can read on pages 24 and 122–125, thanks to the efforts of Vision Zero SF—a city and community effort to eliminate all traffic deaths in San Francisco by 2024—your stroll back along Market will be much safer than in previous years. See the directions on page 244.

WALK 17 NEED TO KNOW

TO GET THERE
- BART: Any train going to Embarcadero Station
- Muni: All underground inbound trains, California St cable cars, F-Line, 1, 2, 5, 6, 9, 14, 21, 31, 28, 71
- Golden Gate Transit 4, 56

PARKING
- Best rate: Golden Gateway Garage 250 Clay St at Davis St
- Many other garage options, offering half-day and full-day rates
- Limited metered street parking

PUBLIC RESTROOMS
- Ferry Building
- 221 Market (Main)
- Yerba Buena Gardens
- Public Library (Grove at Market)
- Civic Center (62 Grove at Larkin)

TURN–BY–TURN INSTRUCTIONS
Begin: EMBARCADERO at MARKET ST (Ferry Building)

- Continue on EMBARCADERO northwest past the Ferry Building
- Left on WASHINGTON ST
  - Note the concrete history bunker on the sidewalk as you cross to WASHINGTON ST

DETOUR to Pyramid bldg

- Continue on WASHINGTON ST two blocks past BATTERY ST to the redwood park outside the Pyramid building. Enjoy.
- Then return to BATTERY ST and turn right (south) to rejoin the route

- If you did take the detour, turn left (south) on BATTERY ST

- Follow BATTERY ST as it veers left just before MARKET ST and becomes BUSH ST, and then 1st ST as you cross MARKET ST

- Cross MARKET ST

- Right on HOWARD ST

DETOUR to Yerba Buena Park

- Right on 3rd ST, half a block
- Turn left into the park and explore
- At any point turn left (perhaps go over the pedestrian overpass) and return to Howard St

- Continue southwest on HOWARD ST

- Right on 9th ST

- As 9th ST crosses MARKET ST, bear right onto LARKIN ST

- Left on GROVE ST

- Right on POLK ST, which turns into GOODLETT PL

End: 1 CARLTON B GOODLETT PL, San Francisco City Hall front steps

TO GET BACK
Muni

- Walk between the Asian Art Museum and the Main Library (FULTON ST)
- Turn right on HYDE ST to MARKET and 8th STS
  - Go to underground Civic Center BART/Muni
  - Take any east-bound BART or inbound Muni train
  - Above-ground, take the F-Line (toward the Ferry Building)
- Get off at Embarcadero Station

OPTIONAL WALK-BACK LOOP DIRECTIONS
Distance: 1.8 miles, 3,600 steps, 35 minutes

Rating: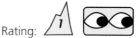

There are two walk-back strategies, one for those completing the official 49 Mile Scenic Route and a second, shortcut route for those who want to stay in the more "tourist-friendly" part of downtown.

Both routes take you back to the Ferry Building via Market Street, SF's wide tree-lined shopping boulevard bustling with trams, buses, cars, and people. Closer to the Civic Center, homeless people sit outside the mix of old stores and new restaurants, with hardly a chain store. Then at Powell and 5th Streets, where the shortcut route-back begins, the shopping opportunities blossom into a dazzling display of every retail store possible, from Nordstrom and Bloomingdale's to the Apple Store and art galleries. Head toward Union Square for more upscale shopping at Tiffany's, Neiman Marcus, and Maiden Lane boutiques. You can watch the tourists line up for a cable car ride at Powell—or join them for a ride to Fisherman's Wharf (see how to ride a cable car on page 253).

As you continue down Market, you'll pass ornate, historic buildings, like the Palace Hotel, before passing back through the Financial District skyscrapers and your final destination at the bay.

WALK-BACK NO. 1:

- Walk between the Asian Art Museum and the Main Library (FULTON ST)
- Continue straight across U.N. Plaza
  - Farmers' Market: Wednesdays and Sundays
- Left on MARKET ST, continue all the way to the Ferry Building

SHORT WALK-BACK NO. 2:

The Short Walk-Back skips the rougher sections of rescue missions, panhandlers, and intoxicated people along 6th ST and 9th ST. You can always come back and do Walk 1 for a spin around the Civic Center another day if you haven't done so already.

- From HOWARD ST or MISSION ST, turn Right on 5th ST
- Right on MARKET ST
- Walk/bus/cab back to the Ferry Building

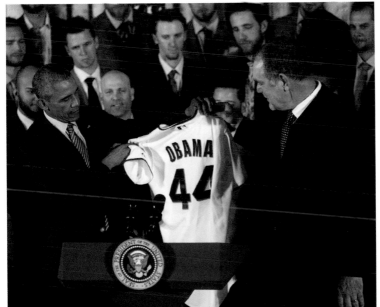

President Obama honoring the World Series Champion San Francisco Giants while manager Bruce Bochy gives the president a custom "44" Giants jersey.

THE DAILY CRAB

San Francisco Historical Times   Vol. 17

PROTECT THE BREASTS

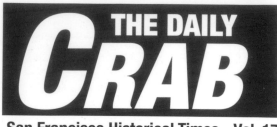

Jasper O'Farrell's 1847 plan to expand Market Street into a grand 120-foot-wide boulevard infuriated the 400 landowners who owned the property in the path of the grand new boulevard. They threatened to lynch O'Farrell and decried the new Market Street running toward Twin Peaks as both an "abominable width" and an arrow aimed straight at the "breasts of the maiden" (Twin Peak's Spanish name: Los Pechos de la Chola). Jasper had to flee town for a while, but his plans survived—and as luck would have it, the expanded Market Street was finished just in time to accommodate the hordes of people and traffic rushing in for the Gold Rush.

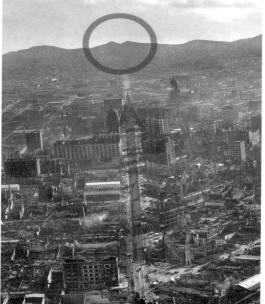

[Public domain] via Library of Congress

Market Street's path to Twin Peaks shows clearly in this picture—as does the destruction caused by the 1906 San Francisco earthquake and fire. George R. Lawrence captured this, his best-known photo, by suspending his camera on a kite, which he then flew 1,000 feet above the city.

GRAND LADY REVIVED

Built in 1898, the Ferry Building ruled for 40 years as the transportation hub for anyone coming to SF from across the bay by train, foot, or car. She survived the 1906 earthquake, and by the 1920s, she was the busiest passenger terminal in the United States, second busiest in the world, serving 50 million passengers a year. When automobile traffic left her in favor of the new Bay Bridge in 1937, she fell into disuse and neglect and was eventually blocked from view by the Embarcadero Freeway. Then the Loma Prieta quake of 1989 gave her a second chance! The quake temporarily ended car traffic on the Bay Bridge—reviving the need for ferry service. The quake also led to tearing down the Embarcadero Freeway, which led to a remodel of the Ferry Building. Now, once again, she's holding court at the end of Market Street—her status as grand lady of San Francisco fully restored. A true San Francisco Phoenix story!

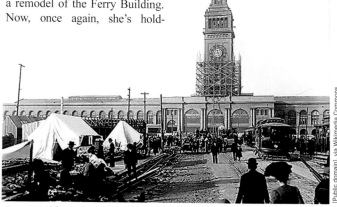

[Public domain], via Wikimedia Commons

Ferry Building, San Francisco, after the 1906 earthquake

TOOR FIGHT
Don't Mess with Old People!

Yerba Buena Gardens took more than three decades to complete (1950s to the 1990s). Much of that delay was due to the large population of poor, elderly tenants in the area who were fighting not to be displaced from their low-rent housing unless decent housing options could be found. These **TOOR** activists (Tenants and Owners in Opposition to Redevelopment) also insisted the Gardens' plan include activities for neighborhood kids, not just the "black-tie and evening gown" crowd. In the end, relatively few residents received the court-ordered new housing. But perhaps we have them to thank for the many recreation areas, such as the bowling alley and open green picnicking space, that were added to **Yerba Buena Gardens** for us all.

VERY GOOD HERB!

Another childhood myth shattered: The yerba buena (or "good herb") that gave San Francisco its original name was *wild mint, not marijuana*.

TRANSAMERICA PYRAMID QUIZ

Which one of these Fun Facts is *not* true?

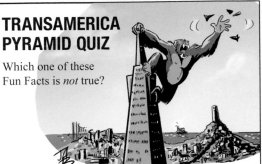

by Jett Atwood

1. Most of its 3,678 windows can be pivoted 360° to be washed from the inside.
2. Top floor (48th floor) conference room can be booked for $600 an hour.
3. Public observation deck on floor 27 was closed after 9/11.
4. Spire on top is 20 stories high and hollow.
5. Universal Studios requested using it for a new King Kong movie.
6. Its tapered shape is due in part to Transamerica CEO John R. Beckett wanting to allow more natural light on the street below.
7. It's covered in crushed white quartz
8. You are welcome to come sit in the ½-acre redwood tree grove at the base (during business hours).
9. The original 1,000-foot-higher building design was denied because it would have interfered with views of the bay from Nob Hill.
10. It sits nearly on top of a buried Gold Rush ship, *The Niantic*.
11. The entire professional urban design community loudly objected to the building, decrying it as a public eyesore.

VALUABLE UNDERWATER REAL ESTATE FOR SALE

In the mid-19th century SF's vast area of scrubland and sandy hills was considered uninhabitable. Ships were the fastest way for products and people to come into or out of California—making shipping the most lucrative industry.

To generate revenue, **Governor Stephen Kearny**, and then the City of San Francisco, drew imaginary lines on the city map to extend the city's existing streets far into Yerba Buena Cove and later Mission Bay, and auctioned off water lots.

The most valuable "land" in San Francisco became a "lot" of water.

The pursuing mad rush to buy, sell, trade, and barter water lots led to legislative corruption, fraudulent sales, shoddy construction, and wild real estate speculation. This also left half of early San Francisco a wharf city of planks, sheds, and businesses built on trembling docks—subject to devastating fires.

As the rickety wharves and their buildings fell into the Bay, and an estimated 500 ships were abandoned and run aground during the Gold Rush, the city began filling in the area.

Unfortunately, water lots are difficult to survey, and many lots had three or four claimants. Scandals and court battles ensued. Probably the people with the most money and political clout ended up with the new land. Sounds like business as usual.

Correct answer: 5

SAN FRANCISCO PARKING AND MUNI BASICS

If you don't drive, park or travel by San Francisco's municipal railway (Muni) in the city often, here are some rules, tips and guidelines to help make your hikes stress-free.

PARKING BASICS

NOTE: These were the rules and rates as of the date of publishing. Always be sure to check street signs and info on meters, or SFMTA.org for current info.

METERS

All meters operate:

- **Every holiday except three: Thanksgiving, Christmas Day, New Year's Day**

Most (not all) meters operate:

- **9 a.m. to 6 p.m. Monday through Saturday**
  - **On Sunday meters operate at** Fisherman's Wharf area, The Embarcadero, five off-street parking lots, "Special Event Area" around AT&T Park during special events.
- **Two-hour time limit.** "Feeding the meter" (adding more coins to extend the two-hour limit) may result in a citation.
- **Rates:** $2.00 to $3.50 per hour for cars and $0.40 to $0.70 per hour for motorcycles.

- **Pay by:** coin, PayByPhone, the SFMTA parking card, credit card

You can prepay meters for the time you need even if you arrive before the meter begins to be enforced— you will not be charged until the meter begins operation (e.g., at 9 a.m.).

Broken meters: Call 311 to report it and then you can park there for the posted time limit or two hours, whichever is shorter.

Restricted meters: Check for time limits. You may be able to park there Sundays or nonbusiness hours.

- **Green-capped meters:** 15- or 30-minute time limit.
- **Yellow-capped meters:** commercial loading
- **Red-capped meters:** commercial loading for vehicles with six or more wheels

PAY BY PHONE

PayByPhone enables customers to add time without returning to the meter. It also sends a reminder message when time is almost up. Cost: 45¢ fee per transaction.

- Call 866-490-7275 or download the app at PayByPhone.com.
- After registering, enter the meter location number and desired length of stay.
- Meter display will not change (e.g., if the meter was expired, it will still flash "expired" after payment). Parking control officers see the payments on their wireless handheld devices.

CURB COLORS

Blue and red curbs: NEVER.

- Blue curbs: valid disabled parking permit only, 24/7
- Red curbs: no parking 24/7

White, green, and yellow curbs: SOMETIMES. Check the curb or signs for restricted hours.

- White curbs: passenger loading/ unloading. 5-minute time limit
- Green curbs: short-term parking. less than 10 minutes
- Yellow curbs: commercial loading/unloading

PARKING LEGALLY

Most neighborhoods limit street parking to two hours, from 9 a.m. to 6 p.m. In some neighborhoods the two-hour limits go until 9 p.m. However, one-, three-, and four-hour parking still exist in some neighborhoods. Read the parking signs.

- Look 100 feet in both directions for parking restriction signs.
- Watch for tow-away zones.
  - Some parking zones become tow-away zones during commute hours.
  - There are crazy, nearly indecipherable rules in areas near, and even seemingly far, from AT&T Park during Giants home games. Good luck.

REAL-TIME PARKING INFORMATION

SF*park*.org helps you find a parking space in San Francisco—*and adjusts price by demand.* Free SF*park* app available for iPhone and Android.

Garages and Lots
SFMTA.com > Getting Around > Parking > Finding a Garage > Search by location near you

TIPS TO AVOID PARKING TICKETS

- **Curb your tires on hills.** When facing downhill, turn your wheel toward the curb; when facing uphill, turn your wheel away from the curb. Where there is no curb uphill or downhill, angle your front wheel toward the roadside.
- **18 inches from the curb.** When parallel parking (the side of your car is against the curb), your wheels must be within 18 inches of the curb
- **Don't repark in the same place in permit zones.** When your time is up do not repark near your former spot. Move to the other side of the street, or at least 500 feet away.

- **Parking *is* allowed *after* street sweeping.** Once the street-sweeping truck has swept the curbside, you may park your vehicle there, even if the posted sweeping hours have not expired.

Info adapted from the San Francisco Municipal Transportation Agency: SFMTA.com.

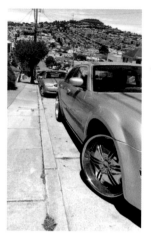

Curb your wheels. We learned the hard way. Carolyn's first parking ticket in San Francisco was for not curbing her wheels.

MUNI BASICS

Walking the 49 Mile Scenic Drive is a San Francisco adventure—and part of that adventure is riding Muni, San Francisco's extensive municipal transit system.

If you are new to Muni, here are the basics of how to use Muni on your hikes.

1. **Plan your trip.** In each walk segment we provide the route info for you to get from the end back to the start. If you have a different destination, we've also provided other bus lines in the area to help you get to where you're going. Remember **511.org**

is a great tool for planning your trip and includes all the Bay Area transit services. Google also does a great job of finding route info.

511.org, NextBus.com: You can use your smart phone to find out when the next bus arrives.

2. **Get to your stop.** At the end of each hike follow the directions to the bus stop that will take you back to the starting point. The

directions include the directional corner of the street where you will find your bus stop. Bus stops may have a shelter or may be a bright yellow painted sign on a pole.

3. **Board and pay—and get a transfer.** Allow off-boarding passengers to exit before you board. Muni accepts cash in exact change or prepaid transit passes.

   ○ Bills and coins are fed into the cash machine upon boarding.
   ○ Electronic passes must be held against the reader right inside the front or back door (it will "ding" when the card registers).
   ○ Activate you MuniMobile app as you board.
   ○ You may enter from the rear if you have an electronic pass.
   ○ At time of publishing, the fare is $2.25 for adults, $1.00 for seniors 65+, riders with disabilities, and youth 5–17. Children under 4 are free.
   ○ **Make sure you keep your fare receipt, which is also a transfer good for 90 minutes.**

Show the driver your receipt to board your transfer bus.

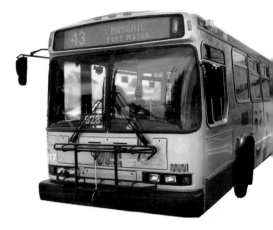

4. **Passport, Clipper® card, Muni-Mobile app.** You can buy visitor passports for one, three, or seven days, or you can buy a monthly Muni pass. A great alternative for people who visit the city often is an electronic pass called a Clipper card. A Clipper card allows you to load value to the card so you don't need to carry cash and is accepted across all Bay Area buses, trains, and ferries. Finally, the MuniMobile app lets you use your

Muni Basics (511.org is your friend)
- Bus stops may have a shelter or may simply be a **yellow-painted band on a pole.**
- **Exact change** (in cash) required: $2.25 for adults.
  - *Bills and coins are fed into the cash machine upon boarding.*
  - *Or activate your MuniMobile app as you board (itunes).*
  - *Or press your Clipper Card up to the Clipper Card reader (clippercard.com)*
- You may board through the backdoor if you have a Clipper Card (use reader on back stairs).
- Take and **keep your receipt/transfer** (you can use it for 90 minutes to ride other buses).
- Watch for your stop.
- Pull the cord or push the button on a pole to signal the driver to stop.
- Exit by the rear door.
  - *Step down and push the handles or the red button on the pole to open the door.*

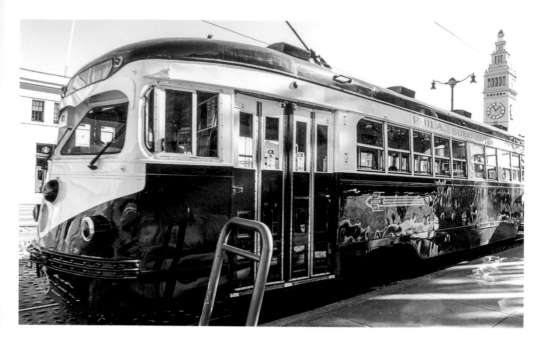

smartphone to buy and pay fares for you or your whole family on a single phone (itunes store).

5. **Find a place to sit or stand.** To keep on schedule, the buses will not wait for you to sit, so move quickly to a nearby seat or grab a rail. Always show consideration to the elderly, people with disabilities, pregnant women, or people with small children. Hold on. Buses may make sudden stops.

6. **Finding your stop and exiting.** If you are not familiar with the route, you can ask the driver upon boarding about the stop you are looking for and listen for stop announcements. However, don't rely on hearing the announcement. It's safer to watch out the window or even count the number of stops you'll be passing. Pull the yellow cord to request the stop. Wait until the bus comes to a full stop and exit through the rear door if possible. The doors will open when you press on the bars on the door or the red button on the pole.

7. **Pets.** Many restrictions apply, including limited to off-peak hours, one pet per vehicle, and muzzles and fares required. See SFMTA.com.

8. **More tips.** For more information on accessibility, strollers, bikes, and safety, go to SFMTA.com.

HOW TO RIDE A CABLE CAR

1. **Find your stop.** Riders can board at any cable car turntable (the beginning/end of each route) or anywhere on the route where the brown and white cable car stop sign is posted.

2. **Wave to stop it.** Wait on the sidewalk (do not run in front of the cable car) and wave to request the grip operator to stop. Wait for the cable car to come to a complete stop before you board. You can enter on either end or side of the car.

3. **Pay $7, one way.** All visitor passes, Clipper cards, monthly passes, MuniMobile, and cash (paid in small bills, directly to the conductor at the rear) are accepted for cable car rides. Cable car tickets do not work as transfers to Muni.

4. **Hang on the sides at your own risk.** Riders may stand on the running boards and hang onto the outer poles as the car moves.

Riders do so at their own risk. Hold on tight and do not let go at stops (a sudden start can throw you off).

5. **Crowded, not wheelchair accessible.** Cable cars are not wheelchair accessible, and owing to limited space, they do not have room for strollers.

6. **Don't stand in yellow areas or block the driver.** Grip Operators (driver or "gripman") are located in the front of the car and are responsible for propelling and stopping the 15,500-pound vehicles—that's three times heavier than a pickup truck! They need to move around to do their job, so make sure to give them plenty of room to work.

7. **Don't get off a moving cable car!** Wait for the cable car to come to a complete stop before you step off or stand to exit. The conductor or grip operator will announce when it is safe to exit.

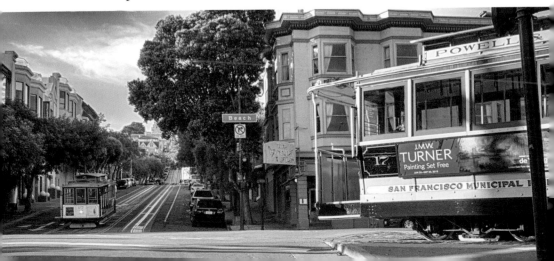

49 MILE ROUTE *DRIVING* DIRECTIONS: FULL AND SHORTER "HIGHLIGHTS" ROUTE

The complete driving instructions are below, including three shortcut options to chop one to two hours off the three- to four-hour driving time.

Hints:

- Do not drive the route Mon.–Fri. during rush hour: 6–9 a.m. or 3–7 p.m.
- Saturday and Sunday traffic is better downtown but worse in Golden Gate Park
- Best time to drive: Mon.–Fri. before 11 a.m., Sat.–Sun. begin by 9 a.m. (6 a.m. great!).
- Never, ever drive anywhere near the Golden Gate Bridge on Christmas Day.
- Some great stops: 10 a.m. tour of City Hall, Golden Gate Bridge (go very early for parking), Visitors Center at Lands End, Japanese Tea Garden at Golden Gate Park, Twin Peaks, and Mission Dolores.

FULL ROUTE

Begin: San Francisco City Hall, 1 CARLTON B GOODLETT PLACE (MCALLISTER and POLK STREETS)

- South on GOODLETT toward GROVE
- Left on GROVE
- Left on LARKIN
- Left on GEARY
- Right on WEBSTER
- Right on POST
- Left on GRANT
- Left on CALIFORNIA
- Right on TAYLOR
- Right on WASHINGTON
- Right on POWELL
- Left on CLAY
- Left on KEARNY
- Left on COLUMBUS
- Right on GRANT
- Left on LOMBARD
- Right on MASON
- Left on JEFFERSON
- Left on HYDE
- Right on BEACH
- Left on POLK
- Right on NORTH POINT
- Left on VAN NESS
- Right on BAY
- Right on LAGUNA

- Left on MARINA
  - Bear right to stay on MARINA
- Right into MARINA GREEN PARKING AREA
  - Follow road around edge of parking area to exit at the other side
  - NOTE: The 49 Mile sign is missing
- As you exit the parking lot, continue straight across the street (MARINA) onto SCOTT
- Right on BEACH
- Left on BAKER
- Left on BAY
- Right on BRODERICK
- Right on CHESTNUT
  - Cross RICHARDSON
- Left on LYON
- Right LOMBARD into the Presidio
- Right onto PRESIDIO
  - PRESIDIO turns into LINCOLN
- Left on FUNSTON
- Right on MORAGA
- Bear right onto INFANTRY TERRACE
- Bear left onto SHERIDAN
- MERGE onto LINCOLN
  - LINCOLN goes under the Golden Gate Bridge
  - LINCOLN turns into EL CAMINO DEL MAR at 25th
- Follow EL CAMINO DEL MAR
  - Veer left with EL CAMINO DEL MAR at the T
- As you hit LINCOLN PARK, continue up to LEGION OF HONOR

- Left on LEGION OF HONOR which turns into 34th
- Follow 34th out of the park
- Right on GEARY
- At 42nd, bear right to join POINT LOBOS
- Follow POINT LOBOS downhill as it curves around the CLIFF HOUSE and becomes GREAT HIGHWAY

SHORT-CUT OPTION NO. 1

- At GREAT HIGHWAY and LINCOLN, left on LINCOLN
- Left on 41st (at stop sign) into the park, which becomes CHAIN OF LAKES

FULL ROUTE CONTINUES

- Continue on GREAT HIGHWAY
  - GREAT HIGHWAY runs into SKYLINE
- Right on SKYLINE as it heads around Lake Merced
- Left on JOHN MUIR as it heads around the lake
- Left onto LAKE MERCED as it heads around the lake
- Continue around the lake on LAKE MERCED
- Right on SUNSET into GOLDEN GATE PARK
- Left on MARTIN LUTHER KING JR (MLK)
- Right on CHAIN OF LAKES
  - **SHORT-CUT OPTION NO. 1 rejoins main route here**

- Right on JOHN F. KENNEDY (JFK)
- Right on TRANSVERSE (no street sign but there is a 49 Mile marker)
- Next stop sign, at the intersection with MIDDLE
- Left to continue on TRANSVERSE
- Next stop sign, left on MLK
  - Continue on MLK across CROSSOVER (19th)
  - Pass the playground on your left
  - At the T intersection with STOW LAKE you'll see the 49 Mile marker

SHORT-CUT OPTION NO. 2
Skip Stow Lake, continue along MLK

FULL ROUTE CONTINUES
- Left on STOW LAKE
- Circle the lake clockwise
  - Just past the boathouse
- Right on STOW LAKE, EAST
  - This curves around the lake back to the bottom of the hill
- Sharp left back onto MLK
  - **SHORT-CUT OPTION NO. 2 rejoins main route here**
- Left on NANCY PELOSI (formerly Middle Drive, backside of the academy)
- Right on BOWLING GREEN
- Left on MLK

- Left on KEZAR, which leads you to the edge of the park
- Right on STANYAN
- Right on PARNASSUS
- Left on 7th
  - 7th turns into LAGUNA HONDA, just past the subway station and Laguna Honda Hospital
- Turn left at the light, which turns into WOODSIDE
  - Continue on WOODSIDE to the top of the hill
- Left on PORTOLA
- Left on TWIN PEAKS
  - Follow the signs and winding road to the top
- Right on CHRISTMAS TREE POINT into Twin Peaks parking lot and view point
  - Follow the viewing platform walkway around the towers, out of the parking lot
- Right on TWIN PEAKS
- Right on CLARENDON (the T at the bottom of TWIN PEAKS)
- Merge left onto CLAYTON
- Right on 17th
- Left on ROOSEVELT
  - NOTE: Be sure to veer right with ROOSEVELT and not go straight onto Loma Vista
- Right on 14th to MARKET

SHORT-CUT OPTION NO. 3

Skip the Mission and the Embarcadero. These are great areas, but if you're tired or running late, or the kids can't take any more, skip them and head straight back to City Hall via the directions below, or head back to your hotel.

- Left on MARKET
- Left on FRANKLIN
- Right on MCALLISTER
- Right on POLK (GOODLETT)

FULL ROUTE CONTINUES

- Cross both CHURCH and MARKET, veering left to stay on 14th
- Right on DOLORES
- Left on CESAR CHAVEZ
- Left on INDIANA
  - NOTE: At INDIANA the official 49 Mile route markers direct automobiles to the 280 freeway. You have two options: (1) Take the freeway, get off at 3rd, (2) Keep going straight down INDIANA to follow the scenic walking route.
- Right on 22nd
- Cross 3rd
- Left on ILLINOIS
- Right at TERRY A FRANCOIS BLVD (MARIPOSA)
  - FRANCOIS eventually curves left and runs into 3rd
- Right on 3rd
- Cross the (cantilever) bridge

- Right on KING (WILLIE MAYS PLAZA),
  - Where it curves to meet the shore, it becomes EMBARCADERO
- Follow EMBARCADERO passed the Ferry Building
- Left on WASHINGTON
- Left on BATTERY
- Follow BATTERY as it veers left just before MARKET, becoming BUSH (then 1st STREET as you cross MARKET)
- Cross MARKET
- Continue on 1st
- Right on HOWARD
- Right on 9th
- As 9th crosses MARKET bear right onto LARKIN
- Left on MCALLISTER
- Left POLK, which turns into GOODLETT
  - **SHORT-CUT OPTION NO. 3 rejoins main route here**

END: 1 CARLTON B GOODLETT PLACE, San Francisco City Hall front steps

ACKNOWLEDGMENTS

Thank you to the many, many people who so graciously supported this effort—from test-walking the routes to many other practical and emotional actions—including: Abraham Hanif, Amy Johnson, Austin Mader-Clark, Ben Keim, Bill Lowell, Brian Tognotti, Curt Engelhard, Dave Stevenson, David Feldman, Deborah Hall, Deborah Schweizer, Donald Martin, Dorothy Webster, Ellen Miller, Eric Barnes, James Camarillo, Jeff Becker, Jett Atwood, Jim Oerther, Joselle Monarchi, June Bonacich, June Brown, Karen Noll, Lawrence Turner, Lisa Eller, Lisa Shaner, Lorri Ungaretti, Mark Poirier, Melissa Karam, Michael Hamlin, Cindy Eidson Reich, Paul Stoner, Richard Davis Lowell, Sabrina Wong, Scott Turco, Scott Walton, Shannon Martinez, Skip Purdy, Sue Mennear, Tom McElroy, Tom Sharp, Tony Clark, Travis Cheng, Vin Eiamvuthikorn, Natalie Burdick, Katharine Holland, Amy Gladin, Stephanie Lynne Smith, and the fellow artists from our Artist's Way groups.

Thanks also to the John Daly and Westlake branches of the Daly City Public Library for the quiet, comfortable desk space where much of the book was written.

RESOURCES

Want to learn more about San Francisco History?

» **SF History Resources**
SF History Association, SF Museum and Historical Society, California Historical Society (CHS), FoundSF, Western Neighborhoods Project

» **SF Photos and Maps**
Calisphere, OpenSF History, San Francisco Historical Photograph Collection of the San Francisco Public Library, David Rumsey Historical Map Collection

» **SF Walking Tours**
City Guides, Think Walks, Precita Eyes Muralists

City of San Francisco Resources

- ParkMe.com
- 511.org
- NextBus.com
- San Francisco Municipal Transportation Agency (SFMTA)
- San Francisco Recreation & Parks Department

CREDITS

Map Design
Carolyn Eidson

The Daily Crab
Design: Kristine Poggioli

Photos as credited

Illustrations: Carolyn Eidson, Jett Atwood (cartoonist, storyboard artist, animator, collaborator on a comic book series, "iPlates.")

Architectural Illustrations
Clay Seibert.com

Photo Credits
Photography: Carolyn Eidson

Additional photos used by permission from: Michael Hamlin, Kristine Poggioli, Scott Walton, Andy Honess, Robin Allen, San Francisco Scooter Girls, Piyawan Rungsuk, San Francisco Historical Photograph, Collection of the San Francisco Public Library, OpenSF History, Golden Gate National Regional Area Park Archives, anonymous private collectors, Lorri Ungaretti, Dennis O'Rorke, Hoodline.com, IT'S IT Ice Cream

Photos without credits are works in the public domain via Wikimedia, Creative Commons, U.S. National Archives and Records Administration, Library of Congress, or Pixabay CC0 licensed photos.

Wikimedia and Creative Commons are non-profits who benefit us all and would appreciate your donations. wikimediafoundation.org, creativecommons.org/donate/

Creative Commons Licenses
https://creativecommons.org/share-your-work/public-domain/cc0/

https://creativecommons.org/licenses/by/2.0/legalcode

https://creativecommons.org/licenses/by-sa/3.0/legalcode

https://creativecommons.org/licenses/by-sa/4.0/legalcode

Walk 1
Batkid key to city cropped by Shelly Prevost cc by 2.0: *https://commons.wikimedia.org/wiki/File%3ABatkid_key_to_city_cropped.jpg*

Harajuku Style Fans at J-Pop Summit 2013, Union Square by Gary Stevens cc by 2.0: *https://commons.wikimedia.org/wiki/File%3AHarajuku_Style_Fans_at_J-Pop_Summit_2013%2C_Union_Square_(9387450129).jpg*

America's Greatest City By The Bay at Union Square, San Francisco, CA by Ltleelim cc by-sa 3.0: *https://commons.wikimedia.org/wiki/File%3AAmerica's_Greatest_City_By_The_Bay_at_Union_Square%2C_San_Francisco%2C_CA.jpg*

Walk 2
Chinatown Souvenir Shop By Christina Spicuzz cc by-sa 2.0: *https://www.flickr.com/photos/spicuzza/4799587004*

Coit Tower City Life mural by Sailko cc by-sa 3.0: *https://commons.wikimedia.org/wiki/File%3AArnautoff_self_portrait_-_crop_from_Coit_Tower_City_Life_mural.JPG*

Walk 4
Crissy Field Overlook San Francisco, CA By Paxson Woelber cc by-sa 3.0: *https://commons.wikimedia.org/wiki/File%3ASan_Francisco%2C_California.jpg*

Walking for Health
Bring your own big wheel 2011 By Niki Dugan Pogue cc by-sa 2.0: *https://commons.wikimedia.org/wiki/File%3ABring-your-own-big-wheel-2011.jpg*

Carnaval San Francisco 2006 By Jmedia.org/wiki/File%3ACarnaval_San_Francisco_2006.jpg*

Pillow Fight By Christopher Michel cc by 2.0: *https://commons.wikimedia.org/wiki/File%3APILLOW_FIGHT_(4357968349).jpg*

Walk 10
Dry Branch Fire Squad By Grey3K cc by-sa 3.0: *https://commons.wikimedia.org/wiki/File%3ADry_Branch_Fire_Squad.JPG*

SF Architecture
The Painted Ladies, San Francisco By Alex Promos cc by 2.0: *https://commons.wikimedia.org/wiki/File%3AThe_Painted_Ladies%2C_San_Francisco_(7664260110).jpg*

Walk 17
Parrots of telegraph hill By Eliya cc by 2.0: *https://commons.wikimedia.org/wiki/File%3AParrots_of_telegraph_hill.jpg*

INDEX

ABOUT THE AUTHORS

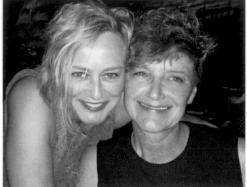

Authors Kristine Poggioli (r), Carolyn Eidson (l)

In 2013, **Kristine Poggioli** and coauthor **Carolyn Eidson** became the first people known to have walked San Francisco's historic 49 Mile Scenic Drive—which launched them into a new healthy lifestyle and resulted in a combined 75-pound weight loss. But perhaps more importantly, they had a blast walking the route, discovered new things about San Francisco, and grew closer together through the journey. They knew they had to share the fun with other people who love San Francisco and so they began a new adventure—writing a book together. It was a great fit.

Kristine "KP" Poggioli (pronounced Po-jo'-lee) is a copywriter and storyteller with a B.A. in history from U. C. Berkeley. As a native San Franciscan, she has given people tours around the city she has loved her whole life.

Carolyn Eidson (pronounced Edson) is an award-winning filmmaker, comedian, and passionate Weight Watchers Leader. As a member of the San Francisco Scooter Girls, she leads rides all over the city.

. . . and the adventure continues, Kristine and Carolyn were thrilled to perform at New York's Carnegie Hall in 2016, and can't wait to see what's next.